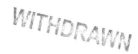

AMYOTROPHIC LATERAL SCLEROSIS

A Guide to Patient Care

Edited by

James T. Caroscio, M.D.
Department of Neurology
Mount Sinai Medical Center
New York, New York

1986
Thieme Medical Publishers, Inc., New York
Georg Thieme Verlag, Stuttgart · New York

Thieme Medical Publishers, Inc.
381 Park Avenue South
New York, New York 10016

Library of Congress Cataloging-in-Publication Data
Amyotrophic Lateral Sclerosis—A Guide to Patient Care

  Includes bibliographies and index.
  1. Amyotrophic lateral sclerosis—Treatment.
I. Caroscio, James T.   [DNLM: 1. Amyotrophic Lateral
Sclerosis.   WE 550 C277]
RC406.A24C37   1986   616.8′3   86-5746
ISBN 0-86577-246-0

Printed in the United States of America

Cover design by Wendy Ann Fredericks

AMYOTROPHIC LATERAL SCLEROSIS—A GUIDE TO
PATIENT CARE
James T. Caroscio, M.D.

TI ISBN 0-86577-246-0
GTV ISBN 3-13-691701-4

5 4

FOREWORD

This book was the inspiration of its guide and primary compiler, Dr. James T. Caroscio, who died just a few days before his fortieth birthday and a short time before the first copies arrived from the presses. It remains, along with the many patients who knew his devoted skillfulness, the most eloquent testimony to his depth of caring for those with a grave debilitating disease. We were close friends, and I am grateful to have been asked by the publisher to contribute this brief tribute.

Dr. Caroscio was a dedicated physician, admired by his colleagues, respected by his students, and trusted by his patients. He was a distinguished member of a small band, those content to let their actions and lives speak for themselves. Just how many lives he touched I have no way of knowing, but I suspect the numbers are a legion. All of us who were privileged to come within the circle of his life and life's work, however, count ourselves as singularly blessed.

Almost immediately after his training, internship, and residency Jim was invited to direct the ALS Clinic at Mount Sinai Medical Center in New York. Before long, he had elicited the loyalty and evoked the talents of an equally dedicated team of associates—social workers, occupational therapists, physical therapists, nurses, psychological and spiritual counselors, and others in the health care profession—to join him in developing a new approach to care for patients. From the first day, he spoke, wrote, studied, developed seminars and protocols, saw and examined patients and recommended treatment with an emphasis on what, in this book, he called "a consistent compassionate approach." Treating the ill and the weak and considering new and more effective ways of treating them was his greatest joy. "I can console myself with one thought," he told me not long before his death. "I've tried to do something substantial with my life. I have always wanted to help others, and I've tried to be true to the ideals I had as a young medical student." He always was true to those ideals. Poor and unknown ward patients received the identical attention he gave eminent statesmen. I saw that for myself, when he invited me to go on rounds with him and to attend clinic meetings. At other times, I heard patients tell his colleagues of Jim's extraordinary manner, his quiet, deep way of demonstrating a quiet, deep concern. His touch was not merely

iii

diagnostic, it was a clear example of one gifted human being reaching out to another.

Before he entered the hospital for the last weeks of his life, his only concern was the successful completion of this book; during the dark and slender weeks before his death, this book was close to his heart. You will find out why as you read, study, and learn from it. I think we can say of him what he said to the New York *Times* of Senator Jacob Javits, a man of substance, as Jim said, and a man whose doctor he was: "He was always available. He seemed totally tireless. In the last few years of his life he became one of the heroes of our time. He showed us that despite disability we can overcome and we can achieve and we can accomplish." This book testifies to much that was rich in his life, and it is a fitting memorial. Nothing, I believe, would give him more joy than that it become the inspiration for more care and more concern for those struggling to endure what still remains a mysterious and incurable illness.

Donald Spoto
July 1986

PREFACE

This book is devoted to all of the things that can be done to assist in the care of patients with ALS.

It is quite simply, as the title suggests, a *guide* for health care professionals, whether they be neurologists, physiatrists, pulmonary specialists, psychiatrists, physical therapists, occupational therapists, speech pathologists, nurses, or social workers.

Some of the chapters in this book are meant to inform the reader about ALS, but the bulk of this volume is concerned with the nitty-gritty of how to handle patients with this disease. The authors of the chapters of this book are members of the ALS Clinics from the Mount Sinai Hospital in New York, the University of Chicago Medical Center, The University of Miami Medical Center, and Hahneman University Hospital in Philadelphia. This book is an extension of a symposium entitled "Caring for Patients with Amyotrophic Lateral Sclerosis" that was held at the Page and William Black Post Graduate School of Medicine on June 3–4, 1985.

The purpose of this volume is to share our experiences, gained from caring for hundreds of ALS patients, with the hope that a high level of care can be brought to ALS patients wherever they may be.

James T. Caroscio, M.D.
March 1986

INTRODUCTION

Few diseases of the nervous system create as great a sense of hopelessness and despair on the part of patients and physicians as does ALS. Striking during the prime of life and selectively destroying the motor elements of the nervous system while leaving the senses intact, it inevitably progresses to the point of total disability. At present, its cause, means of prevention, and cure are unknown.

Since it was first established as a distinctive disorder of the nervous system by Jean-Martin Charcot in 1868, succeeding generations of physicians have struggled with the many problems of ALS. Establishing the diagnosis with certainty as well as finding means of easing the burden of this disease for both the patient and family members are areas of particular concern. In an effort to bring to light the many new concepts and technological findings in medicine for meeting these needs, The National ALS Foundation undertook the development of outpatient clinic facilities committed to this disorder. The first of these was established at Mount Sinai Medical Center in New York City in 1978, under the direction of Dr. James Caroscio. He brought together physicians and paramedical personnel from various disciplines whose efforts resulted in standardizing diagnostic criteria and developing a comprehensive care program for ALS patients. The experience gained from this, as well as similar efforts in other centers throughout the country, was the subject of a national conference held in June 1985 in New York City and is the basis for this publication.

As will be readily evident to the reader, this volume stresses the practical aspects of providing care for the ALS patient. It does not, however, ignore the scientific basis on which these approaches are predicated. Drawing on the experience of those involved in the day-to-day problems encountered in this disorder, the important diagnostic considerations, confirming tests, supportive treatment measures, and ethical issues involved are dealt with in depth.

To a considerable extent what is contained in this volume reflects the concepts Dr. Caroscio espoused and implemented over the past eight years. A skilled clinical neurologist, he combined his understanding of diseases of the nervous system with a compassion and empathy for his patients. Unstintingly, he gave of his time and energy to those afflicted with this disorder. In every sense he emulated the oft quoted adage, ''The care of the patient begins with caring for the patient.'' It is with deep regret and a great sense of loss to report Dr. James Caroscio's death on June 1, 1986. His loss has been felt by all his colleagues and patients, and his guidance in continuing the battle against ALS will be sorely missed.

Melvin D. Yahr, M.D.
Professor and Chairman
Department of Neurology
Mount Sinai Medical Center
New York, N.Y.

CONTENTS

1. Amyotrophic Lateral Sclerosis: The Disease 2

   James T. Caroscio, M.D.

2. The Motor Unit: Normal Properties and Physiologic Changes Associated with Motor Neuron Disease 16

   Albert J. Tahmoush, M.D., Mildred E. Francis, Sc.D., and Terry Heiman-Patterson, M.D.

3. Considerations in the Differential Diagnosis of Amyotrophic Lateral Sclerosis 32

   Jeffrey Allen Cohen, M.D.

4. Respiratory Failure in Amyotrophic Lateral Sclerosis 44

   Mark J. Rosen, M.D.

5. Pulmonary Function and Respiratory Failure in Neuromuscular Disorders with Reference to Amyotrophic Lateral Sclerosis 60

   Albert Miller, M.D.

6. Surgical Management of Feeding Difficulties in Patients with Amyotrophic Lateral Sclerosis 78

   Tomas Heimann, M.D.

7. Etiologic Considerations and Research Trends in Amyotrophic Lateral Sclerosis 84

   Terry Heiman-Patterson, M.D., Mark J. Gudesblatt, M.D., and Albert J. Tahmoush, M.D.

8. Ethical Issues in Amyotrophic Lateral Sclerosis 104

   James T. Caroscio, M.D.

9. Nursing Care of the Patient with Amyotrophic Lateral Sclerosis 113

   Linda Murray, R.N., M.S. and Cynthia F. DeBartolo, R.N., M.S.

10. Nutritional Management of Dysphagia 137

    Linda Slowie, M.S.R.D.

ix

11. Swallowing Difficulties in Amyotrophic Lateral Sclerosis 154

Jill Brooks, M.S., C.C.C.–S.P.

12. Rehabilitation for Patients with Amyotrophic Lateral
Sclerosis 162

Somchat Chiamprasert, M.D.

13. Functional Profiles Based on Clinical Variations of
Amyotrophic Lateral Sclerosis 172

Janet Zawodniak, B.S., P.T.

14. Selection of Assistive Devices for
Amyotrophic Lateral Sclerosis Patients...................... 188

Valerie Takai, B.A., O.T.R.

15. Exercise, Ambulation, and Pulmonary Physical Therapy for
the Amyotrophic Lateral Sclerosis Patient 218

Janet Zawodniak, B.S., P.T.

16. Home Care of the Amyotrophic Lateral Sclerosis Patient 246

Pat C. Heidkamp, M.S., O.T.R.

17. Communication Problems in the Patient with Amyotrophic
Lateral Sclerosis 256

Steven H. Blaustein, M.S., M.Ph.

18. Reactions of Patients, Family, and Staff in Dealing with
Amyotrophic Lateral Sclerosis 266

Philip B. Luloff, M.D.

19. Living and Coping with Amyotrophic Lateral Sclerosis: The
Psychosocial Impact 272

Nurit Ginsberg, C.S.W.

20. Emotional Response to ALS and Its Impact on Management of Patient Care 282

Eliana Horta, M.S., R.N.

21. Role of the Voluntary Health Care Agency in Amyotrophic
Lateral Sclerosis 290

Rochelle L. Moss

Index 297

CONTRIBUTORS

Steven H. Blaustein, M.S., M.Ph.
Department of Speech and Hearing
Mount Sinai School of Medicine
New York, New York

Jill Brooks, M.S., C.C.C.-S.P.
Department of Speech-Language Pathology
Jackson Memorial Hospital/University of Miami Medical Center
Department of Neurology
University of Miami School of Medicine
Miami, Florida

James T. Caroscio, M. D.
Department of Neurology
Mount Sinai School of Medicine
New York, New York

Somchat Chiamprasert, M. D.
Department of Rehabilitation Medicine
Mount Sinai School of Medicine
New York, New York

Jeffrey Allen Cohen, M. D.
Mount Sinai School of Medicine
New York, New York

Cynthia F. DeBartolo, M.S.
Mount Sinai Hospital
New York, New York

Mildred E. Francis, Sc.D.
Department of Neurology
Temple University
Philadelphia, Pennsylvania

Nurit Ginsberg, C.S.W.
Department of Social Services
Mount Sinai Hospital
New York, New York

Mark J. Gudesblatt, M. D.
Mount Sinai Medical Center
New York, New York

Pat C. Heidkamp, M.S., O.T.R.
Department of Neurology
University of Chicago Medical Center
Chicago, Illinois

Tomas M. Heimann, M. D.
Department of Surgery
Mount Sinai School of Medicine
New York, New York

Terry Heiman-Patterson, M. D.
Department of Neurology
Hahnemann University
Philadelphia, Pennsylvania

Eliana Horta, M.S., R.N.
ALS Clinic-Annenberg 3-64
Mount Sinai Hospital
New York, New York

Philip B. Luloff, M. D.
Mt. Sinai School of Medicine
New York, New York

Albert Miller, M. D.
Pulmonary Laboratory
Mount Sinai School of Medicine
New York, New York

Rochelle L. Moss
Executive Director
The ALS Association, Inc.
185 Madison Avenue
New York, New York

Linda Murray, R.N., M.S.
Mount Sinai Hospital
New York, New York

Mark J. Rosen, M. D.
Department of Pulmonary Medicine
Mount Sinai School of Medicine
New York, New York

Linda Slowie, M.S.
Department of Medicine
University of Chicago
Chicago, Illinois

Albert J. Tahmoush, M. D.
Department of Neurology
Hahnemann University
Philadelphia, Pennsylvania

Valerie Takai, B.A., O.T.R.
Department of Occupational Therapy
Mount Sinai Hospital
New York, New York

Janet Zawodniak, B.S., P.T.
Rehabilitation Medicine Department
Mount Sinai Hospital
New York, New York

Amyotrophic Lateral Sclerosis

CHAPTER ONE

AMYOTROPHIC LATERAL SCLEROSIS: THE DISEASE

James T. Caroscio, M.D.

Amyotrophic lateral sclerosis (ALS) is a degenerative disease of the nervous system which was first described by Bell in 1830 and named by Charcot in 1874.[1] It is also known as "Lou Gehrig's disease," after the famous baseball player who was a victim of this malady.

It is a disease whose cause remains unknown and for which there is no known cure. Despite this, experience in caring for over 800 ALS patients in an outpatient setting has shown that ALS is a disease that lends itself to intervention by physicians and ancillary medical personnel. Much can be done from a medical, physical, psychiatric, and social standpoint to enable victims of this disease to lead more comfortable and functional lives despite their disabilities.

PATHOLOGY

The word *amyotrophic* (absence of muscle growth) refers to the muscle atrophy that occurs in ALS as a consequence of degeneration of the anterior horn cells of the spinal cord and the motor cranial nerve nuclei in the lower brain stem (or bulb). These are the so-called lower motor neurons which undergo massive neuronal cell loss with gliosis (Fig. 1–1a). In addition, there are intracytoplasmic acidophilic inclusions in the lower motor neurons of ALS patients called *Bunina bodies*.[2]

The words *lateral sclerosis* refer to the demyelination and gliosis occurring in the cortico-spinal tracts (located in the *lateral* spinal cord), (Fig. 1b), and corticobulbar tracts. This is a consequence of degeneration and drop-out of Betz cells (upper motor neurons) in the motor cortex.

These pathologic changes characterize the sporadic form of ALS that is seen in 95% of patients.

Five percent of patients have a familial form of ALS (usually Mendelian dominant). In some of these cases there are the additional patho-

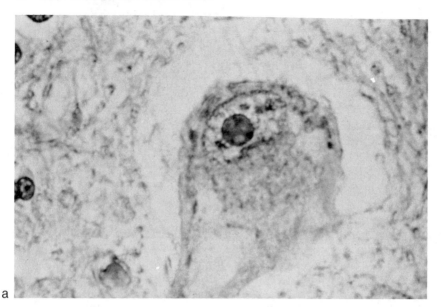

a

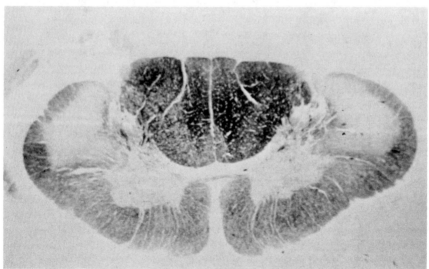

b

Figure 1–1. The pathology of ALS. a. Degenerating anterior horn cells in spinal cord. b. Demyelinated lateral corticospinal tracts in a cross-section of spinal cord.

logic changes of a loss of cells in Clark's column and degeneration of the posterior columns and spinocerebellar tracts.[3]

A third pathologic variant of ALS is called the Guamanian form since it was first described in the Chamorro Indian population of the Island of

Guam.[4] This form has since been described among inhabitants of the Kii Peninsula of Japan,[5] and most recently among the Auyu and Jakai people of West New Guinea.[6] In this form, motor neurons undergo neurofibrillary degeneration and some contain granulovacular bodies.[4] Clinically, the Guamanian form of ALS is indistinguishable from the sporadic form, but the pathologic changes in many Guam cases extend beyond the motor neurons, and there is also evidence of the parkinsonism dementia complex.[7] (It is fascinating to note that in these areas of the world there is a very high incidence of three degenerative nervous system diseases that occur sporadically in the rest of the world: ALS, parkinsonism and Alzheimer's disease.)

ETIOLOGY

Although the etiology of ALS is unknown, there is no lack of theories. Viral theories are spurred by the affinity of the polio virus for anterior horn cells as well as the observation that the natural history and pathology of ALS are consistent with a slow virus etiology.[8] No virus has ever been isolated, however, and attempts to transmit ALS to primates have failed.

The observation that lead poisoning produces a motor neuropathy has given rise to toxic theories and there have been several reports of elevation of lead levels in various ALS tissues. Perhaps the most scientifically sound basis for a toxic theory comes from work with the Guamanian form of ALS.[6] The soil and water in Guam, the Kii Peninsula of Japan, and Western New Guinea are deficient in calcium and magnesium. Yase has postulated that decreased intake of these substances results in a secondary hyperparathyroidism with the consequence that calcium is then increased in the central nervous system where it is protein bound and a metal (lead or aluminum)-induced calcification occurs, manifesting itself as a form of hydroxyapatite. This then causes motor neuron degeneration.[9] This theory finds support in findings of elevated aluminum in neurons of Guamian ALS patients.[10]

The abiotrophy theory holds that ALS is a genetically determined accelerated form of normal aging.[11]

Other researchers have recently proposed other possibilities: that ALS is the result of damage or loss of androgen receptors in motor neurons,[12] that there is a lack of neurotrophic hormone,[13] or that there is an accumulation of abnormal DNA in motor neurons.[14] In addition, a recent report that thyrotropin-releasing hormone (TRH) reverses signs and symptoms in ALS patients[15] has led to speculation that this substance may play a role in the etiology of ALS. A more detailed discussion of etiologic theories in ALS and consequent research trends can be found in Chapter 7.

CLINICAL FEATURES

Since ALS is a disease that affects the upper and lower motor neurons, it is sometimes referred to as motor neuron disease (MND).

The signs and symptoms of upper motor neuron degeneration are muscle weakness, spasticity, and hyperreflexia, and those of lower motor neuron degeneration are muscle weakness, atrophy, fasciculations, hypotonia, and areflexia. In ALS there is upper *and* lower motor neuron degeneration, resulting in the clinical picture of weakness, atrophy, fasciculations, spasticity, and hyperreflexia. Generally, there is bulbar and spinal muscle involvement, but some patients with ALS do not have bulbar involvement. When bulbar muscle weakness (speech and swallowing difficulty) is the major clinical feature of a patient the diagnosis given is progressive bulbar palsy (PBP). When the clinical picture is one of pure lower MND, the diagnosis is progressive muscular atrophy (PMA), and when a patient has pure upper MND, he is said to have primary lateral sclerosis (PLS).

Thus, the MNDs are ALS, PBP, PMA and PLS, and they can be looked at as a spectrum with PMA or pure lower MND at one end, and PLS or pure upper MND at the other. Amyotrophic lateral sclerosis and PBP are in the middle, with patients demonstrating varying combinations and degrees of upper and lower motor neuron involvement (Fig. 1–2). Amyotrophic lateral sclerosis is by far the most common of the MNDs and for this reason the terms ALS and MND are often used interchangeably. In a series of 397 cases of MND, 324 patients had ALS, 37 PBP, 29 PMA, and there were 7 cases of PLS (Fig. 1–3) (Caroscio JT, Calhoun WF, Smith H: unpublished data).

The incidence of ALS is 1/100,000 population, making it as common as muscular dystrophy and three times more common than myasthenia gravis.

THE "SPECTRUM" OF MOTOR NEURON DISEASES

LOWER MOTOR NEURON	Progressive Muscular Atrophy	Amyotrophic Lateral Sclerosis and Progressive Bulbar Palsy	Primary Lateral Sclerosis	UPPER MOTOR NEURON

Figure 1–2. Degeneration of upper and lower motor neurons results in various clinical presentations. It is the clinical picture that is the basis for defining the various motor neuron diseases. They can be viewed as a spectrum (see text, Clinical Features).

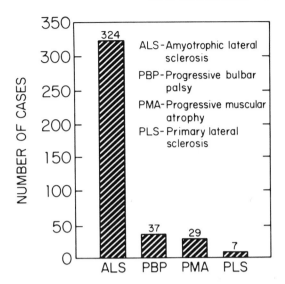

ALS-Amyotrophic lateral sclerosis
PBP-Progressive bulbar palsy
PMA-Progressive muscular atrophy
PLS-Primary lateral sclerosis

Figure 1–3. The various motor neuron diseases and their incidence.

There is a sex predisposition, with 1.5 male cases of ALS to every 1 female case. The disease can occur at any age during adulthood, but two-thirds of patients are between 50 and 70 and the median age of onset is 57 years.

The principal symptom of ALS is weakness; this can occur in any voluntary muscle of the body in a segmental pattern since the pathology is in spinal cord segments and the weakness occurs in muscle groups innervated by these segments. (Weakness does not fit into nerve root or peripheral nerve patterns.) The weakness begins insidiously and progresses at a rate that varies greatly from patient to patient. An important clinical feature of the disease is the asymmetry of the weakness. Generally, the rate of progression remains unchanged throughout the course of the disease, and patients' courses plotted on a graph take the form of a straight line whose slope is variable from patient to patient. There are fast, moderate, and slow progressive cases. Occasionally patients plateau or stabilize at some point and do not progress further and there are rare reports of recovery from this disease.

The first symptom of ALS is weakness in over 90% of patients. A few patients report muscle twitching or cramps as initial symptoms. The area of first weakness is greatly variable. Onset in the lower extremities is slightly more common that in the upper extremities which, in turn, is more common than a bulbar onset. The cranial nerves involved in ALS are the lower motor ones. The oculomotor nuclei are almost always spared. Two-thirds of patients have tongue fasciculations and weakness, facial and palatal weakness, and difficulty in swallowing. About one-third of 272 patients with ALS who were followed never developed bulbar symptoms (Caroscio JT: unpublished data).

The clinical manifestations of upper motor neuron involvement of the cranial nerves is an increased jaw jerk and gag reflex. In addition, the bilateral corticobulbar tract degeneration that occurs in this disease results in a pseudobulbar palsy. This contributes to patients' speech and swallowing difficulty and results in emotional lability. (A curious and potentially disabling situation in which patients will laugh or cry uncontrollably. This occurs either without associated affect or with minimal provocation and is evidently the result of a loss of inhibition of the reflex motor acts involved in laughing or crying.) This symptom occurs in about 43% of ALS patients.

Weakness is the principal symptom of ALS and one would be hard pressed to make a diagnosis in its absence. One hundred percent of 272 patients with ALS had weakness in some muscle group. Ninety-three percent had atrophy and 92% fasciculations. Forty-seven percent of patients had spasticity and about 50% reported muscle cramps as a motor symptom. Babinski's signs were present in 50% of patients, absent in 24%, and neutral in 26% (Caroscio JT: unpublished data).

Weakness in ALS affects all muscles of the limbs and trunk including the neck, intercostals, paraspinals, and diaphragm. Involvement of the muscles of breathing is the most serious problem in ALS, since ineffective cough eventually leads to pneumonias which are one of the most frequent causes of death. Aspiration pneumonia from swallowing difficulties also occurs, but in our clinical experience this is less common. Hypoxic deaths from muscle paralysis alone are common. Pulmonary emboli and congestive heart failure have been less common causes of death in our patients. Dyspnea occurs in ALS, but is somewhat unusual, though occasionally this is a prominent symptom in the absence of much muscle weakness elsewhere. What is more impressive is the absence of respiratory symptoms in patients with severely compromised pulmonary function tests (PFTs). Amyotrophic lateral sclerosis patients have a remarkable ability to maintain normal arterial blood gases despite poor PFTs. A detailed discussion of pulmonary management of ALS patients as well as the use of PFTs can be found in Chapters 4 and 5 of this volume.

Certain functions are preserved in ALS: eye movements, sexual function, and bladder and bowel control. Occasionally urinary frequency occurs in patients with prominent spasticity, but incontinence almost never occurs. Sexual dysfunction can occur due to psychological causes, of course. Constipation is a problem, not from sphincter muscle tone changes, but because of inactivity, poor fluid intake, and inability to bear down from abdominal muscle weakness. (Constipation can be a serious problem in ALS patients. We have seen patients die from the complications of high fecal impactions.)

The reason for preservation of sphincter and sexual function in ALS stems from the remarkable sparing of a group of motor neurons in the sacral anterior horn from pathologic involvement (the *Onufrowicz nucleus*).[16]

Sensation is also spared in ALS and except for posterior column loss in some hereditary cases, the sensory examination should be normal. Occasionally patients will have sensory findings secondary to another process (i.e., radiculopathy or peripheral neuropathy). This absence of sensory deficits may be responsible for the very rare occurrence of bed sores in ALS patients. When they do occur, they are mild and respond readily to treatment.

Mentation in generally spared in ALS as well, though 4.7% of 272 patients had organic mental syndromes. The etiology of these mental changes was variable, but it seems there is a subset of ALS patients who have an Alzheimer-type dementia.

DIAGNOSIS

The diagnosis of ALS is based primarily on clinical criteria; when a patient has a progressive motor weakness with atrophy, fasciculations, and hyperreflexia, and no sensory or sphincter disturbance, the diagnosis of ALS is highly probable. If there are purely motor bulbar signs as well, the diagnosis is virtually certain.

There are, of course, other conditions that enter into a differential diagnosis, and Table 1–1 lists the various categories of misdiagnosis that were found in 52 of 388 patients referred with a diagnosis of ALS.[17] Myelopathies and myeloradiculopathies are by far the most common conditions misdiagnosed as ALS. One helpful rule of thumb is to follow patients in whom the diagnosis of ALS is questionable. Since ALS is almost always progressive, failure to progress may indicate another diagnosis. In addition, in few other conditions as they progress are the findings limited to the motor system, and in many of our misdiagnosed patients the emergence of sensory symptoms, for instance, as the disease process evolved made another diagnosis obvious.

There have been reports of the rare occurrence of an ALS-like syndrome secondary to another underlying disease process. Hexosaminidase deficiency,[18] lead toxicity,[19] and macroglobulinemia[20] are examples of such occurrences. In general, it warrants checking urinary or serum lead levels as well as serum protein electrophoresis in all ALS suspects and hexosaminidase A levels in younger patients.

More common in our experience and that of others[21] is the presence of a cervical myeloradiculopathy mimicking ALS. To rule out this possibility, one can justify performing a cervical myelogram in patients in

Table 1–1. Misdiagnoses in 52 of 388 Patients Referred as Having Amyotrophic Lateral Sclerosis*

Diagnosis	No. Patients
Myelopathy/myeloradiculopathy	15
Clinically probable MS	3
Late progression of poliomyelitis	3
Psychiatric	3
Benign fasciculations	3
Tumors (ependymoma, chordoma)	2
Polyradiculopathy	2
Charcot–Marie–Tooth disease	2
Multifocal neuropathy from diabetes	2
Unspecified neuropathy	2
Parkinsonism	2
Dementia	2
Unclassified CNS disease	2
Guillain–Barre syndrome	1
Chronic relapsing polyneuropathy	1
Lumbar plexopathy	1
Mononeuropathy	1
Brain stem infarct	1
Syringobulbia	1
Olivopontocerebellar degeneration	1
Cramps	1
Hoarsness of unknown etiology	2
Total	52

Abbreviations: CNS, central nervous system; MS, multiple sclerosis.

*This table provides a partial compendium of differential diagnoses for ALS.

whom the signs and symptoms are all "below the neck." Previous reports have linked ALS with a high incidence of cancer,[22] while other reports have failed to confirm such an association.[23] In our experience, the incidence of new cancers in 347 ALS patients followed for a mean of 2.5 years was 0.57%/year, which was not statistically different from the incidence in the age-matched general population (Zisfein J, Caroscio JT: Unpublished data). The clinical lesson here is that costly and exhausting "occult malignancy workups" are not warranted in ALS patients.

All patients with ALS should have an electromyogram (EMG) to confirm the diagnosis. The typical EMG features are spontaneously occurring fibrillations and fasciculations, large or giant motor units on voluntary activity, and a diminished or absent interference pattern. These findings are noted in diffuse muscles. Nerve conduction velocities are usually normal. Electromyography, of course, must be used in conjunction with the clinical picture in confirming a diagnosis. A detailed discussion of the electrophysiology of ALS appears in Chapter 2.

The only frequently noted abnormality on screening blood tests in ALS patients is creatine phosphokinase (CPK) elevations which occur in about 70% of patients. This rarely goes above 500 U/ml, and higher elevations should raise suspicions about the diagnosis (Caroscio JT: unpublished data).

The cerebrospinal fluid in ALS shows no abnormalities of protein, glucose, or cell count.

PROGNOSIS

Amyotrophic lateral sclerosis is generally accorded a grave prognosis[24,25] and there is no question that this can be a malignant disease that generally progresses to death. However, a recent survival study of 397 ALS patients indicates that survival is longer than previously believed; the median survival in this study was 4.08 years (Fig. 1–4). This means that 50% of patients will still be living over 4 years after onset of symptoms. Other conclusions of this study were that there was no statistical difference in survival in patients with ALS, as compared to those with PBP, or to those with onset in bulbar versus spinal muscles; and that there were generally longer survivals for patients with PMA and PLS, shortening of median survival with increasing age of onset, and longer survival time for females (Caroscio JT, Calhoun WF, and Smith H: unpublished data).

TREATMENT

The nature of ALS as a malignant disease whose main symptom, weakness, is readily manifest, added to the facts that the cause is un-

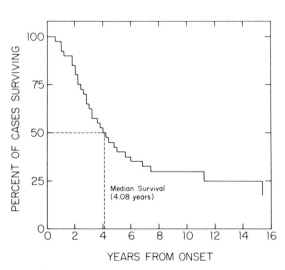

Figure 1–4. Survival analysis of 397 patients with motor neuron disease indicates a median survival of 4.08 years. This is longer than previously reported (Caroscio JT, Calhoun WF, and Smith H: unpublished data).

known, that there is no cure, and that mentation is spared, has made this a very difficult disease for physicians to deal with. Avoidance, identification, rejection, inadequacy, feelings of impotence and loss of control, frustration, anxiety; indeed, all the negative emotional responses described as affecting physicians[26] seem to be brought out by this disease.

Physicians dealing with ALS patients would do themselves and their patients a service by becoming familiar with the coping strategies that are helpful in dealing with their negative responses.[26]

Experience with large numbers of ALS patients has brought to light the common tendency of physicians to avoid telling patients their diagnosis. This has the effect in most instances of heightening patients' anxiety, the nonverbal message being "this is such a terrible disease it cannot even be named." Added to this is the stress applied to family interactions in "keeping the secret" (a ridiculous thought in a disease whose primary symptom is so readily manifest), and the difficulties encountered by ancillary medical personnel in trying to deal realistically and effectively with patients who don't know their diagnosis. The first act in initiating treatment with ALS patients, then, becomes telling them their diagnosis. Indications that survival is longer than was previously believed,[24] add further stress to the importance of intervention on the part of the physician to provide symptomatic and supportive care, for there is ample opportunity for the physician to intervene in improving the quality of life of ALS patients. These and other ethical issues will be discussed in greater detail in Chapter 8.

From a medical standpoint there are several ALS symptoms that are disabling and even life threatening for which there is symptomatic treatment. Saliva pooling is one of these, since it frequently causes choking, especially at mealtimes when there is increased saliva secretion and chance of aspiration is greatest. In almost all patients this symptom can be controlled with atropine 0.4 mg given ½ h before meals and at bedtime. If saliva pooling is still a problem, Pro-Banthine 15 mg can be added to atropine in the same dose schedule; these drugs have the effect of potentiating each other in decreasing saliva secretion. The anticholinergic side effects of tricyclics are also helpful in saliva control in ALS patients and these drugs (imipramine, amitriptyline) have the added effects in small doses of dramatically reducing the symptom of emotional lability, reducing anxiety, and promoting sleep. Another helpful measure in patients with increased secretions is to have a suction machine available in the home.

Swallowing difficulty is, of course, a very serious symptom in ALS, though this function is often amazingly well preserved in even the most advanced cases. This symptom is greatly helped by reducing saliva production with atropine. In our experience, patients refuse to give up the pleasure of oral intake until swallowing is totally impossible. Our policy has been to accede to patients' wishes and intervene only at such times, and our procedure of choice is the feeding gastrostomy tube inserted under local anesthesia. Patients' response to this procedure has been universally positive; it greatly improves the quality of life since meals in ALS patients are sometimes ordeals that take hours and involve frequent episodes of choking. Our experience with surgical management of feeding difficulties in ALS is detailed in Chapter 6.

Because of the nature of ALS as a disease that involves muscle wasting, almost all patients lose weight no matter what their oral intake. This is often of concern to family and patients, but is not necessarily reflective of nutritional deficiency. Our axiom is, "weigh the patient's food, not the patient."

Breathing difficulty is the single most life-threatening symptom in ALS patients. Whenever dyspnea is a prominent symptom, it is an ominous sign and raises medical and ethical problems. When patients present with this complaint, our policy is to perform PFTs, and chest x-ray films to rule out intercurrent disease, and to examine arterial blood gases to ascertain whether there is CO_2 retention (a situation that necessitates immediate intervention when it occurs). If secondary problems are ruled out, the patient and family are counseled that the situation is serious and it is explained that the symptom is likely to progress and that the patient will eventually need mechanical assistance. Patients are then asked to think about what their wish would be if the situation arose, whether in the context of an emergency or otherwise, where mechanical respiratory assistance was deemed necessary for survival. This policy is effective in addressing patients' fears regarding breathing difficulty, and since mentation is spared in ALS, this disease allows the patient to assume responsibility for deciding to use mechanical respiratory assistance, rather than placing the responsibility for such a decision on the physician or family.

Short of tracheostomy and a respirator, other courses of action can help patients with breathing difficulty. Breathing exercises and incentive spirometers can reduce atelectasis. Oxygen can be provided in the patient's home to be taken on a prn basis (patients should never get oxygen at concentrations greater than 2 L/min). Intermittent positive-pressure breathing (IPPB) devices can also help and can even function as respirators of sorts; this is especially effective in patients without bulbar symptoms. Cruiras respirators can also be effective noninvasive alternative respiratory assistive devices; again, these are most helpful in patients without bulbar symptoms. If these measures fail, tracheostomy and the use of portable respirator equipment can enable select ALS patients to live quite comfortably at home. Subsequent chapters will deal with pulmonary management, use of PFTs, pulmonary physical therapy, and ethical issues surrounding life support systems in ALS patients.

There are other less life-threatening, although disabling ALS symptoms for which treatment exists. Spasticity is most safely and effectively treated with baclofen in a dose of 5–25 mg tid. This should be titrated up slowly by patients, increasing the dose by increments of 5 mg tid every 3 days to assess optimim therapeutic results. Nocturnal muscle cramps are frequent and respond readily to quinine sulfate 325 mg hs.

The other way in which the physician can serve the ALS patient is by being aware of and making use of medical support services that are available. In addition, the knowledge that there are other disciplines and sources of support for ALS patients acts as a coping mechanism for physicians in helping them to deal with the disease.

Physical disability is a progressive and ever-changing reality in ALS. A previously independent person can be made helpless by attempting to perform such mundane acts as opening doors, turning keys, cutting meat, and buttoning buttons. This is an area where the occupational therapist can intervene and restore some degree of independence. How this can be accomplished is detailed in Chapters 14 and 16.

Difficulty in walking is another obvious difficulty in ALS. Through exercise, gait training, and use of orthotics and ambulation aids, ambulation can be maintained for as long as possible. Indeed, 50% of patients who presented in a nonambulatory state to our ALS clinic were enabled to walk by physical therapy intervention. A more detailed description of what physical medicine has to offer the ALS patient can be found in Chapters 12, 13, and 15.

Speech difficulty is another disabling ALS symptom, and intervention by a speech pathologist can enable patients to maintain intelligible speech for as long as possible and then prepare them for using nonvocal communmications aids. This is detailed in Chapter 17, as are the functions and services that can be provided by nurses (Chapter 9), psychiatrists (Chapter 18), and social workers (Chapters 19 and 20) to ALS patients. In addition, physicians should be aware of the presence of voluntary health care agencies with services for ALS patients (Chapter 21), and should refer patients to these agencies (e.g., the ALS Association, New York and Sherman Oaks, California, and the Muscular Dystrophy Association, New York).

In summary, much can be done to help the ALS patient, both by the physician directly, and by means of referrals to ancillary professionals. For the physician who can cope with the stresses of dealing with ALS, there is the very real reward of the respect and gratitude of the mentally intact individual who is suffering from the disease.

REFERENCES

1. Rose FC: Clinical aspects of motor neuron disease. In Rose FC (ed.): Motor Neuron Disease, Pittman, London, 1976, pp. 1–13.

2. Hirano A, Iwata M: Pathology of motor neurons. In Tsubaki T, Toyokura Y (eds. Amyotrophic Lateral Sclerosis. University Park Press, Tokyo, 1978, pp. 107–133.
3. Horton WA, Eldrige R, Brody JA: Familial motor neuron disease. Neurology 26:460–465, 1976.
4. Malamud N, Hirano A, Kurland LT: Pathoanatomic changes in amyotrophic lateral sclerosis on Guam. Arch Neurol 5:401–415, 1961.
5. Araki M, Kimura K, Yase Y: A histopathological study on amyotrophic lateral sclerosis in Kii Peninsula. In Bischoff A, Luthy F (eds): Proceedings of the Fifth International Congress of Neuropathology. Excerpta Medica, Amsterdam, 1966, p. 219.
6. Gadjusek DC, Salazar AM: Amyotrophic lateral sclerosis and parkinsonian syndromes in high incidence among the Auyu and Jakai people of West New Guinea. Neurology 32:107–126, 1982.
7. Elizan TE, Hirano A, Abrams BM, et al.: Amyotrophic lateral sclerosis and parkinsonism–dementia complex of Guam. Arch Neurol 14:356–368, 1966.
8. Johnson RT: Virological studies of amyotrophic lateral sclerosis: An overview. UCLA Forum Med Sci 19:173–180, 1977.
9. Yase Y: ALS in the Kii Peninsula: One possible etiological hypothesis. In Tsubaki T, Toyokura Y (eds.): Amyotrophic Lateral Sclerosis. University Park Press, Tokyo, 1978, pp. 307–318.
10. Perl DP, Gadjusek DC, Garruto RM, et al.: Intraneuronal aluminum accumulation in amyotrophic lateral sclerosis and parkinsonism–dementia of Guam. Science 217:1053–1055, 1982.
11. McComas AJ, Upton ARM, Sica REP: Motorneuron disease and aging. Lancet 1477–1480, 1973.
12. Weiner LP: Possible role of androgen receptors in amyotrophic lateral sclerosis. Arch Neurol 37:129–131, 1980.
13. Appel SH: A unifying hypothesis for the cause of amyotrophic lateral sclerosis, parkinsonism and Alzheimer disease. Ann Neurol 10:499–505, 1981.
14. Bradley WG, Krasin F: A new hypothesis of the etiology of amyotrophic lateral sclerosis. Arch Neurol 39:677–680, 1982.
15. Engel WK, Siddique T, Nicoloff JT: Effect on weakness and spasticity in amyotrophic lateral sclerosis of thyrotropin-releasing hormone. Lancet: 273–75, 1983.
16. Iwata M, Hirano A: Sparing of the Onufrowicz nucleus in sacral anterior horn lesions. Ann Neurol 4:245–249, 1978.
17. Caroscio JT, Calhoun WF, Yahr MD: Prognostic factors in motor neuron disease: A prospective study of longevity. In Rose FC (ed): Progress in Motor Neuron Disease. Pittman, London, 1984.
18. Johnson WG, Wigger HJ, Karp HR, et al.: Juvenile spinal muscular atrophy: A new hexosaminidase deficiency phenotype. Ann Neurol 11:11–16, 1982.
19. Boothby JA, deJesus PV, Rowland LP: Reversible forms of motor neuron disease. Arch Neurol 31:18–23, 1974.
20. Rowland LP, Defendini R, Sherman W, et al.: Macroglobulinemia with peripheral neuropathy simulating motor neuron disease. Ann Neurol 11:532–536, 1982.
21. Kasdan DL: Cervical spondylotic myelopathy with reversible fasciculations in the lower extremities. Arch Neurol 34:774–776, 1977.
22. Norris FH, Engel WK: Carcinomatous amyotrophic lateral sclerosis. In Brain R, Norris FH (eds.): The Remote Effects of Cancer on the Nervous System. Grune & Stratton, New York, 1965, pp. 1–10.
23. Bharucha NE, Schoenberg BS, Raven RH, et al.: Geographic distribution of motor neuron disease and correlation with possible etiologic factors. Neurology 32(2):A188, 1982.
24. Rosen AD: Amyotrophic lateral sclerosis. Arch Neurol 35:638–642, 1978.
25. Juergens SM, Kurland LT, Okayaki PH, et al.: ALS in Rochester, Minnesota, 1925–1977. Neurology 30:463–470, 1980.
26. Gorlin R, Zucker HD: Physicians' reactions to patients. N Engl J Med 308:1059–1063, 1983.

CHAPTER TWO

THE MOTOR UNIT: NORMAL PROPERTIES AND PHYSIOLOGIC CHANGES ASSOCIATED WITH MOTOR NEURON DISEASE

Albert J. Tahmoush, M.D.,[1] Mildred E. Francis, Sc.D.,[2] and Terry Heiman-Patterson, M.D.[1]

The motor unit was initially defined in 1925 by Liddell and Sherrington as the motor axon and its adjunct muscle fibers.[1] It was considered to be the functional unit of muscle action. With advances in our knowledge of motor function, the definition of the motor unit has been revised to refer only to the alpha motor neuron, its axon, and its innervated muscle fibers.[2] However, the importance of this functional unit for the understanding of normal and diseased muscle action remains preeminent. Major advances in our understanding of the types of motor units and the principles regulating the activation of motor units have occurred during the last 25 years.[3–6]

The purpose of this chapter is to review the anatomic and physiologic properties of motor units and the changes that occur in amyotrophic lateral sclerosis (ALS). The prognostic value of these changes and their implications for therapy are discussed.

MORPHOLOGY OF LOWER MOTOR NEURONS

The alpha motor neurons are large cells, with soma diameters ranging from about 30 to 70 μm in the cat.[7] The extent of the dendritic tree, the diameter of the axon, and the size of the cell body are closely correlated. Small neurons have fewer dendritic branchings and smaller axons than larger neurons. The number of synapses per unit surface area is relatively constant, with the total number of synaptic endings varying from 20,000 to 50,000.

17

LOCALIZATION OF LOWER MOTOR NEURONS

The motor neurons in the human spinal cord are divided into medial and lateral cell groups. A diagrammatic presentation of the columnar cell groups is given in Figure 2–1. The medial group is present at nearly all cord levels and supplies innervation to the neck, trunk, intercostal, and abdominal muscles. The lateral group is present at cervical (C4–8) and lumbosacral (L2–S2) levels. In the lateral cell group, neurons are spatially distributed so that those projecting to proximal muscles are located ventrolaterally and those projecting to distal muscles are located dorsolaterally. Thus, the shoulder, upper arm, hip, and thigh muscles are innervated by ventrolateral neurons whereas the forearm, hand, leg, and foot muscles are innervated by dorsolateral neurons.

The bulbar and facial muscles are innervated by neurons in the pons and medulla oblongata. The muscles of the tongue are innervated by neurons in the hypoglossal nucleus; the striated branchiomeric musculature of the soft palate, pharynx, and larynx are innervated by neurons in the nucleus ambiguus; and the superficial muscles of the face and scalp are innervated by neurons in the motor facial nucleus.

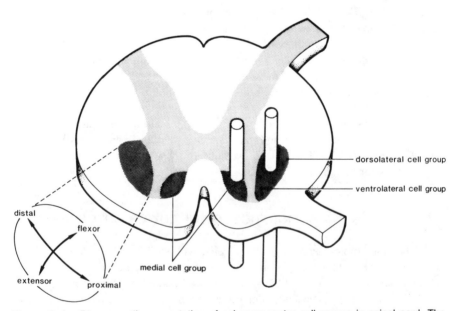

Figure 2–1. Diagrammatic presentation of columnar motor cell groups in spinal cord. The muscle innervation for the lateral cell groups is also shown.

Table 2–1. Types of Motor Units

Motor Unit Characteristics	Type 1	Type 2a	Type 2b
Resistance to fatigue	High	Intermediate	Low
Twitch contraction time	Slow	Fast	Fast
Tetanic tension	Low	Intermediate	High
Adenosine triphosphatase (pH 9.4)	Low	High	High
Oxidative enzymes	High	Intermediate	Low
Phosphorylase (glycolytic)	Low	High	High
Glycogen content	Low	High	High

TYPES OF MOTOR UNITS

The mechanical and histochemical properties of the three types of motor units are presented in Table 2–1. Burke and co-workers defined these properties during their study of cat hindlimb motor units.[2,8,9] With a microelectrode located in a single motor neuron and the gastrocnemius tendon connected to a strain gauge, intracelluar stimulation of the motor neuron permits characterization of the mechanical properties and histochemical profile of the innervated muscle fibers. These studies showed that type 1 motor units maintain the same tension throughout long periods of stimulation. They have slow contraction times, and they develop only small tetanic tensions. Type 1 motor units have a low adenosine triphosphatase (pH 9.4) activity, high oxidative enzyme activity, low glycolytic phosphorylase activity, and low glycogen content. Type 2a motor units show some decrement in maximum tension during long repetitive stimulations. They have fast contraction times, and they develop higher tetanic tensions than type 1 units. Type 2 motor units have high adenosine triphosphatase (pH 9.4) activity, intermediate oxidative enzyme activity, high glycolytic phosphorylase activity, and high glycogen content. Type 2b motor units show rapid decrement in maximum tension during repetitive stimulation. They have fast contraction times and they develop the highest tetanic tensions. Type 2b motor units have high adenosine triphosphatase (pH 9.4) activity, low oxidative enzyme activity, high glycolytic phosphorylase activity, and high glycogen content. The high oxidative enzyme activity and rich capillary supply of muscle fibers in type 1 motor units suggests that they primarily utilize aerobic energy pathways. In contrast, the abundance of glycogen, the low oxidative enzyme activity, and the sparse capillary supply of type 2 motor units suggest that these muscle fibers depend primarily on anaerobic glycolysis for energy.

The muscle fiber distribution of single motor units has been determined in animals by repetitive stimulation of single motor nerve fibers

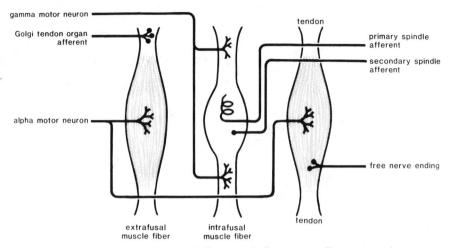

Figure 2–2. Schematic presentation of afferent and efferent nerve fibers to muscle.

and staining for muscle glycogen.[10–12] A diffuse scattering of muscle fibers is noted for each motor unit. For the rat tibialis anterior muscle, 76% of all the muscle fibers in a motor unit are completely separated from other muscle fibers of the same motor unit. Groups of two muscle fibers lying in direct contact occur approximately ten times per motor unit. Groups of three fibers are noted twice per motor unit, and larger groups occur only once in every other unit.

PERIPHERAL INPUTS TO LOWER MOTOR NEURONS

The lower motor neurons receive inputs from several muscle receptors. A schematic presentation of the afferent and efferent nerve fibers to muscle is given in Figure 2–2. The muscle spindles contain primary (annulospiral) and secondary (flower spray) afferent nerve terminals. The primary nerve terminals are the receptors for the group 1a afferent fibers which have large-diameter axons and fast conduction velocities. As presented in Figure 2–3, they make monosynaptic excitatory connections with lower motor neurons that innervate the same muscle from which the group 1a fiber originates. In addition, they make monosynaptic excitatory connections with lower motor neurons that innervate synergistic muscles, and disynapatic connections through an inhibitory interneuron to lower motor neurons that innervate antagonistic muscles. The secondary nerve termi-

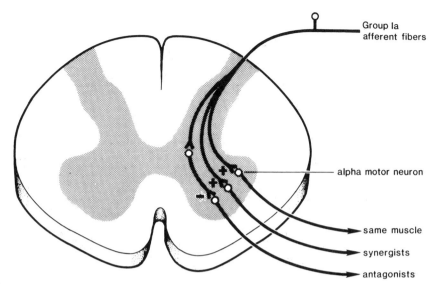

Figure 2–3. Schematic presentation of group 1a afferent fiber connections with spinal cord cells.

nals are the receptors for the group 2 afferent fibers which have smaller diameter axons and slower conduction velocities. These fibers also make monosynaptic excitatory connections with lower motor neurons that innervate the same muscle from which the group 2 afferent fiber originates. In addition, they excite motor neurons to physiologic flexors and inhibit motor neurons to physiologic extensors through polysynaptic pathways.

Golgi tendon organs are located in series with the muscle fibers. They contain Group 1b afferent nerve fibers. As shown in Figure 2–4, they make disynaptic connections through an inhibitory neuron to lower motor neurons that innervate the same muscle from which the group 1b fiber originates. In addition, the group 1b afferent fiber makes disynaptic connections through an inhibitory neuron to lower motor neurons that innervate synergistic muscles, and disynaptic connections through an excitatory interneruon to lower motor neurons that innervate antagonistic muscles.

There are muscle receptors that carry information through myelinated group 3 and unmyelinated group 4 afferent fibers. As shown in Figure 2–5, they make polysynaptic excitatory connections to motor neurons innervating ipsilateral flexor and contralateral extensor muscles, and polysynaptic inhibitory connections to motor neurons innervating ipsilateral extensor and contralateral flexor muscles.

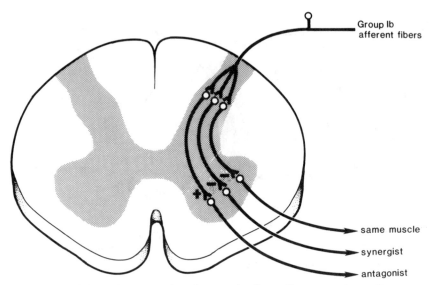

Figure 2–4. Schematic presentation of group 1b afferent fiber connections with spinal cord cells.

SUPRASEGMENTAL INPUTS TO LOWER MOTOR NEURONS

The brain stem nuclei that provide suprasegmental inputs to lower motor neurons are schematically shown in Figure 2–6. Three inputs pro-

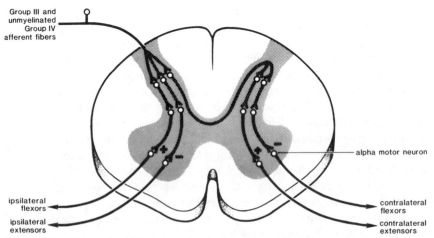

Figure 2–5. Schematic presentation of group 3 and unmyelinated group 4 afferent fiber connections with spinal cord cells.

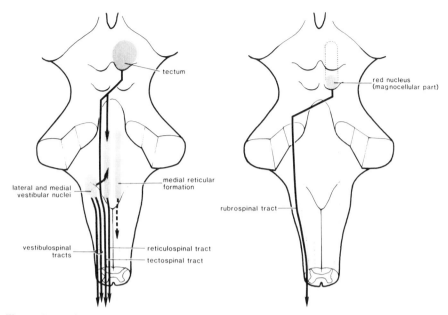

Figure 2–6. Suprasegmental inputs to lower motor neurons from brain stem nuclei. Medial and ventrolateral neurons receive inputs from lateral and medial vestibulospinal, tectospinal, and reticulospinal tracts. Dorsolateral neurons receive brain stem input from the rubrospinal tract.

ject to the medial and ventrolateral neurons of the spinal cord: (1) the lateral and medial vestibulospinal tracts which originate in the lateral and medial vestibular nuclei and carry information for the reflex control of equilibrium from the vestibular labyrinth; (2) the tectospinal tract which originates in the superior colliculus and carries information for the coordination of eye and head movements; and (3) the reticulospinal tracts which originate in the reticular formation of the pontine and medullary tegmentum and carry information for the control of muscle tone. The dorsolateral spinal cord neurons receive input from the rubrospinal tract which originates in the magnocellular portion of the red nucleus and carries information for the control of muscle tone.

As shown in Figure 2–7, the corticospinal tracts originate from three major cortical areas: (1) the precentral gyrus of the frontal lobe (area 4 of Brodmann) contributes approximately 30% of the corticospinal nerve fibers; (2) area 6 of Brodmann (frontal lobe) also contributes about 30% of the corticospinal tract fibers; and (3) the parietal lobe (especially the somatic sensory cortex) contributes the remaining 40%. The corticospinal tract fibers that cross the midline in the pyramidal decussation form the

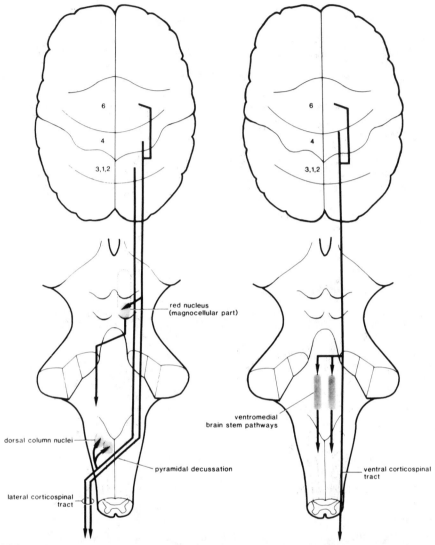

Figure 2-7. Cortical inputs to lower motor neurons. The lateral corticospinal tract projects to dorsolateral neurons and the ventral corticospinal tract projects bilaterally to medial and ventrolateral neurons.

lateral corticospinal tract, whereas those that do not cross form the ventral corticospinal tract. The lateral corticospinal tract projects to sensory neurons in the dorsal horn and to motor neurons innervating distal muscles. The ventral corticospinal tract projects bilaterally to motor neurons innervating axial and proximal muscles.

PHYSIOLOGY OF LOWER MOTOR NEURONS

Henneman and co-workers correlated the three types of motor units with the types of motor neurons present in the cat lumbosacral cord.[7,13-18] Recordings from pairs of motor axons were performed. These studies showed that smaller neurons fire first and drop out last when an excitatory input is given. These small neurons were found to innervate type 1 motor units which have relatively small numbers of muscle fibers and produce low maximum tetanic tensions. Larger motor neurons were found to innervate type 2a and 2b motor units which have larger numbers of muscle fibers and produce higher maximum tetanic tensions.

Why is the excitability of a motor neuron related to its size? It is unlikely that the size principle is due to preferential presynaptic inputs to small motor neurons. It appears to be a biophysical consequence of the properties of the cell membrane. Small neurons have fewer conductance channels than large neurons. Therefore, they have a higher resistance. The same excitatory input produces a larger postsynaptic potential (from Ohm's law $V = IR$) which brings the small neuron closer to discharge than a large neuron.

The size principle and the functional properties of the three types of motor units can account for graded muscle performance. For a small contraction, the motor neurons receive a small excitatory input which predominantly fires small neurons. These neurons innervate type 1 motor units which produce low sustained tensions. For larger contractions, increased excitatory inputs fire larger neurons. These neurons innervate type 2a and type 2b units which have large numbers of muscle fibers and produce higher tensions. With the contraction completed, the neurons cease firing in reverse order.

MOTOR UNITS IN AMYOTROPHIC LATERAL SCLEROSIS

Human motor units are examined by several methods in most clinical electrophysiology laboratories.[19,20] Nerve conduction studies, F-wave amplitude measurements, conventional needle electromyography, repetitive nerve stimulation, and single-fiber electromyography are useful methods for the study of human motor units.

In nerve conduction studies, distal nerves are supramaximally stimulated and the evoked muscle response recorded. The amplitude of the evoked muscle response is an index of the number of motor units. This method is most commonly used to study the median-nerve-innervated abductor pollicis brevis (APB) muscle, the ulnar-nerve-innervated abductor digiti minimi (ADM) muscle, the peroneal-nerve-innervated extensor digitorum brevis (EDB) muscle, and the posterior-tibial-nerve-innervated abductor hallucis (AH) muscle. A quantitative technique for estimation of the number of motor units has been developed using finely graded incremental stimuli applied to the motor nerve with computer analysis of the evoked muscle action potential increments.[21]

Supramaximal stimulation of a distal nerve often elicits a late response called the F wave.[19,20] This response is due to antidromic discharge of some of the lower motor neurons by the electrical stimulus. The amplitude of the F wave provides an index of motor neuron excitability.[19,20,22] As discussed in Physiology of Lower Motor Neurons, above, motor neuron excitability is determined by both the size principle and an algebraic summation of peripheral, segmental, and suprasegmental inputs.

Conventional needle electromyography permits examination of most muscles.[19,20] With the muscle at rest, no electrical activity should be detected. The electrical abnormalities most commonly detected in a relaxed muscle are fibrillations and positive waves (the spontaneous discharge of denervated single muscle fibers), fasciculations (the spontaneous discharge of a motor unit), and iterative discharges (spontaneous, regularly firing, time-locked multispikes). When a muscle contraction is performed, the motor unit potential characteristics (amplitude, duration, phases) and the pattern of motor unit recruitment can be examined. An orderly increase in both the firing rates and the number of motor units recruited should be evident as the patient increases contraction.

Repetitive nerve stimulation is performed by applying supramaximal stimulation to distal nerves at rates varying from 3 to 50 stimuli/s and measuring changes in the evoked muscle potential amplitude.[19,20] A defect in neuromuscular transmission will result in a change in the evoked muscle potential amplitude. A decrement of greater than 10% between the first and the lowest of the next four evoked potential amplitudes is commonly seen in myasthenia gravis.

Single-fiber electromyography permits examination of muscle fibers within the same motor unit.[23] The single fiber electrode has a recording diameter of 25 to 30 μm which makes possible extracellular recording of single muscle fiber action potentials. The variability (jitter) of the interpotential interval between two or more single muscle fibers belonging to the same motor unit can be determined by this technique.

In ALS, nerve conduction studies show a wide range of values for the evoked muscle response.[24-26] The amplitude of the evoked response generally decreases as the muscle atrophy increases. The F-wave amplitude tends to increase if spasticity occurs without significant muscle atrophy.[22] Conventional needle electromyography generally shows fibrillations, positive waves, and fasciculations in several muscles. In addition, the motor unit potentials may be of large amplitude and long duration, with an increased number of phases.[23-26] The motor unit recruitment is reduced. The diffuse neuropathic changes of ALS can be differentiated from those of focal neuropathic disorders if abnormalities occur in the muscles of at least three extremities or of two extremities and a cranial-nerve-innervated muscle. Repetitive nerve stimulation may show a decrement in the evoked muscle response similar to that found in myasthenia gravis.[27,28] Single-fiber electromyography may show an increase in jitter.[29]

MOTOR UNIT EVALUATION IN THE CARE OF THE AMYOTROPHIC LATERAL SCLEROSIS PATIENT

Since changes in the characteristics and numbers of motor unit potentials provide an indirect index of the changes and loss of motor neurons, electrodiagnosis may provide helpful insights into the care of the

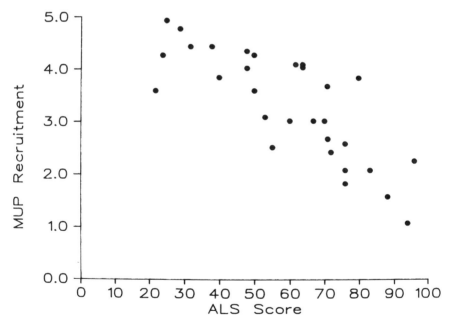

Figure 2–8. Scattergram of ALS scores and motor unit potential (MUP) recruitment scores for 30 patients with ALS. A MUP recruitment score of 0 signifies a normal pattern and a score of 5 signifies a maximum loss (no units). Spearman's coefficient of rank correlation, r_s, is $-.80$ ($p<.01$).

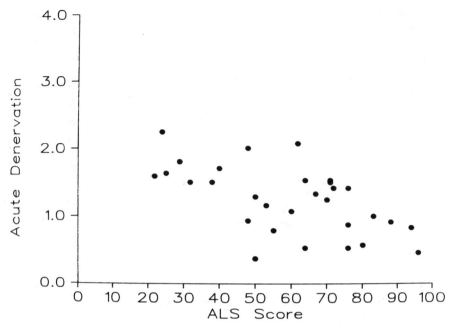

Figure 2–9. Scattergram of ALS scores and acute denervation scores for 30 patients with ALS. An acute denervation score of 0 signifies no fibrillations or positive waves and a score of 4 signifies abundant fibrillations and positive waves in all examined muscle areas. Spearman's coefficient of rank correlation, r_s, is $-.59$ (p<.01).

ALS patient. If the amount of acute denervation (fibrillations and positive waves), fasciculations, or decrease in motor unit potential recruitment were highly correlated with functional disability due to ALS, these electrical parameters would be helpful in assessing disease severity and prognosis. In order to test the correlation between motor unit abnormalities and functional disability from ALS, 30 patients from the Hahnemann University Amyotrophic Laterial Sclerosis Clinic consented to have a standardized electrodiagnostic study (Tahmoush AJ: unpublished results) and an assessment of functional disability.[30] Electrical measures were performed by conventional needle electromyography in 12 muscles (the deltoid, biceps, flexor carpi ulnaris, flexor digitorum indicis, vastus lateralis, and tibialis anterior bilaterally). Spearman's coefficient of rank correlation[31] was calculated to describe the relationship between the ALS score and each of the electrical activity measures. A scattergram of the ALS scores and the motor unit potential recruitment scores is presented in Figure 2–8. The value of the rank correlation coefficient r_s is $-.80$, which is statistically significant. A scattergram of the ALS scores and acute denervation

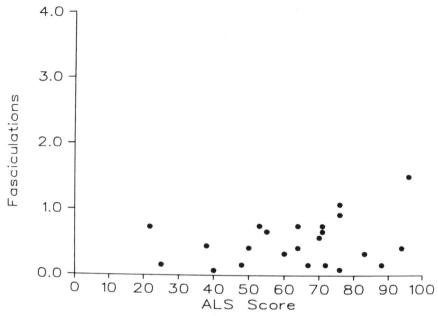

Figure 2–10. Scattergram of ALS scores and fasciculation scores for 30 patients with ALS. A fasciculation score of 0 signifies no fasciculations and a score of 4 signifies many fasciculations in most muscles. Spearman's coefficient of rank correlation, r_s, is .27 (p>.05).

scores is presented in Figure 2–9. The rank correlation coefficient, r_s, is $-.59$, which is statistically significant. These negative values indicate that patients with the most severe functional disability (i.e., low ALS scores) have fewer motor units and more acute denervation. A scattergram of ALS scores and fasciculation scores is presented in Figure 2–10. Although some positive correlation between the variables is present ($r_s = .27$) the rank correlation coefficient is not significant at the .05 level. Therefore, functional disability is most highly correlated with decrease in motor unit potential recruitment.

REFERENCES

1. Liddell EGT, Sherrington CS: Recruitment and some other factors of reflex inhibition. Proc R Soc Lond Ser B 97:488–518, 1925.
2. Burke RE: Motor units: Anatomy, physiology, and functional organization. In Brookhart JM, Mountcastle VB, Brooks VB (eds): The Nervous System. Motor Control. Handbook of Physiology. American Physiological Society, Bethesda, MD, 1981.

3. Brookhart JM, Mountcastle VB, Brooks VB: In Brookhart JM, Mountcastle VB, Brooks VB (eds): The Nervous System. Motor Control. Handbook of Physiology, American Physiological Society, Bethesda. MD, 1981.
4. Schmitt ED, Worden FG: The Neurosciences. Third Study Program. MIT Press, Cambridge, MA, 1974.
5. Desmedt JE: Motor Control Mechanisms in Health and Disease. Advances in Neurology, Vol. 39. Raven Press, New York, 1983.
6. Desmedt JE: Spinal and supraspinal mechanisms of voluntary motor control and locomotion. In Progress in Clinical Neurophysiology, Vol. 8. Karger, Basel, 1980.
7. Henneman E, Mendell LM: Functional organization of motorneuron pool and its inputs. In Brookhart JM, Mountcastle VB, Brooks VB (eds): The Nervous System. Motor Control. Handbook of Physiology. American Physiological Society, Bethesda, MD, 1981.
8. Bruke RE, Levin DN, Zajac FE, et al.: Mammalian motor units: Physiological-histochemical correlation in three types in cat gastrocnemius. Science 174:709–712, 1971.
9. Burke RE, Levin DN Tsairis P, et al.: Physiological types and histochemical profiles in motor units of the cat gastrocnemius. J Physiol 234:723–748, 1973.
10. Edstrom L, Kugelberg E: Histochemical composition, distribution of fibres and fatigability of single motor units. Anterior tibial muscle of the rat. J Neurol Neursurg Psychiatry 31:424–433, 1968.
11. Kugelberg E: Properties of the rat hindlimb motor units. In Desmedt JE (ed): New Developments in Electromyography and Clinical Neurophysiology, Vol 1. Karger, Basel, 1973, pp. 2–13.
12. Brandstater ME, Lambert EH: Motor unit anatomy. In Desmedt JE (ed): New Developments in Electromyography and Clinical Neurophysiology, Vol 1. Karger, Basel, 1973, pp. 14–22.
13. McPhedran AM, Wuerker RB, Henneman E: Properties of motor units in a homogeneous red muscle (soleus) of the cat. J Neurophysiol 28:71–84, 1956.
14. Wuerker RB, McPhedran AM, Henneman E: Properties of motor units in a heterogeneous pale muscle (M. gastrocnemius) of the cat. J Neurophysiol 28:85–99, 1965.
15. Henneman E, Somjen G, Carpenter DO: Functional significance of cell size in spinal motorneurons. J Neurophysiol 28:560–580, 1965.
16. Henneman E, Olson CB: Relations between structure and function in the design of skeletal muscles. J Neurophysiol 28:581–598, 1965.
17. Henneman E, Somjen G, Carpenter DO: Excitability and inhibility of motoneurons of different size. J Neurophysiol 28:599–620, 1965.
18. Luscher HR, Ruenzel P, Henneman E: How the size of motoneurons determines their susceptibility to discharge. Nature 282:859–861, 1979.
19. Kimura J: Electrodiagnosis in Diseases of Nerve and Muscle. Davis, Philadelphia, 1983.
20. Goodgold J, Eberstein A: Electrodiagnosis of Neuromuscular Diseases. Williams & Wilkins, Baltimore, 1983.
21. Hansen S, Ballantyne JP: A quantitative electrophysiological study of motor neurone disease. J Neurol Neurosurg Psychiatry 41:773–783.
22. Eisen A, Odusote K: Amplitude of the F wave. A potential means of documenting spasticity. Neurology 29:1306–1309, 1979.
23. Stalberg E, Trontelj J: Single Fiber Electromyography. The Miravelle Press, Old Woking, England, 1979.
24. Lambert EH: Electromyography in amyotrophic lateral sclerosis. In Norris FH, Kurland LT (eds): Motor Neurone Diseases. New York, Grune & Stratton, 1969.
25. Lambert EH, Mulder DW: Electromyographic studies in amyotrophic lateral sclerosis. Proc Staff Meet Mayo Clin 32:441–447, 1957.
26. Daube JR: EMG in motor neuron disease. American Association of Electromyography and Electrodiagnosis (AAEE). Minimonograph No. 18. AAEE, Rochester, MN, 1982.
27. Mulder DW, Lambert EH, Eaton LM: Myasthenic syndrome in patients with amyotrophic lateral sclerosis. Neurology 9:627–631, 1959.
28. Denys EH, Norris FH: Amyotrophic lateral sclerosis. Impairment of neuromuscular transmission. Arch Neurol 36:202–205, 1979.

29. Stallberg E, Schwartz MS, Trontelj JV: Single fiber electromyography in various processes affecting the anterior horn cell. J Neurol Sci 24:403–415, 1975.
30. Norris FH, Calanchini PR, Fallat RJ, et al.: The administration of guanidine in amyotrophic lateral sclerosis. Neurology 24:721–728, 1974.
31. Snedecor GW, Cochran WC: Statistical Methods, Ed. 7. Iowa State University Press, Ames, 1980.

CHAPTER THREE

CONSIDERATIONS IN THE DIFFERENTIAL DIAGNOSIS OF AMYOTROPHIC LATERAL SCLEROSIS

Jeffrey Allen Cohen, M.D.

The diagnosis of amyotrophic lateral sclerosis (ALS) is made by the presence of upper motor neuron (UMN) signs (spasticity, increased reflexes, mild weakness, pathologic reflexes), lower motor neuron (LMN) signs (atrophy, fasciculation, loss of reflexes, weakness), and the absence of significant sensory deficits. Additional features include its sporadic occurrence, usually in the fifth to seventh decade of life, lack of sphincter involvement, and its progressive course.[1]

The diagnosis may be confirmed by normal nerve conduction studies, in particular normal sensory nerve action potentials (Fig. 3–1) and electomyographic examination of at least three limbs and/or tongue and facial musculature that demonstrates diffuse anterior horn cell pathology (active denervation, fasciculations, and neuropathic motor unit potentials

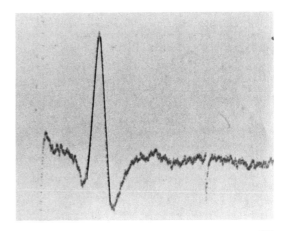

Figure 3–1. Normal sensory nerve action potential recorded with surface electrodes from the sural nerve orthodromically. Calibration: 10 μV/2 μms.

that recruit incompletely).[2,3] Radiographic examinations, myelography to the level of the foramen magnum, computed tomography (CT) of the spine, and now, Magnetic Resonance Imaging (MRI) of the spinal cord may be necessary to exclude structural pathology of the spinal cord.

The purpose of this chapter is to discuss the differential diagnosis of ALS; specifically, the situation where there are atypical features that make the certainty of an ALS diagnosis doubtful. It is easiest to examine features that may give the physician a clue to another diagnosis, one pointing to a cause that is possibly treatable.

LOWER MOTOR NEURON FINDINGS

A form of ALS, progressive muscular atrophy (PMA) is characterized by a more benign course and the selective involvement of the LMNs without clinical UMN signs. Predominant involvement of the LMNs may occur in other conditions.

In motor neuropathies, there is LMN pathology that may give a clinical picture similar to PMA. Some features may be present that help to differentiate this condition from PMA. These may include: distal symmetrical nature, predominance in the lower extremities, and lack of bul-

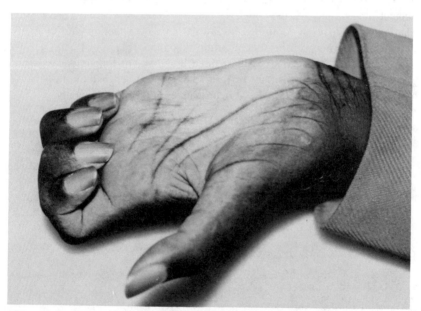

Figure 3–2. Photograph of a patient with distal wasting representative of a motor neuropathy.

bar musculature involvement[4] (Fig. 3–2). Motor neurpathy may be associated with neoplasia as a paraneoplastic syndrome, in particular with lymphoma.[5] The course of the motor neuropathy is independent of the course of the malignancy. Postmortem examination reveals pathologic involvement of the anterior horn cells.[5]

Additionally, marked LMN findings may be associated with the neuropathies of the acquired immune deficiency syndrome (AIDS),[6] paraproteinemias[7-9] (Fig. 3–3), and heavy metal intoxication[10] (lead, mercury, and arsenic, though sensory findings are usually present).

The occurrence of this condition with lymphoma and AIDS has raised the possibility of an opportunistic viral infection selective for anterior horn cells, although such a viral association has not been proven.[5] Recently, specific immunoglobulins that are selectively destructive to peripheral nerve myelin have been isolated in patients with paraproteinemias (see Testing for Associated Abnormalities, below).[7,9]

Therefore, slowly progressive LMN findings warrant certain testing. Sensory nerve action potentials should be carefully performed (sural nerve in particular), as well as complete blood counts, sedimentation rate, blood chemistries, special serum immunoelectrophoresis, and evaluation for the presence of heavy metals (urine, hair samples, and nail clippings). In patients complaining of systemic symptoms, for example, severe weight loss, fevers, and lymphadenopathy, further immunologic, hematologic, and ra-

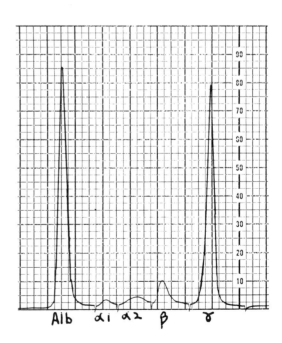

Figure 3–3. Serum protein electrophoresis demonstrating a spike γ.

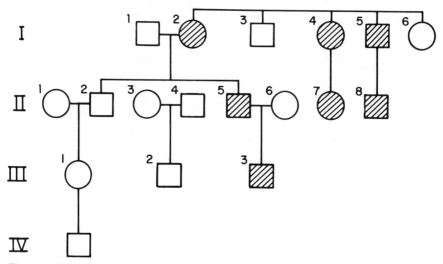

Figure 3–4. Pedigree of a family with a hereditary motor neuropathy, dominant inheritance. (Boxes are males, circles females, Roman numerals indicate generations, Arabic numerals indicate family members. Shaded figures indicate presence of disease.)

diographic (chest x-rays films, CT scan of body, bone survey) investigations may be necessary.

Chronic relapsing inflammatory polyneuropathy may be difficult to recognize despite the presence of sensory findings and its clinical course.[11] The nerve conduction studies should reveal a demyelinative process (markedly slowed conduction velocities), while lumbar puncture demonstrates an elevated protein level. Treatment with steroids and plasmapheresis may be of benefit to these patients.[11,12]

There are also hereditary forms of LMN involvement, the hereditary motor neuropathies (HMN).[13] The usual onset is in childhood but adult forms have been described. The illness must "run true" within the family as to the pattern of inheritance (autosomal dominant, recessive, or sex-linked) (Fig. 3–4). The distribution of weakness may be either proximal or distal. Involvement of the bulbar musculature in the adult form is uncommon. By definition, UMN involvement and sensory deficits are rare. The differentiation of HMN from PMA is difficult. Family history must be scrupulously investigated and family members should be neurologically examined and electrophysiologic testing performed if the diagnosis is unclear.

Additionally, LMN findings may be restricted to a single limb, the focal atrophies. These may be manifest at birth or become observable at a later age. Some of these focal atrophies may be familial.[13] The use of nerve conduction studies and electromyography should help confirm the clinical impression of the focal LMN findings.

UPPER MOTOR NEURON FINDINGS

The presence of pure UMN signs may be seen in the slowly progressive condition of primary lateral sclerosis (PLS).

Diagnostic confusion may arise with other conditions that primarily demonstrate muscle tone changes. Multiple sclerosis and other white matter disorders may rarely present with only UMN findings. In this situation, abnormal evoked potential testing (visual, brain stem, and somatosensory) may be of assistance, though abnormalities in ALS have been reported.[14] MRI of the head demonstrating multiple plaques can be useful. Additionally, cerebrospinal fluid (CSF) examination for oliogoclonal banding, IgG synthetic rate, and myelin basic protein may help to establish the diagnosis of multiple sclerosis (MS).[15]

Parkinsonism in its atypical forms may be confused with ALS, especially if amyotrophy is present. Again, nerve conduction velocity studies (NCVs) and electomyograms (EMG) are of importance, usually demonstrating restricted distal anterior horn cell findings. Clinical course and the response to a trial of antiparkinsonian medications may assist in diagnosis.

In the multisystem atrophies, UMN signs (as well as LMN signs) may be present, though there is always the presence of other neurologic dysfunction (autonomic, brain stem, cerebellar, and so forth). Specific enzyme testing (glutamic dehydrogenase, as in the olivopontocerebellar atrophies) may be useful[16] (Fig. 3–5).

Familial spastic paraplegia (FSP) may be difficult to distinguish from PLS, especially when the family history is unobtainable. This condition is usually characterized by predominate lower extremity involvement, but progression to upper extremity involvement is also seen.[17] In some instances urinary disturbance, evidenced by spasticity of bladder musculature may be present clinically (frequent urination in small amounts) and documented by cystometric studies.

SENSORY DISTURBANCE

It is widely held that the diagnosis of ALS cannot be made with the presence of significant sensory disturbance. The word *significant* is of great importance, since distal vibratory loss of the lower extremities may be present without an identifiable cause. Prior investigators have reported the existence of sensory deficits in ALS patients.[18] Additionally, there has been documentation of nerve fiber loss in sural nerve biopsies performed in ALS patients. It has been our experience and that of others that despite the clinical presence of sensory abnormalities, standard sensory nerve conduction studies (with the limb maintained at room temperature) are of

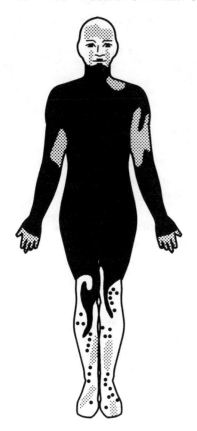

Figure 3–5. Sweat test, showing areas of anhidrosis, shown unshaded, in a patient with multisystem atrophy. The patient had lower motor neuron, optic nerve, cerebellar, and autonomic nervous system findings on examination. (Courtesy of Robert Fealy, M.D., Mayo Clinic.)

normal amplitude and latency. If abnormalities are documented then the diagnosis of ALS should be reconsidered. A situation that demands attention is sensory loss and/or weakness that occurs in multiple specific nerve distributions. This picture is consistent with the diagnosis of mononeuritis multiplex. Typically, mononeuritis multiplex is asymmetrical and of sudden onset; it may be associated with connective tissue disease[19] (rheumatoid arthritis, systemic lupus erythematosus, periarteritis nodosa, Lyme's disease),[20] sarcoidosis,[21] or diabetes[22] (Fig. 3–6). In connective tissue disease the arthritis may be active: swollen inflamed joints, and perhaps other system involvement (kidney, cardiac, pulmonary) may be present, but a nonsystemic mononeuritis multiplex has also been observed.

Additionally, plexopathies of any etiology (diabetic,[23] idiopathic, familial,[13] or radiation[24]) may present as either a predominantly sensory or LMN involvement. Again, history, laboratory testing (glucose, glycosylated hemoglobin), and EMGs and NCVs are of great use for ability to confirm the diagnosis.

A final note should be added concerning one of the most difficult

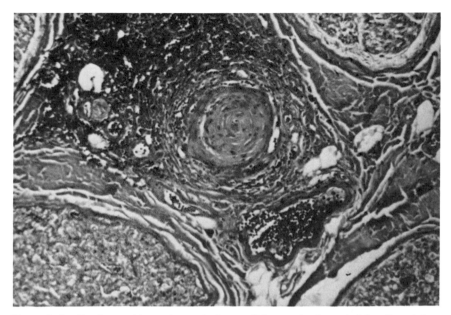

Figure 3–6. Sural nerve biopsy demonstrating medial necrosis of an arteriole with an inflammatory cell infiltrate. (Courtesy of Peter J. Dyck, M.D., Mayo Clinic.)

situations within clinical neurology. The findings of cervical arthritis with severe spondylitis and possible spinal cord impingement may be demonstrated radiographically. There is always the question of whether the clinical picture is the result of radiographic abnormalities.[25] If there is a sensory level or marked bladder or bowel dysfunction, then the presence of cervical myelopathy with the need for surgical consultation is raised.[26] On the other hand, with a paucity of sensory findings and normal bladder and bowel function, the clinical significance of the radiographic changes may be unclear. Unnecessary spinal surgery for cervical arthritis should be avoided by careful clinical and complete radiographic examinations supplemented by NCVs and EMGs. Repeated clinical and electrophysiologic examinations may be necessary (Fig. 3–7).

PROGRESSION, AGE, AND FAMILY HISTORY

The progression of ALS is inexorable. With the exceptions of PLS and PMA, it is unusual for the disease to progress slowly or plateau.[27] When present, additional possibilities must be examined (see Testing for Associated Abnormalities, below).

Age of onset is usually the fifth to seventh decade. 80.6% of patients from the Mount Sinai Hospital ALS Clinic fell within this group; while

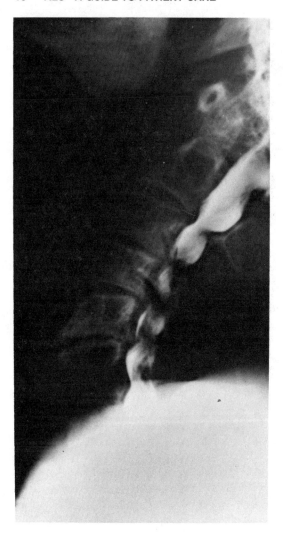

Figure 3–7. Cervical myelogram of a 50-year-old male with progressive spasticity of the lowe extremities and fasciculations o the upper extremities. Note the impingement on the spinal cord.

less than 5% of patients had age of onset before 35 years.[26] Additionally, family clustering of ALS is uncommon, though there is an autosomal-dominant form of ALS, as mentioned in Chapter 1.[28]

Abnormalities of GM_2 ganglioside metabolism due to hexosamini-dase A (Hex A) deficiency have been associated with ALS pheno-types.[29–31] The clinical features described in these ALS patients with Hex A deficiency included the atypical features noted above: early onset, family history, and/or long disease duration. As a result, the records of the Mount Sinai Amyotrophic Lateral Sclerosis Clinic were reviewed to select those patients with these atypical features. Hexosaminidase A deficiency was not found in any of the "atypical" ALS patients.

TESTING FOR ASSOCIATED ABNORMALITIES

It is suggested that ALS may be the common clinical picture of many different etiologies. As a result, rather than simply undertaking extensive investigation of only atypical ALS patients, it is also necessary to carefully investigate all ALS patients and to look for patterns of abnormalities.

As an example, abnormalities in immunoglobulins have been associated with peripheral neuropathies.[7-9] Specific myelin antibodies (anti-mag) have been found in patients with typical ALS.[6,7] Unfortunately, the exact role of these immunologic abnormalities is unclear and the effect of therapy has not been dramatic.[6]

As to abnormalities of calcium and selenium, these findings have not been widely reproducible nor have therapeutic measures employed changed the course of illness.

OTHER DIFFICULTIES

The presence of fasciculations alone is not sufficient to establish the diagnosis of ALS. There have been reports of differences between "benign" fasciculations and the fasciculations associated with ALS.[32] It is important to use caution when examining and discussing diagnosis with patients whose presenting complaint is fasciculation. It is not uncommon that these patients are either medical personnel or family members of patients with ALS. Electromyography is of great utility in this situation since many patients with benign fasciculations have normal EMGs and in those patients in whom fasciculations are present, there is evidence of widespread denervation typical of ALS. If necessary, follow-up clinical examinations usually help to confirm the benign nature of the fasciculations.

In our experience there have rarely been difficulties in differentiating between psychiatric illness and ALS. Occasionally, patients present with a thorough knowledge of ALS symptomatology and insist they have the disease, though clinical examination reveals no atrophy, fasciculations, tone changes, or hyperreflexia. Electromyography is recommended in such cases to rule out organic disease, since it should be realized that a patient with ALS may present with concurrent psychopathology. Psychiatric consultation is essential in both of the above situations.

LATE PROGRESSION OF POLIOMYELITIS

The occurrence of progressive weakness after a long period of clinical stability in patients with prior poliomyelitis has been described.[33-35] There is not a consensus of opinion as to the existence or etiology of this condition. Attempts have been made to explain late progression of poliomyelitis (LPOP) as: progressive anterior horn cell dropout, "fatigue" of surviving motor units, joint deformities, or general senescence.[33,35] There has been no documentation of reactivation of polio virus within the CSF of these patients.[33] The evaluation of patients with prior poliomyelitis and progressive weakness should include a complete history with explicit documentation of the loss of functional abilities. Confirmation by friends and relatives is also helpful. Structural spinal pathology should be investigated wtih radiographic examinations, and other possible causes should be considered (diabetes, alcohol, and so forth). Physical medicine evaluation is necessary to assess the need for therapy and/or assistive devices. Electromyography may be of limited use in documenting the presence and extent of anterior horn cell pathology.[34] Further investigation of these patients is necessary for our better understanding of LPOP.

ACKNOWLEDGMENT
The secretarial assistance of Andrea Payne is greatly appreciated.

REFERENCES

1. Mulder DW: Motor neuron disease. In Dyck PJ, Thomas PK, Lambert E, et al. (eds): Peripheral Neuropathy, Vol. 2. Saunders, Philadelphia, 1984, pp. 1525–1536.
2. Denys EH: Motor nerve conduction studies. In Molder DW (ed): The Diagnosis and Treatment of Amyotrophic Lateral Sclerosis. Houghton Mifflin, Boston, 1980, pp. 105–117.
3. Lambert EH: Electromyography in amyotrophic lateral sclerosis. In Norris FH, Kurland LT (eds): Motor Neuron Diseases. Grune & Stratton, New York, 1969, pp. 135–153.
4. Schaumburg H, Spencer PS, Thomas PK: Disorders of Peripheral Nerves. Davis, Philadelphia, 1983, pp. 7–25.
5. Schold SC, Cho E, Somasundasam M, et al.: Subacute motor neuropathy. A remote effect of lymphoma. Ann Neurol 5:271–287, 1979.
6. Levy RM, Bredesen D, Rosenblum, M: Neurological manifestations of the acquired immunodeficiency syndrome (AIDS): Experience at UCSF and review of the literature. J Neurosurg 62:475–495, 1985.
7. Latov N, Sherman W, Nemnl R, et al.: Plasma cell dyscrasia and peripheral neuropathy with a monoclonal antibody to peripheral nerve myelin. N Engl J Med 303:618–621, 1980.
8. Rowland LP, Defendini R, Sherman W, et al.: Macroglobulinemia with peripheral neuropathy simulating motor neuron disease. Ann Neurol 11:532–536, 1982.
9. Shy ME, Trojaborg W, Smith T, et al.: Motor disease and plasma cell dyscrasia. Neurology (Suppl) 35:107, 1985.
10. Windebank AJ, et al.: Metal neuropathy. In Dyck PJ, Thomas PK, Lambert E, et al. (eds): Peripheral Neuropathy, Vol. 2. Saunders, Philadelphia, 1984, pp. 2133–2161.

11. Dyck PJ, Lais A, Ohta M: Chronic inflammatory polyradiculoneuropathy. Mayo Clin Proc 50:621–637, 1975.
12. Server A, Lefkowith J, Braine H, et al.: Treatment of chronic relapsing polyradiculoneuropathy by plasma exchange. Ann Neurol 6:258–261, 1979.
13. Harding AE: Inherited neuronal atrophy and degeneration predominantly of lower motor neurons. In Dyck PJ, Thomas PK, Lambert E, et al. (eds): Peripheral Neuropathy. Saunders, Philadelphia, 1984, pp. 1537–1556.
14. Oh SJ, Sunwoo I, Kim H: Cervical and cortical somatosensory evoked potentials differentiate cervical spondolytic myelopathy from amyotrophic lateral sclerosis. Neurology (Suppl) 35:147, 1985.
15. Caroscio JT, Kochwa S, Sacks H, et al.: Cerebrospinal fluid IgG and albumin indices in multiple sclerosis and other neurological disease. Arch Neurol 40:409–413, 1983.
16. Plaitakis A, Nicklas W, Desnick R, et al.: Glutamate dehydrogenase deficiency in three patients with spinocerebellar syndrome. Ann Neurol 7:297–303, 1983.
17. Bundey S: Genetics and Neurology. Churchill Livingstone, New York, 1985, pp. 241–253.
18. Dyck PJ, Stevens J. Mulder D, et al.: Frequency of nerve fiber degeneration of peripheral motor and sensory neurons in amyotrophic lateral sclerosis. Neurology 25:781–787, 1975.
19. Conn DL, Dyck PJ: Angiopathic neuropathy in connective tissue disease. In Dyck PJ, Thomas PK, Lambert E, et al. (eds): Peripheral Neuropathy, Vol. 2. Saunders, Philadelphia, 1984, pp. 2027–2043.
20. Pachner AR, Steeve A: The triad of neurologic manifestations of Lyme Disease: Meningitis, cranial neuritis and radiculoneuritis. Neurology 35:47–53, 1985.
21. Delaney P: Neurologic manifestations of sarcoidosis. Ann Intern Med 87:337–345, 1977.
22. Mulder DW, Lambert E, Bastron J, et al.: The neuropathies associated with diabetes mellitus: A clinical and eletromyographic study of 103 unselected diabetic patients. Neurology 11:275–284, 1961.
23. Bastron, JA, Thomas TE: Diabetic polyradiculopathy. Mayo Clin Proc 56:725–738, 1981.
24. Kori SH, Foley K, Posner, J, et al.: Brachial plexus lesions in patients with cancer: 100 cases. Neurology 31:45–50, 1981.
25. Kasden DL: Cervical spondylotic myelopathy with reversible fasciculations in the lower extremities. Arch Neurol 34:774–776, 1977.
26. Iwata M, Hirano A: Sparing of the Onufrowicz nucleus in sacral anterior horn lesions. Ann Neurol 4:245–249, 1978.
27. Caroscio JT, Calhoun, WF, Yahr MD: Prognostic factors in motor disease: A prospective study of longevity. In Rose FC (ed): Progress in Motor Neurone Disease. Pittman, London, 1984, 34–43.
28. Horton WA, Eldrige R, Brody JA: Familial motor neuron disease. Neurology 26:460–465, 1976.
29. Johnson WG: The clinical spectrum of hexosaminidase deficiency diseases. Neurology 31:1453–1456, 1981.
30. Johnson WG: Hexosaminidase deficiency: A cause of recessively inherited motor neuron disease. In Rolwand LP (ed): Human Motor Neuron Diseases. Raven Press, New York, 1982, pp. 159–164.
31. Johnson WG, Wigger HJ, Karp HR, et al.: Juvenile spinal muscular atrophy: A new hexosaminidase deficiency phenotype. Ann Neurol 11:11–16, 1982.
32. Trojaborg W, Buchthal F: Malignant and benign fasciculations. Acta Neurol Scand 44:251–254, 1965.
33. Alter M, Kurland LT, Molgaard C: Late progressive muscular atrophy and antecedent poliomyelitis. Adv Neurol 36:303–309, 1982.
34. Cruz-Martinez A, Ferrer MT, Perez-Conde MC: Electrophysiological features in patients with nonprogressive and late progressive weakness after paralytic poliomyelitis. Electromyogr Clin Neurophysiol 24:469–479, 1984.
35. Dalakas M, Elder G, Cunningham G, et al.: A 9-year follow-up study of patients with late postpoliomyelitis muscular atrophy (PPMA). (suppl) Neurology 35:106, 1985.

CHAPTER FOUR

RESPIRATORY FAILURE IN AMYOTROPHIC LATERAL SCLEROSIS

Mark J. Rosen, M.D.

One of the most serious complications of amyotrophic lateral sclerosis (ALS) is the development of respiratory failure. Weakness of the respiratory muscles sufficient to interfere with adequate ventilation, and cough usually occurs late in the course of the disease, but is the most common cause of death among patients with ALS. Rarely, ventilatory failure may be the initial symptom of ALS.[1] This chapter will discuss the pathophysiology of respiratory failure in ALS, and review the options for treatment.

THE RESPIRATORY MUSCLES

The primary function of the respiratory muscles is to provide the driving force to sustain ventilation. Contraction of the diaphragm and sternocleidomastoid, scalene, and internal intercostal muscles expands the chest cage, providing the negative intrathoracic pressure necessary to inflate the lungs. With quiet breathing, this task is carried out almost exclusively by the diaphragm, with exhalation occurring passively due to the elastic recoil of the lungs and chest wall. However, with increased ventilatory demands, such as during exercise or with intrinsic lung diseases, the "accessory" inspiratory muscles increase their contribution to ventilatory efforts. The expiratory muscles, which include the internal intercostal and abdominal muscles, are usually not active during quiet breathing, but may serve to increase expiratory flow with increased ventilatory demands. Effective contraction of these muscles is also necessary to provide high expiratory flow rates during cough.[2]

Respiratory muscles may be characterized by their strength and endurance.[3] Strength, or the ability of a muscle to generate an expected force, depends upon an adequate neural drive, a normal number of contractile elements, and integrity of cellular structures. The force of muscular con-

45

Table 4–1. Maximal Respiratory Pressures (Mean ± SD): Normal Values According to Sex and Age Groups

	9–18 Years	*19–49 Years*	*50–69 Years*	*≥ 70 Years*
Males				
PI_{max} (cm H_2O)	-96 ± 35	-127 ± 28	-112 ± 20	-76 ± 27
PE_{max} (cm H_2O)	170 ± 32	216 ± 45	196 ± 45	133 ± 42
No. patients	13	80	27	6
Females				
PI_{max} (cm H_2O)	-90 ± 25	-91 ± 25	-77 ± 18	-66 ± 18
PE_{max} (cm H_2O)	136 ± 34	138 ± 39	124 ± 37	108 ± 28
No. patients	12	121	28	12

Source: Arora NS: Pulmonary Research Laboratory, Charlottesville, Va. With permission.

traction is also modified by the length of the muscle at the onset of contraction and by the velocity at which it shortens during contraction.[4] Respiratory muscle strength may be assessed clinically by simply measuring the inspiratory and expiratory pressures developed during maximal efforts against a closed airway.[5] In normal individuals, maximal inspiratory and expiratory pressures (PI_{max} and PE_{max}, respectively) are greater in men than women, and decline with age (Table 4–1).

Respiratory muscle strength can also be assessed using an intraesophageal balloon catheter to measure changes in intrapleural pressure, or using both esophageal and gastric balloon catheters to determine transdiaphragmatic pressure generation. However, these techniques are more invasive and require sophisticated equipment. Therefore, their major use is in clinical research.

Endurance, or the ability of a muscle to maintain an expected force with repeated contractions,[6] depends first upon the strength of the muscle, such that a weaker muscle will fatigue faster than a stronger one. Furthermore, in a given muscle, any imbalance between the supply of oxygen and glucose to the muscle and the rate at which these substrates are consumed causes fatigue.[7] Finally, the energy demands of respiratory muscles grow with the increase in the work of breathing associated with an increase in airway resistance or decrease in pulmonary compliance. Substrate supply to contracting muscles may be impaired by reduction of oxygen transport caused by reduced cardiac output, severe anemia or hypoxemia, or by reduction of blood concentrations of glucose or fatty acids.[7]

RESPIRATORY MUSCLE DYSFUNCTION IN AMYOTROPHIC LATERAL SCLEROSIS

Any disease that affects the respiratory muscles reduces both their strength and endurance. In ALS, degeneration of the anterior horn cells of the spinal cord leads to atrophy of the respiratory muscles, rendering them weaker and more subject to fatigue. In patients with severe weakness, even the work of breathing at rest may cause fatigue, leading to a decrease in resting minute ventilation and diminished ability to excrete carbon dioxide.

Respiratory muscle weakness may be quantitated in patients by measuring PI_{max} and PE_{max}, which closely correlates with changes in transdiaphragmatic pressures.[8] These measurements are more sensitive than reductions in vital capacity and tidal volume, which become impaired later in the course of the disease as muscular weakness worsens. As weakness progresses, the arterial PCO_2 ($PaCO_2$) rises and PO_2 falls reciprocally, but this does not usually occur until PI_{max} and PE_{max} are less than 30% of the predicted normal values, suggesting that hypercapnia occurs only when weakness is severe.[8]

In addition to the reduction in strength and endurance caused by the underlying disease, many patients with ALS are also significantly undernourished, which further impairs respiratory muscle function. Arora and Rochester demonstrated that malnutrition decreases the mass of the diaphragm, even out of proportion to the reduction in body weight.[9] Even in the absence of intrinsic neuromuscular disease, poorly nourished patients have significant impairment in respiratory muscle strength and endurance, with an approximately 60% reduction in PI_{max} and PE_{max}.[10] The weakness and fatigue of a patient with impaired respiratory muscle function due to ALS is compounded if adequate nutrition is not maintained.

RESPIRATORY FAILURE COMPLICATING AMYOTROPHIC LATERAL SCLEROSIS

When respiratory muscle strength falls below a critical level, then the generated inspiratory pressures are inadequate to maintain alveolar ventilation, and $PaCO_2$ begins to rise and PaO_2 falls. In ALS, the degree of $PaCO_2$ elevation is proportional to the reduction in vital capacity.

In addition to muscle weakness, other factors may further impair gas exchange (Fig. 4–1). Reduction in expiratory muscle strength interferes with the generation of an effective cough, leading to retention of respiratory tract secretions and subsequent atelectasis and pulmonary infection.[2] These problems are aggravated in patients who have coexistent bulbar paralysis and impairment in swallowing reflexes, in whom repeated episodes of aspiration occur.

Pulmonary infection and atelectasis lead to hypoxemia and, in many patients, worsening of CO_2 retention and acidosis. Hypoxemia, hypercapnia and acidosis may, in turn, cause further reductions in respiratory muscle strength.[11,12] In addition, atelectasis and pneumonia both decrease

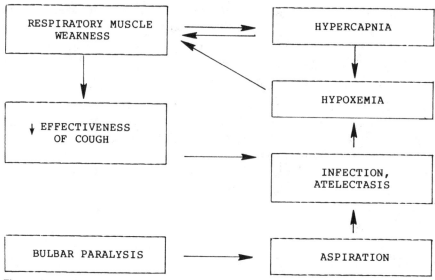

Figure 4–1. Mechanisms of respiratory failure in amyotrophic lateral sclerosis.

pulmonary compliance, increase the work of breathing, and hasten the development of respiratory muscle fatigue. Thus, a cascade of untoward events is established whereby muscle weakness and fatigue cause atelectasis and pneumonia, which in turn further impair muscle function. The end result may be the development of frank respiratory failure, with marked hypercapnia, acidosis, and hypoxemia, often complicated by massive atelectasis or overwhelming pneumonia.

CLINICAL RECOGNITION OF RESPIRATORY MUSCLE FAILURE

Obviously, it is desirable to recognize the development of impairment in respiratory muscle strength and to intervene before life-threatening complications arise. In patients with ALS, respiratory muscle strength should be evaluated with routine spirometry and measurements of maximum voluntary ventilation, PI_{max} and PE_{max} at the time that the diagnosis is established, and serial measurements should be obtained at appropriate intervals. Until a critical level of impairment is reached, a patient has no subjective respiratory complaints. Later, he may become dyspneic in a setting of increased ventilatory demand, such as with exercise or respiratory infection. The onset of CO_2 retention may be heralded by the appearance of headaches due to cerebral vasodilation caused by hypercapnia. Headaches are often present upon arising, since $PaCO_2$ is higher during sleep, when central respiratory drive normally diminishes and the work of the diaphragm to displace abdominal contents is increased by the recumbent position.[3] It has been our observation that the occurrence of nightmares can also be the warning sign of CO_2 retention.

As the disease progresses, or during periods of increased ventilatory demands, impending respiratory failure can be recognized by a sequence of clinical signs that can be easily detected at the bedside. Before frank CO_2 retention occurs, the respiratory rate increases in an attempt to compensate for the reduced tidal volume and restore minute volume to normal.[13] As fatigue becomes more severe, abnormal respiratory patterns emerge. Normally, an individual breathing quietly in the supine position has outward movement of the abdomen during inspiration, with little if any discernible movement of the rib cage. This is due to the diaphragm displacing the abdominal contents as it descends. As the diaphragm fatigues, the accessory muscles of inspiration become more active, and the patient begins to inspire by displacing the rib cage. At first, "respiratory alternans" or alternation between abdominal and rib cage movements, is seen. Later, "abdominal paradox," or paradoxical inward motion of the diaphragm during inspiration, occurs (Fig. 4–2). This indicates that the diaphragm is not contracting effectively during inspiration, and the negative intrathoracic pressure generated by the inspiratory accessory muscles is transmitted across the diaphragm to the abdomen, inwardly displacing the abdominal wall. These abnormal respiratory movements are easily detected by simple observation of the patient, and portend the development of CO_2 retention.[13]

With progressive elevations in $PaCO_2$, particularly when occurring rapidly over a short period of time, the patient may report the onset of

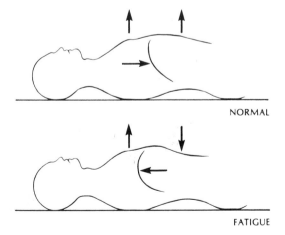

NORMAL

FATIGUE

Figure 4–2. "Paradoxical" breathing pattern. Normally, the diaphragm descends with inspiration, displacing the abdominal contents and moving the abdominal wall outward. When the diaphragm is fatigued, the accessory muscles of inspiration cause the diaphragm to move passively cephalad, and the abdominal wall moves inward. (From Rochester DF, Arora NS: Respiratory muscle failure. Med Clin N Am 67:573–597, 1983. With permission.)

headaches. With further elevations of $PaCO_2$, the syndrome of CO_2 narcosis occurs, which begins with mild sedation and may progress to frank coma. Hypercapnia also causes systemic vasodilation, with increased blood flow to the skin and conjunctivae, as well as an increase in sympathetic tone, manifested by tachycardia and hypertension. As the $PaCO_2$ rises, the PaO_2 falls, and severe hypoxemia may produce further alterations in mental status and increase in sympathetic tone. Cyanosis is usually seen only when hypoxemia becomes severe, and therefore measurement of arterial blood gases is essential in establishing the presence of abnormalities in gas exchange before they reach a critical stage.

In many patients with ALS, the onset of ventilatory failure may be slow and insidious, with progressive increases in $PaCO_2$ over several months as the respiratory muscles gradually lose their strength. In these individuals, there is ample time for compensatory mechanisms to assure homeostasis of acid-base balance. When $PaCO_2$ is chronically elevated, augmented renal excretion of hydrogen ions leads to an increase in serum bicarbonate concentration and relative preservation of arterial pH. One clue to the presence of chronic CO_2 retention is the finding of an otherwise unexplained elevation in serum bicarbonate in the routine determination of serum electrolytes. Hypercapnia may then be confirmed by an arterial blood gas analysis.

Alternatively, some patients with ALS develop acute respiratory failure following an episode of aspiration or with respiratory infection. Demands on the respiratory muscles abruptly increase, and they are incapable of augmenting minute ventilation. In this situation, there is a far more dramatic clinical presentation, with rapid deterioration of gas exchange progressing to lethargy and coma.

TREATMENT OF ACUTE RESPIRATORY FAILURE IN AMYOTROPHIC LATERAL SCLEROSIS

Mechanical Ventilation

Because respiratory failure in patients with ALS is usually a consequence of weakness and fatigue of the respiratory muscles, the major thrust of treatment is directed at correcting life-threatening hypercapnia and hypoxemia, and later at attempting to improve respiratory muscle function and decrease the work of breathing.

With any form of muscle fatigue, the best treatment is rest. In patients with respiratory failure, the mainstay of supportive therapy is the use of mechanical ventilation. In addition to rapidly correcting hypercapnia and hypoxemia, the ventilator assumes the work of breathing for the patient, permitting the respiratory muscles to rest.

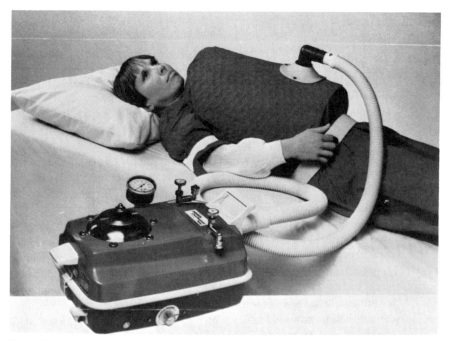

Figure 4–3. Cuirass ventilator. The patient's thorax is placed in a rigid shell. Intermittent negative pressure is applied, providing the driving force for inhalation. (Courtesy of J.H. Emerson Co., Cambridge, MA. With permission.)

Several types of mechanical ventilators are available for ventilatory support. They may be classified as negative-pressure or positive-pressure ventilators, depending on the type of pressure that is applied to the respiratory system. The "iron lung" used extensively during poliomyelitis epidemics of the 1940s and 1950s exemplifies the negative-pressure ventilator. The patient was placed into a rigid cylinder with the head protruding through a hole with an airtight seal around the patient's neck. Intermittent negative or alternating negative and positive pressure within the container could then be applied to the patient's chest by the mechanical pump. This pressure was transmitted to the pleural space, providing the driving force for ventilation. The disadvantages of this type of ventilator were that it was cumbersome, did not permit good nursing care, and was uncomfortable for most patients. The design of the early negative-pressure ventilation has been subsequently modified, leading to Cuirass ventilators that are in common use today. These devices cover only the patient's chest or chest and abdomen, providing intermittent negative-pressure ventilation by means of an attached pump or a specially modified vacuum cleaner (Fig. 4–3). Although the Cuirass ventilators are not suitable for acutely ill patients in whom access to the airway and strict control of tidal volume and respiratory rate are desirable, these devices are very useful in patients with chronic respiratory failure, particularly when this occurs as a complication of neuromuscular disease.

In patients who are acutely or critically ill, positive pressure ventilation delivered via a cuffed endotracheal tube is preferred. This technique has several advantages over support with a Cuirass ventilator. The endotracheal tube permits access to the lower respiratory tract, facilitating clearance of secretions by suctioning in patients who are too weak to cough effectively. In patients with bulbar disease, the cuffed tube also represents a barrier to aspirated secretions. Positive-pressure ventilators permit precise adjustments of respiratory rate and tidal volume, and are much more likely than negative-pressure ventilators to assure adequate gas exchange in critically ill patients.

Once the decision to institute mechanical ventilatory support is made, an endotracheal tube is inserted by either the oral or nasal route. The cuff is inflated to assure an adequate seal, the trachea is suctioned, and the endotracheal tube is tightly fitted to the ventilator tubing. Generally, supraphysiologic tidal volumes of 12 to 15 ml/kg body weight are employed to prevent or reverse areas of atelectasis, and the respiratory rate should be adjusted to provide that level of $PaCO_2$ that achieves an arterial pH in the range of 7.35 to 7.45. Repeated determinations of arterial blood gases are essential, since it is impossible to predict the effect of a change in respiratory rate or tidal volume on $PaCO_2$. More emphasis should be placed on correcting the arterial pH than on aiming for a specific level of $PaCO_2$, since many patients with ALS have chronic hypercapnia and hyperbicarbonatemia. In these patients, providing a $PaCO_2$ in the ''normal'' range of 34 to 45 mm Hg may provoke severe alkalosis, arrhythmias and seizures.

Since one object of assisted ventilation in patients with ALS is to allow the respiratory muscles to rest, either the ''control'' or ''assist-control'' modes of ventilation should be employed. In contrast to intermittent mandatory ventilation (IMV), where the patient breathes spontaneously between ventilator-provided breaths, these modes allow the ventilator to assume the work of breathing completely, allowing total rest of the respiratory muscles. Once the patient has achieved adequate gas exchange, full ventilatory support should probably be continued for at least 24 to 48 h to allow the chronically fatigued respiratory muscles a sufficient rest period.

Supplemental oxygen should be also provided, initially at an inspired fraction of oxygen (FiO_2) of 0.4 to 0.6. The concentration of oxygen may then be adjusted based on PaO_2 measurements.

If an acute problem occurs, such as infection or atelectasis precipitating acute respiratory failure, weaning from the ventilator should be considered when these complications resolve. Once the inciting cause of respiratory failure is eliminated, even patients with chronic respiratory muscle weakness may reassume the work of breathing and avoid the commitment to chronic ventilatory support. Unfortunately, and for reasons that are poorly understood, once a patient with chronic, compensated hypercapnia is begun on ventilatory support, it is often difficult or impossible to discontinue this form of therapy, even after the factors causing the acute decompensation are corrected. Therefore, before starting mechanical ventilatory support in any patient with ALS, it must be understood by the patient, family, and medical team that the patient may become permanently ventilator-dependent.

Pharmacologic Treatment

Although mechanical ventilation represents the major mode of therapy of respiratory failure complicating ALS, recent studies have shown that at blood levels conventionally used to effect bronchodilation, theophylline increases the strength and suppresses fatigue of the diaphragm in normal individuals and patients with chronic obstructive pulmonary disease.[14,15] Although no controlled studies have yet demonstrated its effectiveness in patients with ALS, it is reasonable to use this drug as adjunctive therapy in individuals with chronic respiratory muscle weakness in an attempt to avoid or postpone the need for mechanical ventilation.

Additional Treatment of Acute Respiratory Failure

Metabolic factors such as dehydration, electrolyte abnormalities, and hypophosphatemia may contribute to muscle weakness, and should be treated when present. Patients should be evaluated for respiratory tract infections, and treated with appropriate antibiotics. Because of poor clearance of secretions due to an ineffective cough, respiratory therapy assumes a vital importance in patients with ALS. Occasionally, routine suctioning is inadequate to clear secretions, especially in the left lower lobe, and fiberoptic bronchoscopy may have to be employed to treat persistent areas of atelectasis. However, vigorous respiratory therapy usually makes bronchoscopic clearance of secretions unnecessary.[16]

Efforts at correction of nutritional deficiencies are important in the restoration of muscular strength. Whenever possible, nasogastric tube feedings should be instituted promptly in patients with ventilatory failure in an attempt to maintain or increase respiratory muscle mass, particularly when patients are malnourished before the onset of the acute decompensation. Larca and Greenbaum have demonstrated that nutritional repletion of ventilator-dependent patients may result in successful weaning from mechanical ventilation.[17]

CHRONIC RESPIRATORY FAILURE IN AMYOTROPHIC LATERAL SCLEROSIS

Many patients with ALS who develop acute respiratory failure cannot successfully resume the work of breathing after mechanical ventilation is begun. Furthermore, since ALS causes progressive deterioration of respiratory muscle strength, irreversible respiratory failure is a threat to all patients with ALS if their course is prolonged. Therefore, patients must face the prospect of requiring permanent mechanical ventilatory support in order to survive. Decisions regarding whether to undertake ventilatory support should be carefully considered by the patient, family, and medical team, hopefully long before a crisis arises. Once begun, mechanical ventilation "literally locks a patient into his disease with no short-term means of escape."[18] Sivak and associates point out that the cognitively competent patient has the best persepctive on the desirability of this form of therapy, but cannot foresee the true impact of this decision until after support measures are undertaken.[18] Many patients opt to forego hospitalization and life-supporting measures when the disease becomes far advanced, while others choose to go on to chronic ventilatory support.

Once the decision to proceed with further life-sustaining measures is made, several options are available. Many patients with neuromuscular diseases requiring mechanical ventilation do quite well for long periods of time using negative-pressure devices such as the Cuirass shell.[19-21] These patients avoid the discomfort and potential hazards of tracheostomy and prolonged endotracheal intubation, and may even lead productive lives by using the ventilator only intermittently or while asleep.[19] However, most patients with ALS whose disease has progressed to the point of requiring mechanical ventilation also have bulbar weakness predisposing them to repeated bouts of aspiration. In these patients, a tracheostomy and postive-pressure ventilation through a cuffed endotracheal tube afford them airway protection and the ability to suction secretions, and provide the most effective and reliable method of ventilation. However, this course of action carries with it the potential discomfort and complications associated with tracheostomy, is a more complex level of care, and requires greater effort and expense.

One promising area of active investigation involves the intermittent use of mechanical ventilation in patients with chronic respiratory muscle weakness. Since rest is the preferred treatment of muscle fatigue, Braun and co-workers evaluated the use of intermittent ventilatory support on 35 patients with chronic hypercapnia due to a variety of disorders.[8] Despite maximal medical management, these patients required repeated hospitalization for respiratory decompensation. After starting on a program of ventilatory support for periods of 4 to 10 h daily at home, it was found that respiratory muscle function and arterial blood gases were significantly improved when measured 5 months later. This was associated with lower $PaCO_2$, decreased frequency of hospitalization, and increase in functional activity. In another study, Braun and colleagues used nighttime ventilatory support in nine patients with sequelae of poliomyelitis.[8] Those patients with chronic hypercapnia also experienced increases in respiratory muscle strength and normalization of daytime $PaCO_2$. It is possible that in patients with ALS, instituting periodic rest periods using mechanical ventilation may delay the development of respiratory muscle fatigue, permitting a greater degree of function when breathing spontaneously.

The patient, family, and health care team must collectively decide whether chronic ventilatory support is to be provided in the hospital, in a specialized respiratory care facility, or in the patient's home. In our experience, ventilation with a Cuirass shell can be started either in the hospital or the home, since these devices require minimal training to operate effectively. However, most patients with ALS who go on to require chronic ventilatory support eventually undergo tracheostomy and positive pressure ventilation, which must be started in the hospital.

Sophisticated respiratory care can be easily rendered in intensive care units, but chronic care in this setting is unacceptable because of the enormous expense and unpleasant surroundings. Chronic ventilatory support on a general hospital ward is also extremely expensive.

Two major alternatives are becoming increasingly available to patients who require chronic ventilatory care. The first is the prolonged or chronic respiratory care unit, designed for patients who require extensive respiratory support but who cannot be maintained at home or on a general hospital ward. An example of such a unit is the Bethesda Lutheran Medical Center in St. Paul, Minnesota.[22] This 24-bed unit is run by a medical director, associate director of nursing, and technical director of respiratory therapy, and employs 20 full-time nurses and 7 full-time respiratory therapists. This type of unit has been demonstrated to be cost-effective, providing sophisticated chronic ventilatory support at approximately one-third the daily cost of an intensive care unit. Many similar units exist throughout the country, making chronic inpatient care available at a greatly reduced cost.

For many patients, respiratory care at home represents the most desirable alternative. Advances in technology have made positive-pressure ventilators smaller, easier to operate, and portable. With proper training and education, the well-motivated patient and family can continue chronic ventilatory support outside the hospital.[18,22-24] This may vastly improve the quality of life of ventilator-dependent patients by allowing them to live at home and continue their personal and professional lives. Furthermore, by presenting an alternative to hospitalization for months or years, this type of care can potentially save society millions of dollars in health care expenditures.

Success of a home mechanical ventilation program hinges on appropriate selection of patients by individuals from many disciplines. Evaluation by a team of physicians, nurses, social workers, and respiratory therapists is necessary to assure that the patient and family can assume the great personal and financial responsibilities associated with home respiratory care.[25] First, the patient must be alert and deemed medically stable. The patient's condition should be such that intercurrent infections have been eradicated, and the ventilator settings and medication regimen have not required frequent adjustments. Both the patient and support personnel must be well motivated, physically and emotionally capable of providing respiratory care for the rest of the patient's life, and financially capable of paying for the expense of home care. They must also be fully informed that even though home care may be a desirable alternative, it does carry an increased risk compared with chronic hospitalization.

If the health care team, patient, and family agree to pursue mechanical ventilation at home, a detailed period of instruction in the hospital is required. We have found a "contract" between the health care team, patient, and family to be helpful in outlining the responsibilities of all parties, as well as in providing a medico-legal framework for this type of program (see Appendix 4–1).

The patient and caregivers are taught the principles of respiratory therapy including tracheostomy care, endotracheal suctioning, and operation and maintenance of the ventilator and other equipment. This educational process must also have the input of physicians, nurses and respiratory therapists. The social worker plays a vital role by assisting in the mobilization of community resources to assist the family, and by providing support and counsel regarding the adjustment to home care.

Once the educational process is complete, provision is made for a "practice" period in the hospital.[25] This gives the patient and family the opportunity to assume total responsibility for care and increases their self-confidence while the patient is still hospitalized. Nursing and respiratory therapy personnel are available for whatever assistance or supervision is necessary until all parties are comfortable with the prospect of discharge from the hospital. A comprehensive checklist for discharge planning has been devised, which may be modified depending on the needs of the patients.[26]

Appendix 4–1. *Statement of Participation in and Contract for Home Ventilator Training Program*

The philosophy of the Mount Sinai Home Ventilator Program is that the patient and his/her primary caregiver are solely responsible for learning the process of ventilator care. As much as medically possible, the patient will be expected to be an active participant in the training process.

The patient and his/her primary caregiver(s) will be trained by the Mount Sinai Hospital staff to:

- understand the principles of mechanical ventilation
- manage the mechanics of the ventilator
- monitor the patient's status and record necessary information
- perform all aspects of care required to sustain the patient on mechanical ventilation
- recognize complications, how to deal with them and whom to report to in reference to these complications

The patient and his/her primary caregiver(s) are expected to make commitments in the following areas:

- to follow the directions of the Mount Sinai Hospital staff very carefully and specifically in terms of monitoring care and techniques of care
- to cooperate with staff responsible for their training
- to contact appropriate personnel for any problems that may arise
- to contact the respiratory care company which is responsible for the functioning of equipment, for providing supplies and for resolving questions regarding equipment
- to work with home care agencies and approved respiratory care company involved in maintaining optimal care at home

Because of the nature of home ventilator support and our responsibility to help you maintain the appropriate level of care, we reserve the right to terminate this training program if:

a) it is deemed necessary for medical reasons;
b) you or your caregiver do not demonstrate the commitment outlined or are unable to follow through;
c) there exists a condition we consider potentially harmful to you.

We have read and understand the information outlined and agree to participate in this program under these terms:

Patient's Signature   Caregiver's Signature

Physician's Signature   Nurse's Signature

Date

Prior to discharge from the hospital, arrangements are made with visiting nurses, respiratory therapists, and medical equipment providers to assure that adequate support services are available. It is crucial that emergency services are available in the event of an acute medical crisis or the equipment malfunctions. Special arrangements for emergency services by power and telephone companies are also necessary. Telephone numbers should be provided for the patient and family to call when questions arise after the transition from home to hospital is made.

The home should be visited by a visiting nurse service and respiratory therapy supplier prior to the patient's discharge. Equipment is delivered and installed with views toward electrical safety, accessibility, and simplicity of use.[25] After discharge from the hospital, periodic visits by respiratory therapists and visiting nurses facilitate the continuity of patient care. These individuals should provide the responsible physician with pertinent follow-up information.

Although chronic respiratory failure is a serious consequence of ALS, many patients have successfully resumed productive and rewarding lives at home using mechanical ventilatory support. It is incumbent upon society to encourage this form of care in those individuals who desire it by providing the financial support necessary for home care. In addition to improving the quality of life of these individuals, home care has the potential for enormous savings in health care costs compared with chronic hospitalization.

ACKNOWLEDGMENTS

This work was supported by a grant from the Catherine and Henry Gaisman Foundation.

REFERENCES

1. Fromm GB, Wisdom PJ, Block AJ: Amyotrophic lateral sclerosis presenting with respiratory failure. Chest 71:612–614, 1977.
2. Irwin RS, Rosen MJ, Braman SS: Cough: A comprehensive review. Arch Intern Med 137:1186–1191, 1977.
3. Rochester DF, Arora NS: Respiratory muscle failure. Med Clin N Am 67:573–597, 1983.
4. Rochester DF: Respiratory muscle function in health. Heart Lung 13:349–354, 1984.
5. Black LF, Hyatt RE: Maximal respiratory pressures: Normal values and relationship to age and sex. Am Rev Respir Dis 99:696–702, 1969.
6. Edwards RHT: Physiological analysis of skeletal muscle weakness and fatigue. Clin Sci Mol Med 54:463–470, 1978.
7. Braun NMT: Respiratory muscle dysfunction. Heart Lung 13:327–332, 1984.
8. Braun NMT, Faulkner J, Hughes RL, et al.: When should respiratory muscles be exercised? Chest 84:76–84, 1983.
9. Arora NS, Rochester DF: Effect of body weight and muscularity on human diaphragm muscle mass, thickness and area. J Appl Physiol 52:64–70, 1982.
10. Arora NS, Rochester DF: Respiratory muscle strength and maximal voluntary ventilation in undernourished patients. Am Rev Respir Dis 126:5–8, 1982.
11. Roussos CH, Fixley M, Gross D, et al.: Fatigue of the inspiratory muscles and their synergic behavior. J Appl Physiol 46:897–904, 1979.
12. Juan G, Calverley P, Talamo C. et al.: Effect of carbon dioxide on diaphragmatic function in human beings. N Engl J Med 310:874–879, 1984.
13. Cohen CA, Zagelbaum G, Gross D, et al.: Clinical manifestations of inspiratory muscle fatigue. Am J Med 73:308–316, 1982.
14. Aubier M, DeTroyer A, Sampson M, et al.: Aminophylline improves diaphragmatic contractility. N Engl J Med 305:249–252, 1981.
15. Murciano D, Aubier M, Lecocguic Y, et al.: Effects of theophylline on diaphragmatic strength and fatigue in patients with chronic obstructive pulmonary disease. N Engl J Med 311:349–353, 1984.

16. Marini JJ, Pierson DJ, Hudson LD: Acute lobar atelectasis: A prospective comparison of fiberoptic bronchoscopy and respiratory therapy. Am Rev Respir Dis 119:971–978, 1979.
17. Larca L, Greenbaum DM: Effectiveness of intensive nutritional regimens patients who fail to wean from mechanical ventilation. Crit Care Med 10:297–300, 1982.
18. Sivak ED, Gipson WT, Hanson MR: Long-term management of respiratory failure in amyotrophic lateral sclerosis. Ann Neurol 12:18–23, 1982.
19. Garay SM, Turino GM, Goldring RM: Sustained reversal of chronic hypercapnia in patients with alveolar hypoventilation syndromes. Am J Med 70:269–274, 1981.
20. Curran FJ: Night ventilation by body respirators for patients in chronic respiratory failure due to late state Duchenne muscular dystrophy. Arch Phys Med Rehab 62:270–274, 1981.
21. Splaingard ML, Jefferson LS, Harrison GM: Survival of patients with respiratory insufficiency secondary to neuromuscular disease treated at home with negative pressure ventilation (NPV) (Abstr). Am Rev Respir Dis 125:139(S), 1982.
22. Indihar FJ, Walker NE: Experience with a prolonged respiratory care unit—revisited. Chest 86:616–620, 1984.
23. Fischer DA, Prentice WS: Feasibility of home care for certain respiratory-dependent restrictive or obstructive lung disease patients. Chest 82:739–743, 1982.
24. Splaingard ML, Frates RC, Harrison GM, et al.: Home positive-pressure ventilation: Twenty years' experience. Chest 84:376–382, 1983.
25. Kopacz MA, Morrarty-Wright R: Multidisciplinary approach for the patient on a home ventilator. Heart Lung 13:255–262, 1984.
26. Kettrick RG, Donar ME: The ventilator-dependent child: Medical and social care. In Critical Care: State of the Art. Society of Critical Care Medicine, Fullerton, CA, 1985, pp. VI(F) 1–38.

CHAPTER FIVE

PULMONARY FUNCTION AND RESPIRATORY FAILURE IN NEUROMUSCULAR DISORDERS WITH REFERENCE TO AMYOTROPHIC LATERAL SCLEROSIS

Albert Miller, M.D.

MECHANISMS FOR RESPIRATORY FAILURE IN NEUROMUSCULAR DISORDERS

The basic impairment in all neuromuscular diseases is reduced generation of muscular force by the ventilatory pump. Although the lungs are the organ of *respiration,* the organ of *ventilation* is the ventilatory musculature. In the broad spectrum of neuromuscular disease, the failure of force generation may reside within central nervous system nuclei or pathways, in peripheral nerves activating the respiratory musculature, at the motor end-plate, or in the muscles themselves. In amyotrophic lateral sclerosis (ALS), the most important lesions are in the anterior horn cells which activate the various respiratory muscles; this results in atrophy of the muscles as well.

In respiratory failure secondary to neuromuscular disease and in ALS, with rare exceptions, both the inspiratory and expiratory muscles are affected. Loss of the diaphragm results in failure to develop negative intrapleural pressure necessary for inspiration and indirectly for expiration, since expiration is normally passive and results from recoil of the lung which had been inflated during inspiration. However, loss of expiratory muscle function results in failure of the cough mechanism since development of positive intrapleural pressure is necessary to generate a cough.

Weakness of inspiratory muscles may be of a lesser degree which allows tidal ventilation to take place but which results in failure of the sigh mechanism. Failure of sigh, with ventilation at fixed and often re-duced tidal volumes (monotonous ventilation), reduces the pulmonary compliance. Failure of cough results in inability to clear secretions, bringing about the respiratory complications of aspiration of secretions and foreign materials, atelectasis, and pneumonia. These all in turn cause hypoxemia, in addition to any hypoxemia present from hypoventilation. This addi-tional hypoxemia is due to imbalance between ventilation and perfusion (increased venous admixture) and is recognized as an increase in the al-veolar–arterial difference in oxygen tension (ΔA–aPO$_2$).

PULMONARY FUNCTION IN AMYOTROPHIC LATERAL SCLEROSIS: RESTRICTIVE IMPAIRMENT DUE TO REDUCED FORCE GENERATION

Classification of Restrictive Ventilatory Impairment

Restrictive ventilatory impairment or ''restriction'' is simply defined as a reduction in lung volumes, including the most easily measured lung volume, the vital capacity (VC).

Restrictive impairment may result from intrapulmonary or thoracic cage disorders (Table 5–1). Intrapulmonary causes include diffuse pul-monary disease, generally interstitial in nature, and resection of lung tis-sue or destruction of lung equally involving parenchyma, airways, and vasculature, a process that has been called *autopneumonectomy*. Chest bellows disorders may reside in the skeleton, in the soft tissues of the thorax, or in the pleura (of which the most important example is fibro-thorax). Obesity is another type of chest bellows insufficiency in which the main mechanism is increased abdominal pressure against which the diaphragm must work. Neuromuscular diseases are often classified as a

Table 5–1. Classification of Restrictive Ventilatory Impairment

I. Diffuse pulmonary disease
   A. Interstitial
   B. Alveolar filling
II. Lung resection and autopneumonectomy
III. Chest wall (or chest bellows) disorders
   A. Skeletal deformities: kyphosis and/or scoliosis, Morquio's syndrome, ankylosing spondylitis, thoracoplasty
   B. Nonskeletal disorders of the chest cage: myositis ossificans, scleroderma involving the thorax, Klinefelter's syndrome
   C. Pleural disease: fibrothorax (fibrous pleuritis), pleural neoplasia, large pleural or pericardial effusions, plombage
   D. Increased abdominal pressure: obesity
IV. Reduced force generation: neuromuscular diseases

chest bellows disorder; however, the mechanism is reduced activation rather than reduced mobility of the chest bellows.

There are findings on pulmonary function testing that are common to all restrictive disorders, to those of chest bellows origin, and to neuromuscular disease.

Findings in All Restrictive Impairments

By definition, any restrictive impairment means that the lung volumes are "restricted" or reduced. The most easily measured and most readily available lung volume is the VC, since it requires only a simple spirometer to be measured. Because the VC may be reduced in obstructive airways disease as a result of air trapping, a reduction in VC by itself cannot be equated with restrictive impairment. Of course, knowledge of the clinical situation, for example, that a patient has ALS and/or has no evidence of airways disease, is useful in deciding whether a reduction in VC is due to air trapping or to restriction. Many laboratories require that in addition to the VC, the total lung capacity (TLC) must be reduced in order to classify an impairment as restrictive. The measurement of TLC is not available in clinics or smaller hospitals and requires more extensive equipment and prolonged testing. In lung disease resulting in restrictive impairment, the residual volume (RV, or volume of air remaining in the lungs at the end of a forced expiration) may be reduced to a lesser degree than the VC or may be normal; in chest bellows or neuromuscular disorders, the RV may be increased (see Static Lung Volumes, below). As a result, the TLC, which is the sum of the VC and RV, is less reduced than the VC or indeed may be within normal limits. Therefore, it may be misleading to require a reduction in TLC to classify an impairment as restrictive. It is sufficient to have a reduction in VC in the presence of a TLC that is *not increased*.[1] When airway obstruction results in air trapping, the RV, the functional residual capacity (FRC), and the TLC are increased and numerous measurements of airflow such as the forced expiratory volume—1s/forced vital capacity ratio, (FEV_1/FVC) are reduced.

Findings in Chest Bellows Disorders. Most chest bellows disorders are apparent *clinically*. Separation from restrictive impairment of the pulmonary type is therefore not difficult even though VC (and often TLC) are reduced in both types. *Physiologically,* this distinction can generally be made on the following grounds:

1. The maximum voluntary ventilation (MVV) is more likely to be reduced, often pari passu with the decrease in VC.

2. The diffusing capacity (D_L) for carbon monoxide, a test of gas exchange in the lung parenchyma, is well maintained; diffusing capacity adjusted for lung volume (D_L/V_A) is high.

3. Lung compliance, a complicated measurement requiring intubation of the

esophagus to obtain pressures that are similar to those in the pleura, is relatively normal. Although lung compliance may be reduced due to long-standing decrease in lung volumes and in tidal volumes, it is not reduced to the degree seen in interstitial lung disease (ILD). Dynamic compliance (quiet breathing) ranged from 0.045 to 0.097 L/cm H_2O in six patients with kyphoscoliosis studied by Sinha and Bergofsky.[2] It increased 70% after a 5-min period of intermittent positive-pressure breathing (IPPB), although FRC did not increase. The increase in compliance was maintained for 3h. The authors suggested that brief applications of IPPB might decrease the work of breathing in patients with kyphoscoliosis, and by extension, in those with neuromuscular disease.

4. Retention of CO_2 develops at an earlier stage of the disease. Indeed, chest cage disorders are classic causes of alveolar hypoventilation.

Findings in Neuromuscular Disorders: Maximal Static Respiratory Pressures

The tests that are most useful for the diagnosis of ventilatory impairment due to neuromuscular disease are the maximal static respiratory pressures, inspiratory (PI_{max}) and/or expiratory (PE_{max}).[3] These are illustrated in Figure 5–1. The two pressures are often summed to provide a single index of respiratory muscle strength.

Low quadriplegia and high paraplegia are accompanied by predominant weakness of abdominal muscles, primarily concerned with expiration. Maximal expiratory pressure is disproportionately reduced and expiratory flow rates and expiratory reserve volume (ERV) are low. Because of the decrease in ERV, weakness of expiratory muscles results in an increased RV. Abdominal muscle weakness additionally limits inspiration since the diaphragm needs the contracting abdominal muscles in order to generate pressure.

When spinal involvement is higher or generalized weakness is present as in diffuse ALS, polyneuropathy, or primary muscular disease, the diaphragm is affected, both inspiratory and expiratory forces are reduced, and the ERV is also low. Loss of anterior horn cells at the C_3–C_5 level in ALS is associated with diaphragmatic (inspiratory) weakness, causing a decrease in inspiratory capacity (the volume inspired after a normal resting expiration).

Factors that limit the clinical use of maximal respiratory pressures:

1. It is often more difficult to obtain reproducible results for PE_{max} than for PI_{max}. This may be because it is difficult for the subject with facial muscle weakness to affect a seal with his lips around the tube through which he is blowing when he generates a positive (expiratory) pressure.

2. The tremendous effect of learning and/or fatigue in these wholly effort-dependent tests; some investigators repeat the measurements ten times!

The apparatus necessary for measuring maximal static respiratory pressures is simple. The patient puts his lips around a tube containing a

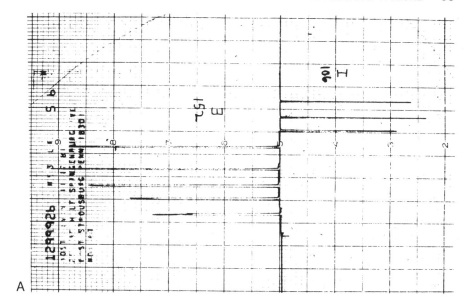

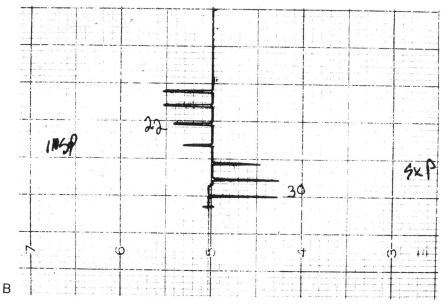

Figure 5–1. Maximal static inspiratory pressures (PI_{max}) and expiratory pressures (PE_{max}) measured at the mouth (actual tracings). A. Normal subject: PI_{max} 106 cm H_2O, PE_{max} 152 cm H_2O. B. Patient with ALS: PI_{max} 22 cm H_2O, PE_{max} 30 cm H_2O.

pinhole air leak and pressures are measured by a mechanical gauge or electronic transducer; the leak eliminates artifact due to fluctuations in buccal pressure. PE_{max} is generally measured at peak inspiration (or total lung capacity) and PI_{max} at peak expiration (or residual volume). PI_{max} may also be measured at the resting ventilatory level, that of a normal expiration (or functional residual capacity).

Maximum static respiratory pressures are often reduced when other pulmonary function tests are still normal in neuromuscular disorders. They may be reduced as a result of lung disease and in the absence of primary neuromuscular disease, as a result of muscle wasting and mechanical disadvantage, but in such situations they are not reduced to the extent seen in neuromuscular disease and, of course, other findings of pulmonary disease are evident.

These measurements help explain why patients with neuromuscular disease may complain of dyspnea (indeed, dyspnea has been an occasional presenting complaint in neuromuscular disease). The prevailing explanation of dyspnea is that it is perceived when there is an imbalance in the relationship of ventilatory drive to ventilatory volume achieved. Since central nervous system drive is maintained in neuromuscular disease while the volume achieveable is reduced, such diseases are a prime example of this imbalance. In these diseases there is a decrease in the maximal pressures available for ventilation, so that the patient must use a large proportion of these maxima to ventilate normally. It has been observed that dyspnea results when more than 20% of the maximal inspiratory pressure is used, and fatigue at more than 80%.[4] Therefore, dyspnea may be seen either when high ventilatory pressures are called for during the stress of progressive exercise even though maximal pressures are normal, or when barely normal or less than normal pressures are generated to sustain barely adequate or less then adequate ventilation when maximal pressures are decreased.

Other Pulmonary Function Findings in Amyotrophic Lateral Sclerosis

Spirometry and Inspiratory-Expiratory Flow-Volume Curves.

Measurements derived from the volume–time or flow-volume curves are not as useful as maximal static respiratory pressures in detecting respiratory involvement in neuromuscular disease. They are less sensitive, that is, they are abnormal in a smaller percentage of patients (although they are abnormal in most patients), and they are reduced to a lesser de-

Table 5–2. Prevalence of Abnormal Pulmonary Function in 194 Patients at First Visit to Mount Sinai Medical Center Amyotrophic Lateral Sclerosis Clinic

Test	Mean Value	Prevalence of Abnormality (%)
FVC	61.2*	73
FEV₁	81.8*	49
FEV₁/FVC	0.86	4
MMF†	75.6*	53
MET†	0.60 s	18
MVV†	57.0*	73
PE_max†	34.9*	97
PI_max†	47.4*	83

*Percentage predicted.
†Not all patients had these measurements.

gree than are the static pressures. This may be seen from Table 5–2, which presents our pulmonary function findings on first visit in 194 patients presenting to the Mount Sinai Medical Center Amyotrophic Lateral Sclerosis Clinic. The mean age of these patients was 58 years. The FVC was reduced in 73%*, with a mean value of 61% of predicted. The FEV_1 was reduced in a smaller percentage of patients, namely 49%*, with a higher mean value of 82% of predicted. The ratio of FEV_1 to FVC, which when reduced reflects obstruction, was reduced in only 4% of patients with a mean value of 0.86, higher than normal. In contrast, the PE_{max} was reduced in 97% of patients* with a mean value of 35% of predicted, while the PI_{max} was reduced in 83%* with a mean value of 47% of predicted.

Spirometic values are extremely useful in following the course of patients with ALS, as will be discussed below. Spirometric values may be graphically recorded as a spirogram (volume versus time) or as maximal expiratory flow-volume (MEFV) curves (flow versus volume).

In ALS, spirometric results (including MVV) at first examination correlate better with prognosis than does the neuromuscular examination. Decrease in inspiratory capacity reflects weakness of the diaphragm, while decrease in ERV reflects weakness of the expiratory and abdominal muscles. Ventilatory impairment manifested by a reduction in FVC (and MVV) as low as 50% of predicted is often not appreciated by the patient or the physician.[6] *The lesson from this is to evaluate pulmonary function routinely in patients with neuromuscular disorders.*

In patients with neuromuscular weakness, the decrease in VC is greater

---

*For FVC and FEV_1, an abnormal value was defined as <80% of Miller et al.'s modification of Morris's predicted values,[5] and for PE_{max} and PI_{max}, an abnormal value was defined as <75% of the predicted values of Black and Hyatt.[3]

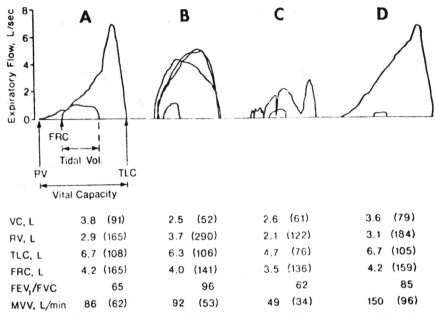

VC, L	3.8	(91)	2.5	(52)	2.6	(61)	3.6	(79)
RV, L	2.9	(165)	3.7	(290)	2.1	(122)	3.1	(184)
TLC, L	6.7	(108)	6.3	(106)	4.7	(76)	6.7	(105)
FRC, L	4.2	(165)	4.0	(141)	3.5	(136)	4.2	(159)
FEV$_1$/FVC	65		96		62		85	
MVV, L/min	86	(62)	92	(53)	49	(34)	150	(96)

Figure 5–2. Characteristic maximal expiratory flow-volume (MEFV) curves in ALS. A. Airway obstruction still apparent early in course (VC normal); FEV$_1$/FVC ratio is reduced. B. Early termination of expiration; FEV$_1$/FVC ratio is increased. C. Erratic expiratory effort; sudden decreases in flow to zero result in low FEV$_1$/FVC ratio. Patient had bulbar involvement and likely occlusion of the glottis by discoordinated muscles. D. Normal MEFV curve in early disease. High RV is attributable to reduced ERV (500 ml). (From Fallat RJ, Jewitt B, Bass M, et al.: Spirometry in amyotrophic lateral sclerosis. Arch Neurol 36:77, 1979. With permission.)

than that predicted from theoretical pressure–volume curves[7,8] or from curves in normal curarized subjects. This has been explained by decrease in lung compliance as a result of ''monotonous'' ventilation with small volumes and by increase in elastance of the chest wall.

An abrupt termination of the MEFV curve has been described as characteristic of ALS[6,9] (Fig. 5–2). This is attributed to expiratory muscle weakness or to discoordination of contraction of the diaphragm leading to premature inspiration or of muscles in the upper airway leading to its occlusion. It is difficult to separate the ALS curve from the common performance artifact brought about by early termination of effort. In addition, we have observed similar abruptly ending MEFV curves in other restrictive disorders, including interstitial lung disease, and in normal adolescents. Many patients with ALS show a marked discoordination of the entire expiratory effort, resulting in totally erratic curves (Fig. 5–2).

It can be appreciated that performing spirometric tests on patients with ALS is difficult since spirometry requires maximum and reproducible effort. The VC reported should be the largest VC, and the FEV_1 the largest FEV_1 even though these two measurements may come from separate efforts. When reproducible tests and identification of a single best effort are not possible, flow rates cannot be reported. It is often difficult for the patient with ALS to use conventional mouthpieces, especially tube-type. Acceptable tests can be obtained using properly fitted masks.

Maximum Voluntary Ventilation

The MVV is the greatest ventilation that a subject can achieve by voluntarily breathing as rapidly and as deeply as he can. It is performed for 10 to 15 s and expressed in liters per minute. Often used as a test of airway function, it is also a good overall index of neuromuscular function. Several studies have found it to be more sensitive than spirometry in such conditions as quadriplegia and paraplegia[10] and ALS.[6] It is almost as sensitive as maximal static respiratory pressures, but is less diminished at the onset of disease. Thereafter, further decrease reflects progression of neuromuscular impairment. Table 5–2 shows that 73% of the patients in our clinic had an abnormal MVV (defined as <80% of the predicted values of Kory and co-workers[11] for men and Lindall and associates[12] for women), the same percentage of patients that had an abnormal FVC. The degree of abnormality was somewhat greater, 57% versus 61% of predicted.

Braun and Rochester[7] studied 28 patients with various myopathies not associated with lung disease. The relationship between MVV and the summed respiratory forces was linear, demonstrating that MVV can be used as a measure of respiratory muscle strength.

In recording the MVV, the slope of integrated volume against time may flatten during the 10 to 15 s of the test, indicating fatigue. This is characteristic of myasthenia gravis and may be seen in other neuromuscular diseases.

Static Lung Volumes

The FRC is characteristically normal, since there is no change in the compliance of either the lungs or the chest wall. A marked decrease in ERV may result in an increase in RV[13]; this is seen especially in ALS patients with an abrupt termination of the MEFV curve. The weaker the patient, the higher the RV.[9] Such an increase in RV (and RV/TLC ratio) is unlike the increase due to air trapping in obstructive airways disease, in which the FRC and very often the TLC are increased.

Flow Rates

There are many different mean and instantaneous flow rates that can be obtained during the FVC maneuver. The most commonly reported is the maximal mid-expiratory flow (MMF), better called the forced expiratory flow 25–75% ($FEF_{25-75\%}$) since it measures the mean flow over the middle half of the FVC. In general, flows in ALS are well maintained by the normal elastic recoil of the lungs and chest wall, especially at a high lung volume. Therefore, flows (and the FEV_1) are less reduced than the FVC, and the FEV_1/FVC and flow-volume ratios are high. This may be seen from Table 5–2 which shows that 53% of the patients at the Mount Sinai Clinic had a reduction in MMF (defined as less than 75% of the modified Morris value,[5] compared with 73% who had a reduced FVC) and that the mean value was 76% of predicted (compared with 61%). The mid-expiratory time (MET) or forced expiratory time 25–75% ($FET_{25-75\%}$) is lower than normal (normal being 0.65 to 0.80 s) in ALS, a finding similar to the higher than normal FEV_1/FVC ratio. Both these measurements indicate that the reductions in FEV_1 and in MMF in terms of percentage of predicted values are secondary to decrease in the VC and not to independent obstructive disease.

One of the important contributions of spirometric testing in neuromuscular disease is the detection of obstructive airways disease since the complications of atelectasis and pneumonia and abnormal gas exchange are more likely in such patients. Such evidence as a reduced FEV_1/FVC ratio or increased $FET_{25-75\%}$ may be appreciated only at the first encounter with the patient since progressive loss of VC will override the reduc-

Table 5–3. Masking of Airway Obstruction with Progression of Amyotrophic Lateral Sclerosis in a 48-Year-Old-Woman with Asthma*

Test	5/82	8/82	12/82
FVC (cc)	2,710 (67%)	2,200 (55%)	1,300 (34%)
FEV_1 (cc)	1,810 (59%)	1,720 (56%)	1,200 (41%)
FEV_1/FVC	0.67	0.78	0.92
FEV_3/FVC	0.94	0.99	1.00
PFR (L/s)	2.78	2.87	—
$FEF_{25-75\%}$ (L/s)	1.13 (33%)	1.47 (44%)	1.59 (47%)
$FET_{25-75\%}$ (s)	1.20	0.75	0.42
$FEF_{50\%}$ (L/s)	1.35	1.85	—
$FEF_{75\%}$ (L/s)	0.51	0.76	—
MVV (L/min)	47 (48%)	47 (48%)	—
PI_{max} (cm H_2O)	41 (33%)	27 (20%)	24 (20%)
PE_{max} (cm H_2O)	54 (24%)	25 (11%)	16 (7%)

Source: Miller A: Pulmonary Function Tests in Clinical and Occupational Lung Disease. Grune & Stratton, Orlando, FL, 1986. With permission.

Abbreviations: PFR, peak flow rate; other abbreviations as in text.

*Nonsmoker, height 163 cm, weight 55 kg.

tion in FEV_1 and expiratory flows. This may be seen in Table 5–3 which shows the pulmonary function in a 48-year-old woman with asthma over a 7-month course of her ALS. At first visit, when the FVC is only slightly reduced, the $FEF_{25-75\%}$ is severely reduced, and the $FET_{25-75\%}$ is prolonged. With progression of the ALS, the $FEF_{25-75\%}$ increases as the FVC falls and the $FET_{25-75\%}$ becomes first normal and then shortened, consistent with restrictive impairment. It is therefore imperative to obtain spirometric measurements on first encountering patients with ALS since later in the course of this disease evidence of airways obstruction will not be apparent.

Adequate expiratory flow rates are necessary for effective cough and may be present in ALS. However, because of the weakness of expiratory muscles, patients with ALS are unable to develop positive intrapleural pressures which are the other prerequisite for effective cough. Therefore, there is a poor correlation between expiratory flow rates and effectiveness of cough in these patients.

Arterial Blood Gases

These are said to be well maintained in ALS even with severe spirometric impairment, so that arterial gas determinations may not be necessary in ambulatory patients.[6] When respiratory muscle strength is less than 30%, CO_2 retention is likely in myopathy[7] and presumably in ALS. In all diseases affecting ventilatory function, an FEV_1 below a certain value presages CO_2 retention. This value is 600–800 ml in chronic obstructive lung disease, but is probably lower in neuromuscular disease since alveolar dead space is not increased.

It should be noted that CO_2 retention reflects global (alveolar) hypoventilation whereas hypoxemia reflects both global hypoventilation and regional hypoventilation in which local ventilation-perfusion relationships are disturbed. The latter occurs primarily when complications of respiratory muscle weakness supervene such as retention of secretions, atelectasis, and pneumonia. In addition to CO_2 retention, global hypoventilation may be separated from regional hypoventilation by the difference in oxygen tension between alveolar and arterial values; in global hypoventilation the $A-aPO_2$ difference is normal, that is, less than 20 mmHg.

Correlations of Pulmonary Function with Clinical Features of Amyotrophic Lateral Sclerosis

There is often a poor correlation of pulmonary function with weakness of other muscles. A useful clue on clinical evaluation is elevation of the diaphragm on chest roentgenogram which indicates weakness of this muscle. Patients generally are not aware of dyspnea. To a large extent this must reflect the decrease in activities that they have undergone. Decrease in FVC and MVV to values below 50% of predicted are often not appreciated by the patient or the evaluating physician, who reported normal breathing scores on neurologic examination in more than 50% of patients whose pulmonary function values were this low.[6] As stated above, this demonstrates the need to perform pulmonary function tests as a routine measure.

Use of Pulmonary Function Tests in Predicting and Following the Course of Amyotrophic Lateral Sclerosis

Both in the Mount Sinai experience and in the reported experience of other workers,[6] the course of ventilatory impairment in ALS is diverse. Many patients show a progressive downhill course with marked loss in VC and MVV within periods of 6 months to 1 year. Thus, the patient in Table 5–3 lost over 50% of her initial VC in 7 months. The patient in Table 5–4 lost two-thirds of her VC in 13 months while her MVV decreased from 66 L/min, a value only slightly abnormal, to 13 L/min, which is extremely reduced, being 13% of the predicted value. This maximal ventilatory capacity is barely twice the ventilatory requirement of a normal individual at rest, demonstrating the marked reduction in ventilatory reserve in advanced ALS.

The changes in pulmonary function shown by the patient in Table

Table 5–4. Progression of Pulmonary Function Changes over 1 Year in a 62-Year-Old White Female* with ALS

Test	4/82	5/83
FVC (cc)	2,250 (66%)	740 (22%)
FEV_1 (cc)	2,230 (88%)	740 (29%)
FEV_1/FVC	0.99	1.00
FEV_3/FVC	1.00	1.00
PFR (L/s)	4.47	1.33
$FEF_{25-75\%}$ (L/s)	3.91 (142%)	0.76 (28%)
$FEF_{50\%}$ (L/s)	4.38	1.25
$FEF_{75\%}$ (L/s)	2.61	0.71
MVV (L/min)	66 (67%)	13 (13%)
PI_{max} (cm H_2O)	22 (30%)	16 (22%)
PE_{max} (cm H_2O)	30 (22%)	18 (13%)

Source: Miller A: Pulmonary Function Tests in Clinical and Occupational Lung Disease. Grune & Stratton, Orlando, FL, 1986. With permission.

Abbreviations: As in Table 5–3.

*Nonsmoker, height 173 cm, weight 93 kg.

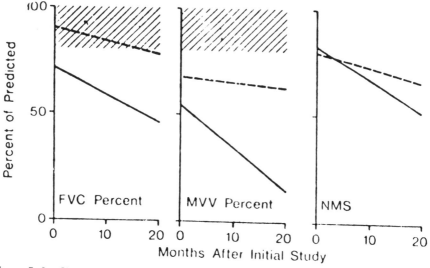

Figure 5–3. Slope of decline in FVC and MVV (as percentage of predicted values) and in neuromuscular score (NMS) in patients who died (solid lines) and in those who remained alive (dashed lines). Note that pulmonary function tests were more reduced at presentation in those with a fatal outcome while NMS was not, and that the slope of decline in MVV was greater than the slope of decline in NMS. (From Fallat RJ, Jewitt B, Bass M, et al.: Spirometry in amyotrophic lateral sclerosis. Arch Neurol 36:76, 1979. With permission.)

5–4 demonstrate another important distinction in the use of pulmonary function tests in ALS. Although maximal static respiratory pressures are useful in *detecting* impairment, they are often not useful in *following* the patient. This is because they are so markedly reduced at the first examination, even when spirometric measurements and MVV are relatively well maintained. Therefore they show little further change during the illness, despite catastrophic reductions in ventilatory function and neurologic score.

There is a strong correlation of pulmonary functional loss with prognosis and mortality in ALS. This correlation is better than that between neuromuscular scores and prognosis. Figure 5–3 shows the different slopes of decline in FVC and MVV between those patients who survived and those who did not survive. Serial tests were available on 103 patients for periods of 1 to 40 months, of whom 31 died.[6] The greater decrement in FVC and MVV than in neuromuscular score at first visit is apparent in those who did not survive. The slopes of losses in pulmonary function in these 31 patients were greater than the slope of loss in overall neuromuscular function. The diversity of course is further demonstrated in Figure 5–4 which shows the slope of pulmonary function in selected patients. The bottom panel demonstrates stable pulmonary function even at levels as reduced as 25 to 50% of predicted. These patients all survived up to 5

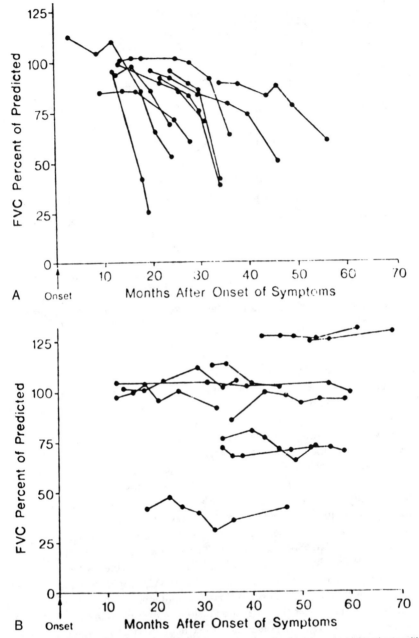

Figure 5–4. Slope of FVC (as percentage of predicted value) in selected patients with ALS. A. Decline in FVC in ten fatal cases; note accelerated decline later in course. B. Stable function in ten subjects who survived for a long period of time, three of whom had values <75% of predicted. Initial values were similar in both groups. (From Fallat RJ, Jewitt B, Bass M, et al.: Spirometry in amyotrophic lateral sclerosis. Arch Neurol 36:79, 1979. With permission.)

Table 5–5. Loss of Pulmonary Function Within 12 Months of First Visit* in 77 Patients at the Mount Sinai Medical Center Amyotrophic Lateral Sclerosis Clinic

Pulmonary Function Test	*Mean Loss Expressed as Percentage of Predicted Values*	*Percentage of Patients Whose Function Decreased >5%*	*Percentage of Patients Whose Function Decreased ≥25%*
FVC	−12.4	57	26
MMF†	−4.4	45	29
MVV†	−14.9	49	27
PI$_{max}$†	−9.3	57	17
PE$_{max}$†	−6.0	55	14

*Mean duration from first visit.
†Not all patients had these measurements.

years. In those who did not survive, there was progressive loss of pulmonary function in all patients. The slope of decline was steeper as death neared. Often there was little change in FVC during the earlier course of the disease. In general, and despite the selected cases shown in Figure 5–4, several of whom died with VC values of about 60% of predicted, death is unlikely in ALS when the FVC and/or MVV are above 30% of predicted.

An important application of pulmonary function tests is to separate the course of neuromuscular impairment as the cause of ventilatory insufficiency from the effect of intercurrent complications, especially aspiration and infections pneumonias. When these complications supervene, there is a precipitous decline in pulmonary function which may be seen to be different from the preceding course. Follow-up within a relatively short time will demonstrate return of pulmonary function with effective treatment of the complication.

Table 5–5 shows the loss of pulmonary function within 12 months of the first visit in 77 ALS patients followed at the Mount Sinai Clinic. Mean loss of MVV was 14.9% percent; that of FVC was 12.4%. Declines in static respiratory pressures were less. Roughly half of all patients showed a *significant* (greater than 5%) decline in all measurements. A greater proportion (26 to 29%) showed a *marked* (≥25%) decline in spirometric measurements or MVV compared with static respiratory pressures (14 to 17%). Thus, more than one-fourth of patients showed a marked decline in pulmonary function within a 1-year follow-up from first visit.

VENTILATORY FAILURE IN AMYOTROPHIC LATERAL SCLEROSIS

Ventilation in ALS is reduced primarily because of failure to generate force. Additional mechanisms include reduction in pulmonary compliance because of monotonous ventilation at low tidal volumes, retention of secretions and aspiration, intercurrent infection, and discoordination of ventilatory efforts. This is seen as discoordination of expiration on the expiratory flow-volume curve, resulting in extremely erratic expiratory efforts with sudden decreases in flow to zero, thought to be caused by occlusion of the glottis by discoordinated muscles (Fig. 5–2), which is especially a problem in bulbar disease. In addition, the initiation of inspiratory effort may be premature because of early discoordinated contraction of the diaphragm or because of premature termination of expiration resulting from discoordinated contraction of muscles of the upper airways or weakness of the expiratory muscles. The net result of all these mechanisms is decreased tidal volumes and minute ventilation. In the absence of massive aspiration or infectious complications, death is usually due to alveolar hypoventilation. This occurs when the inspiratory capacity and/or the VC is reduced below one-third of normal.

It is interesting that the ventilatory failure in ALS is rarely accompanied by clinical or hemodynamic evidence of pulmonary hypertension and cor pulmonale. Indeed, at postmortem examination, medial thickening of the pulmonary arteries is rarely seen. This sparing of the lesser circulation and right ventricle probably is a consequence of the relatively short course of respiratory failure in ALS compared with diseases of the airways, lung parenchyma, or thoracic skeleton.

An interesting question is whether the respiratory center is normally responsive in ALS since brain stem involvement may occur in this disease. It is impossible to assess responsiveness clinically since the end points are increased minute ventilation and/or increased inspiratory pressure as the stimulus to ventilation (usually progressive hypercapnia due to rebreathing) is applied. Both of these reflect the neurologic deficit in ALS rather than the function of the respiratory center.

SUMMARY

This chapter has reviewed the mechanisms for dyspnea and respiratory failure in ALS, and placed the pulmonary function findings in this disease within the pattern of a restrictive impairment of the chest bellows resulting from reduced force generation (despite normal respiratory center drive). This pattern consists of a reduced VC, reduced MVV, well-maintained flow-volume ratios, and predominant reduction in maximal inspiratory and expiratory pressures which are easily measured at the mouth. The use of clinical pulmonary function tests in the initial evaluation, follow-up, and prediction of prognosis of patients with ALS is discussed, citing relevant data from the experience at the Mount Sinai Medical Center. These data showed that VC was reduced in 73% of 194 patients on first presentation (mean value 61% of predicted), that MVV was reduced in 73% (mean 57% of predicted), that PE_{max} was reduced in 97% (mean 35% of predicted), and that PI_{max} was reduced in 83% (mean 47% of predicted). Decline in pulmonary function is the strongest correlate of mortality.

REFERENCES

1. Miller A: Patterns of impairment. In Miller A (ed): Pulmonary Function Tests in Clinical and Occupational Lung Disease. Grune & Stratton, Orlando, FL, 1986.
2. Sinha R, Bergofsky EH: Prolonged alteration of lung mechanics in kyphoscoliosis by positive pressure hyperinflation. Am Rev Respir Dis 106:47–57, 1972.
3. Black LF, Hyatt RE: Maximal static respiratory pressures in generalized neuromuscular disease. Am Rev Respir Dis 103:641–650, 1971.
4. Bowie DM, LeBlanc P, Killian KJ, et al. Can the intensity of breathlessness be predicted from the inspiratory flow rate? Am Rev Respir Dis 129:A239, 1984.
5. Miller A, Thornton JC, Smith H Jr, et al.: Spirometric "abnormality" in a normal male reference population: Further analysis of the 1971 Oregon Survey. Am J Indust Med 1:55–68, 1980.
6. Fallat RJ, Jewitt B, Bass M, et al. Spirometry in amyotrophic lateral sclerosis. Arch Neurol 36:74–80, 1979.
7. Braun NMT, Rochester DF. Muscular weakness and respiratory failure. Am Rev Respir Dis 119 (Part 2):123–125, 1979.
8. Gibson GJ, Pride NB, Newsom Davis J, et al.: Pulmonary mechanics in patients with respiratory muscle weakness. Am Rev Respir Dis 115:389–395, 1977.
9. Saunders NA, Kreitzer SM: Diaphragmatic function in amyotrophic lateral sclerosis. Am Rev Respir Dis 119 (Part 2):127–130, 1979.
10. Keltz H: The effect of respiratory muscle dysfunction on pulmonary function. Am Rev Respir Dis 91:934–938, 1965.
11. Kory RC, Callahan R, Boren HG, et al.: The Veterans Administration–Army cooperative study of pulmonary function. 1. Clinical spirometry in normal men. Am J Med 30:243–258, 1961.
12. Lindall A, Medina A, Grismer JT: A re-evaluation of normal pulmonary function measurements in the adult female. Am Rev Respir Dis 95:1061–1064, 1967.
13. Nakano K, Bass H, Tyler HR, et al.: Amyotrophic lateral sclerosis: A study of pulmonary function. Dis Nerv Syst 37:32–35, 1976.

CHAPTER SIX

SURGICAL MANAGEMENT OF FEEDING DIFFICULTIES IN PATIENTS WITH AMYOTROPHIC LATERAL SCLEROSIS

Tomas M. Heimann, M.D.

Patients with advanced amyotrophic lateral sclerosis (ALS) often have severe swallowing difficulties leading to malnutrition and occasionally to aspiration pneumonia. These symptoms are usually combined with muscular weakness and sometimes respiratory insufficiency. A feeding gastrostomy provides a conduit through which the patient may be nourished without the necessity of swallowing the food. Although there is still production of saliva, some of which must be swallowed, anticholinergic drugs can reduce the amount to a manageable level.

Performance of a feeding gastrostomy in a patient with ALS presents special problems. Due to weakness of the bulbar muscles, many of these patients will not tolerate lying supine even for short periods of time since they develop upper airway obstruction. Therefore, the feeding gastrostomy must usually be performed with the patient in a semisitting position. Also, general anesthesia should be avoided whenever possible for the same reasons. Other factors that can often make this operation technically difficult are the moderate to marked colonic distention that occurs in nearly 50% of patients, and the severe spasticity of the abdominal muscles that is present in over 30% of the patients. This operation must therefore be performed under local anesthesia, the duration should be short, and the amount of gastric manipulation should be minimal.

SURGICAL TECHNIQUE

The standard surgical technique for a permanent feeding gastrostomy consists of the creation of a gastric flap which is then fashioned into a tube. This gastric tube is then brought out through the abdominal wall

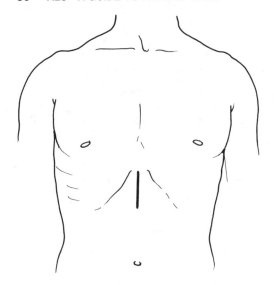

Figure 6–1. This view shows the location of the incision for creation of a feeding tube gastrostomy.

and sutured to the skin. This operation is called a *Depage–Janeway gastrostomy.*[1,2] Unfortunately this type of gastrostomy requires a moderate-sized abdominal incision and quite extensive manipulation of the stomach to create the gastric tube. This operation would be difficult to perform in a patient with ALS and would frequently require general anesthesia.

A modified technique for creation of a permanent feeding gastrostomy with a simple gastric tube has been employed successfully in this group of patients.[3] The patient is brought to the operating room without any premedication. He is placed in a semisitting position on the operating table and the operation is performed under local anesthesia. An anesthetist is present in order to monitor respiratory function and provide tracheal suction when required. If necessary, a small amount of intravenous sedation may be given at this time. The abdomen is entered using a 5-cm midline incision starting at the xyphoid (Fig. 6–1). Once the peritoneum is opened, a long Babcock clamp is used to identify the stomach and bring it into the operative field. Often the stomach is not easily visible due to distention of the transverse colon. Occasionally, the left lobe of the liver must be retracted in order to locate the stomach. Once the stomach is identified, a portion of the body between the greater and lesser curvatures is brought into the area of the incision. A pursestring suture is then placed, the stomach is opened, and a no. 30 Malecot catheter is inserted (Fig. 6–2). A second pursestring suture is then placed about 2 cm proximal to the first one, everting the stomach and thereby creating a simple gastric tube (Fig. 6–3). The stomach is then anchored to the abdominal wall by placing the sutures so the gastric tube is outside the peritoneal cavity. Fre-

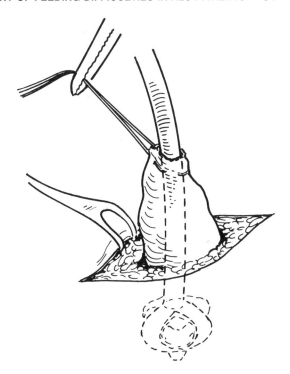

Figure 6–2. The stomach is brought into the incision and a large Malecot catheter is inserted after placing the first pursestring suture.

quently further sutures in the fascia are not necessary due to the small size of the incision. The skin is then closed and the gastrostomy tube is secured in place with a heavy silk tie.

RESULTS

A feeding gastrostomy can be performed under local anesthesia in approximately 90% of patients with ALS. In the remaining group, severe spasticity and colonic distention make the exposure of the stomach extremely difficult and general anesthesia becomes necessary for a short period of time. The complications related to the operative procedure have been minimal.[4,5] Skin excoriation is not usually a problem, and most patients are able to tolerate a 2,000-calorie tube feeding diet within 1 week of insertion of the gastrostomy tube. There have not been any wound infections even though the tube is brought out through the abdominal incision.

Since using the feeding gastrostomy requires a liquid diet, the standard formula contains approximately 1 calorie/ml. Patients are placed on a 2,000-calorie blenderized tube feeding diet and if they are unable to

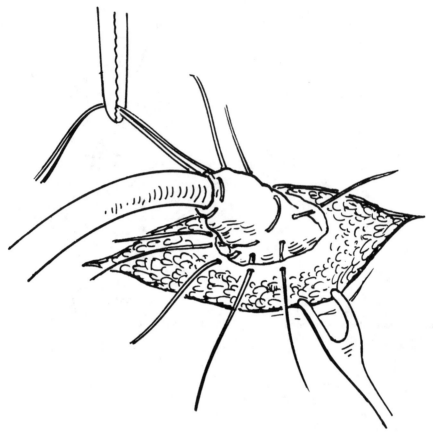

Figure 6–3. This view shows the gastric tube created by the placement of the two pursestring sutures being anchored to the abdominal fascia. The gastric tube remains in the subcutaneous space. Separate closure of the fascial incision is not usually necessary.

prepare their own food, then a commercial preparation is used (Compleat B). The feeding regimen usually consists of five meals of 400/ml each over a period of 12 h. If patients are unable to tolerate this amount, then more frequent smaller meals are given. It is necessary to aspirate the stomach before each feeding to insure that there is no residual material from the previous feeding. The patient must also be kept upright during and for at least 1 h following each feeding. Vomiting and aspiration of gastric contents is a constant threat in patients with bulbar muscle weakness and therefore the aforementioned precautions are extremely important.

Patients with severe swallowing difficulties have uniformly benefited from the insertion of a feeding gastrostomy. Although weight gain is often difficult to achieve due to progression of the disease and continued muscle wasting, their nutritional status improves. Occasionally the disease has progressed to a point where there is simultaneous severe swallowing and respiratory difficulty. These patients are usually able to tolerate the operation for feeding gastrostomy but often develop respiratory insufficiency within the following weeks. It seems possible that gastric distention during feedings may aggravate the precarious respiratory condition. Approximately 10% of patients have required tracheostomy and respiratory support within 3 weeks of insertion of a feeding gastrostomy.

Percutaneous endoscopic insertion of a feeding gastrostomy has recently been advocated in a variety of conditions.[6-8] This operation is performed by placing a small gastrostomy tube percutaneously after inflation of the stomach with a gastroscope. Patients with ALS are not good candidates for this procedure. The insertion of the gastroscope and the necessary gastric dilatation would lead to airway obstruction and respiratory insufficiency in a significant proportion of patients. Also, the colonic distention that is often present makes it more likely that a gastrocolic fistula could occur.[9] This complication would be catastrophic in this group of patients since it requires operative correction. Also, peritonitis from leakage of gastric contents into the peritoneal cavity has been reported.[10] Operative placement of the feeding gastrostomy, on the other hand, is performed under direct vision and the stomach is anchored outside the abdominal cavity. Therefore, gastrocolic fistula and gastric leaks should not occur. The modified operative technique described above seems to be safer and more appropriate for patients with ALS.

REFERENCES

1. Depage A: Nouveau procede pour la gastrostomie. J Chir Ann Soc Belg Chir 1:715, 1901.
2. Janeway HH: Eine neue gastrostomie methode. Munch Med Wochenschr 60:1705, 1913.
3. Heimann TM: A simple technique for permanent feeding gastrostomy in patients with amyotrophic lateral sclerosis. (In press)
4. Shellito PC, Malt RA: Tube gastrostomy: Techniques and complications. Ann Surg 201:180–185, 1985.
5. Wasiljew BK, Ujiki GT, Beal JM: Feeding gastrostomy: Complications and mortality. Am J Surg 143:194–195, 1982.
6. Gauderer MW, Ponsky JL: A simplified technique for constructing a tube feeding enterostomy. Surg Gynecol Obstet 152:82–85, 1981.
7. Gauderer MW, Ponsky JL, Izant RJ Jr: Gastrostomy without laparatomy: A percutaneous endoscopic technique. J Pediatr Surg 15:872–875, 1980.
8. Larson DE, Fleming CR, Ott BJ, et al.: Percutaneous endoscopic gastrostomy: Simplified access for enteral nutrition. Mayo Clin Proc 58:103–107, 1983.
9. Strodel WE, Eckhauser FE, Lemmer JH, et al.: Endoscopic percutaneous gastrostomy. Contemp Surg 23:17–23, 1983.
10. Ponsky JL, Gauderer MWL, Stellato TA: Percutaneous endoscopic gastrostomy: Review of 150 cases. Arch Surg 118:913–914, 1983.

CHAPTER SEVEN

ETIOLOGIC CONSIDERATIONS AND RESEARCH TRENDS IN AMYOTROPHIC LATERAL SCLEROSIS

Terry D. Heiman-Patterson, M.D., Mark J. Gudesblatt, M.D., and Albert J. Tahmoush, M.D.

Research in amyotrophic lateral sclerosis (ALS) is aimed at understanding the pathogenetic mechanism so that specific therapies may be designed. Any pathogenetic theory must explain how the normal functioning of the motor system and its interaction with muscle is altered in order to account for the known clinical and pathologic changes of ALS. In addition, it should explain the selective vulnerability of the upper and lower neurons found in this disorder. Thus, a thorough knowledge of normal structure and function of the motor neuronal system, an understanding of the lower motor neuron interaction with its target organ, muscle, and knowledge of the clinical and pathologic features of ALS are essential to any scientist setting out to study the pathogenesis of ALS. Theories of pathogenesis can then provide the basis for rational clinical treatment strategies.

In this chapter, we will review the most common pathogenetic mechanisms postulated for ALS. Subsequently, we will present the research data that relate to each of these mechanisms. The list of possible etiologic mechanisms includes: the presence of either a slow virus or traditional virus; alteration of the immunologic system; the association with a biochemical defect, including alterations in ability to repair DNA; an abnormality in the trophic interactions between the motor neuron system and its surroundings; and finally, the presence of a toxic substance.

VIRAL FACTORS

Both slow virus and traditional viruses have been implicated in ALS.[1-17] The presence of amyotrophy in Creutzfeld–Jakob disease, a transmissible disorder of latent or slow viral origin, has suggested that a slow virus may be responsible for ALS. However, investigators have been unable to transmit the disease to nonhuman primates in a manner similar to that demonstrated for Creutzfeld–Jakob disease.[2]

Among traditional viruses, polio is most implicated since it preferentially affects anterior horn motor neurons. Furthermore, there exists a late-onset postpolio progressive muscular atrophy syndrome.[3] Amyotrophic lateral sclerosis may be due to a latent or persistent poliovirus illness in a manner similar to measles-related subacute sclerosing panencephalitis (SSPE). Recent research supporting this theory arises from experiments demonstrating poliovirus presistence in immune-suppressed mice and cultured neurons.[4–6] Previous research techniques utilized for detection of polio or other viruses have primarily employed serologic evaluation of antibody titers, viral isolation techniques, and electron microscopy evaluation of ALS tissue.[9–14,16] These studies showed occasional viral particles on electron microscopy of spinal cord or muscle tissue[54,55]; no difference in serum or cerebrospinal fluid (CSF) antibody titers between ALS patients and control subjects for poliovirus[9,14,16] or additional viruses (picornavirus, togavirus, orthomyxovirus, paramyxovirus, rhabdovirus, bunyavirus, reovirus, arenavirus, herpesvirus, adenovirus, rabies, measles, and Lymphocytic Choriomeningitis (LCM)[14–16]; and no isolation of virus from ALS autopsy or culture material aside from adenoassociated virus.[10,11,16] The adenoassociated virus was found in 2 of 11 patients and was felt to be due to environmental factors. Finally, although interferon levels were similar to control subjects, sera from patients with ALS demonstrated antiviral activity.[16] Based on these background studies, newer techniques using C-DNA probes for poliovirus genomic activity have been used to examine RNA extracted from spinal cord tissue of ALS patients and for in situ hybridization to tissues of ALS patients.[6,15–17] These methods are sensitive and able to detect one copy or less of viral genome per cell. One of these studies showed no difference in activity in 11 ALS patients and 3 control subjects using C-DNA probes and extraction of RNA from central nervous system (CNS) tissues.[17] These authors point out that poliovirus may still be the causative agent in an indirect manner; that is, the patient may undergo an immunologic response to viral proteins elaborated in other parts of the body. In fact, polio antigens have been demonstrated in the intestinal wall of ALS patients.[18,19] Other authors have had similar negative results.[6] In situ hybridization experiments have demonstrated poliovirus in some patient material, but also in material from control subjects.[7,15] One of these studies observed more intense staining of ALS neurons.[6] These authors argue that polio remains a possible causative factor and negative results may have several explanations. First, delay in performing experiments may lead to autolysis of tissues leading to inability to detect viral genomic material.[15] Alternatively, poliovirus may be present only early in the illness so that there is little genomic material left in the tissue at death.[6] Furthermore, neurons are markedly decreased at death and these are the likely sites of viral infection.[6] Finally, the viral RNA used to create the C-DNA probes may be divergent enough from wild-type genomic sequences that the C-DNA probe did not recognize the wild-type poliovirus genomic material.[6] Thus, additional studies are necessary before polio and other possible viral pathogens are excluded as etiologic agents in ALS.

IMMUNOLOGIC FACTORS

Several studies have implicated immunologic factors in the pathogenesis of ALS. Since ALS sera inhibits growth of neuronal cell cultures, it was suggested that such toxic effects might be mediated by antibodies toxic to neurons.[20–23] Additional reports of immune complex formation in sera and renal tissues of ALS patients further implicated immune mechanisms.[24]

Research has focused on several aspects. First, there have been attempts aimed at finding specific antibodies to neural antigens. Such recent studies have utilized sophisticated immunoblot techniques, examining sodium dodecyl sulfate (SDS) gels of extracted neural and muscle proteins blotted onto nitrocellulose paper and overlaid with patient sera.[25–27] In the study of Hauser and colleagues,[25] extracted muscle proteins were reacted with immunoglobulin G (IgG) from ALS and control patients. There was no unique binding of ALS sera although 10 of 18 ALS patients and 11 of 14 control subjects, including 3/7 Guillain–Barre patients, demonstrated binding in a 56-kD region.[25] Studies of sera overlaid on blots of homogenized motor neurons, dorsal root ganglia, and muscle demonstrated that 30 of 36 ALS patients and 6 of 30 control subjects had IgG activity against a 140-kD protein of dorsal root ganglia and motor neurons. Two of the six control subjects had significant exposure to ALS patients.[26] A third study that investigated homogenized spinal cord proteins overlaid with sera of 12 ALS patients and 18 control subjects (14 with neurologic disease), demonstrated binding with a 70-kD protein in 12 of 12 ALS patients and 8 of 18 control subjects; and binding with a 50-kD protein in 3 of 12 ALS patients and 1 of 18 control patients.[27] These studies highlight the need to examine immunologic mechanisms. In pursuing these leads, Gurney and co-workers[28,29] have defined an antibody in ALS sera not directed against neural or muscle antigens, but rather against a 56-kD sprouting factor. These authors first demonstrated that sera from 9 of 19 sporadic ALS patients and 2 of 6 familial ALS patients inhibited terminal nerve sprouting in a model system consisting of botulinum-treated mouse muscle. There was no inhibition of sprouting with six control sera and six peripheral neuropathy sera. This inhibition by ALS sera was mediated by an immunoglobulin that recognized a 56-kD protein produced by denervated rat diaphragm. This protein promoted neurite outgrowth in vitro, and antibodies to this protein inhibited neuronal sprouting in botulinum-treated mouse muscle in a similar manner to sera of ALS patients. The 56-kD protein has been labeled as a motor neuron sprouting factor. The role of an antibody to sprouting factor is unclear and may be a primary or secondary event. Several important questions have been raised by Rowland in a recent editorial[1]:

> Why is the abnormality the same in both hereditable and presumably acquired syndrome? Does the antibody have functional importance? Does the antibody affect only nerve terminals, or does it affect the cell body too? If there are indeed antibodies to this nerve growth factor, could it be a nonspecific result of denervation? What can be observed in patients with infantile or juvenile forms of spinal muscular atrophy? Why have others had such difficulty identifying serum antibody activity against motor neurons?

Although some of these questions can be addressed (i.e., zero of 6 peripheral neuropathy sera showed inhibition of sprouting, implying that denervation in itself does not lead to the formation of antibodies to sprouting factors), many of the questions remain unanswered. There is much work still left in investigating these interesting findings and the effect of ALS sera on nerve–muscle trophism.

Another approach has been to examine genetically determined immune factors that might predispose to autoimmune disorders or infectious agents.[23] Specific histocompatibility (HLA) locuses are associated with viral disorders while others are associated with autoimmune disease. Demonstration of specific Human Leukocyte Antigen (HLA) antigens in association with a clinical disease is considered indirect evidence that a given disease is of viral or autoimmune etiology. Histocompatibility locuses have been examined in ALS patients and an increase in HLA-A3 has been demonstrated in both sporadic and familial ALS. HLA-B12 has been correlated with slower disease and HLA-B35 has also been implicated. The importance of these findings remains to be determined, but further studies of multiple affected family members will help to elucidate whether linkage exists between HLA antigens and inheritance of ALS.

A third approach to the assessment of immune factors in ALS has been to examine patients for generalized immune system defects.[23,30,31]

Such defects could pertain to cell (T-cell-mediated) or humoral (B-cell-mediated) mechanisms or immune regulatory mechanisms. No major abnormalities have been demonstrated.[23] B-cell and T-cell suppressor activity appear normal.[23] Although some authors have found a decrease in $T\mu$ cells,[31] others have not been able to demonstrate T-cell subset abnormalities.[23] Responsiveness of mononuclear cells to T-cell mitogens was comparable to age-matched healthy control subjects[23] in some studies, but decreased in others.[32,33] Thus, studies of generalized immune system defects have been generally unrewarding.

A final approach is to assess the association of clinical motor neuron disease with other disorders of presumed immunologic pathogenesis. There have been several reports of ALS associated with monoclonal gammopathy.[34–37] In one review of 210 ALS patients, 13 (6.2%) had M-protein abnormalities.[35] Three patients treated with plasmapheresis from this series did not improve while one patient treated with azathiaprine did.[35] Although other studies have reported similar encouraging results with prednisone and azathiaprine,[34,37] three studies showed plasmapheresis to be ineffective as a treatment modality in ALS.[38,39,105] However, these studies did not note the presence of immune protein electrophoresis abnormalities. One additional study described 18 ALS patients with immune abnormalities, including polyclonal gammopathy, elevation of C4 or C3, or muscle biopsies with evidence of inflammation. After a follow-up of 2 to 8 years, three patients demonstrated sustained remission on treatment with prednisone and Cytoxan.[40] These findings may indicate a subgroup of ALS patients with underlying immune mechanisms who potentially respond to therapy. Furthermore, the finding by one of these authors that an M-protein directed at myelin-associated glycoprotein was associated with the clinical picture of motor neuron diseases raises important questions about distinguishing abnormalities of cell bodies, peripheral neuropathies, and axonal disorders in relation to clinical presentation.[41,137] Thus, these findings bear directly on mechanisms of motor neuron disease.[1]

BIOCHEMICAL FACTORS

Although many biochemical and metabolic factors have been discussed in relation to the pathogenesis of ALS,[42–57] the recent findings of altered DNA synthesis in ALS patients,[46,54,57] and the recent reports of the phenotypic expression of hexosaminidase-A (Hex A) deficiency as motor neuron disease[48–51,54,58–60] will provide the focus for the following discussion. Among other biochemical and metabolic abnormalities reported, there has been increased activity of acetylcholinesterase in progressive muscular atrophy,[53] increased ammonia and ornithine in spinal cords of ALS patients,[52] abnormalities of calcium (Ca) metabolism;[61–71] abnormalities of glucose metabolism[45,55,56] increased muscle protease activity,[42] decreased thiamine and thiamine pyrophosphatase in plasma and CSF,[45] altered levels of neurotransmitters in the blood,[44] and altered neurotransmitter receptors in the spinal cord.[47] Neurotransmitters and neuropeptides will be discussed more fully in Trophic Factors (pg. 91).

First, abnormalities of DNA synthesis that have been postulated could lead to abnormal transcription of RNA which would in turn cause either translation of abnormal proteins or absence of certain essential proteins. This could then lead to premature motor neuronal degeneration and clinical ALS.[46,54,57] Studies have demonstrated reduced RNA content[72–74] and altered base composition[74] in motor neurons of ALS patients. Altered base composition may reflect abnormal transcription of damaged DNA. There was also a decrease in RNA content and protein synthesis in the wobbler mouse, an animal model of ALS.[75] These abnormalities of RNA and the proteins produced could lead to cell death. Furthermore, abnormalities in translation of enzymes responsible for DNA repair mechanisms would speed this process. In fact, using agents that damage DNA, the unscheduled synthesis of DNA (U-DNA) has been measured using [^{3}H]thymidine uptake in fibroblast cultures of six ALS patients and six control subjects. The U-DNA synthesis was significantly decreased.[54] It is postulated that a vicious cycle is present in which a primary defect in DNA repair mechanism exists. Other factors could precipitate this cycle by increasing transcription and translation needs of the cell. Such factors could act in several ways, for example, by increasing DNA damage, decreasing DNA repair enzymes or increasing metabolic demands on the cell. For example, heavy metals inhibit many enzymes and may specifically inactivate DNA repair enzymes.[57] Other factors such as Ca, gastrointestinal, and endocrine abnormalities might increase metabolic demands. Similar arguments have been made for other etiologic factors.[57] Thus, the DNA hypothesis helps to explain how the many implicated etiologic factors could all play a role in the pathogenesis of ALS. Further work in this area is ongoing.

Another exciting new finding is the recent descriptions of Hex A deficiency associated with or presenting solely as motor neuron disease.[48–51,58–60] These patients have low levels of Hex A in serum and leukocytes. Hex A is a lysosomal enzyme catabolizing GM_2 gangliosides. Total absence of Hex A is associated with Tay–Sachs disease. Partial deficiencies have been associated with several neurologic disorders, including spinocerebellar degeneration, seizures, dementia, and motor neuron disease, presenting from adolescence to adulthood.[48–51,58–60] The clinical features of Hex A-associated motor neuron disease include early onset, slow progression, and autosomal-recessive inheritance. It can take the form of either spinal muscle atrophy or ALS. Those patients with both Hex A deficiency and ALS manifest dysarthria, atrophy, fasciculations, spasticity, and Babinski's signs.[48–51,58–60] When ALS is associated with a known enzyme deficiency, there are major genetic implications for the patient and family. It is yet unknown what role these enzymes may play in anterior horn cell function, and why some cases of Hex A deficiency are expressed as Tay–Sachs disease and others as motor neuron disease. Evidence now exists that there are at least two loci (α and β) for hexosaminidase on chromosomes 5 and 15[50] with two alleles. At least nine hexosaminidase compounds are possible,[50] any of which may be deficient. Further elucidation of Hex A at the genomic level and factors regulating its expression are necessary to understand the diverse manifestations of Hex A deficiency and the function of this enzyme within the nervous system.

TROPHIC FACTORS

One theory of ALS pathogenesis postulates that there is a lack of a trophic factor necessary for motor neuron survival and growth. This lack of trophic factor might be due to inadequate supplies, agents that block trophic factor action (e.g., an antibody[29],) impaired transport of the trophic factor, or impaired trophic factor receptor function.

Research into trophic factors has been aided by two important findings. First, a nerve growth factor (NGF) has been identified that promotes growth of sensory neurons from the dorsal root ganglia.[76,77] This factor has been isolated as a purified protein. Similar additional growth factors for other types of neurons may be present and, in fact, a sprouting factor for motor neurons isolated from denervated rat diaphragm has been described.[28,29] Furthermore, muscle extracts have been shown to enhance neurite outgrowth and increase cholinergic activity in cultured rat ventral horn neurons.[78] These studies extensively utilize tissue culture techniques that provide isolated systems in which the effects of a presumed trophic substance can be evaluated. Furthermore, antibodies to these trophic factors can be produced and the effect of such antibodies can be studied both in vitro and in vivo.[28,29]

The second important finding is the occurrence of neuronal attrition related to synaptic development and presence of target organs.[79,80] Neuronal attrition markedly increases if the target organ is absent. This implies that the target organ may supply and release factors important to survival and growth of the innervating neurons.[79] Such factors for motor neuron growth have been isolated from muscle and denervated diaphragm.[28,29,78] Trophic factors need not derive from target organs alone, but may be elaborated by adjacent glia or neuronal contacts; or even distant cells that secrete such factors into the CSF or serum.

Among possible trophic factors that might play a role in ALS, motor nerve sprouting factor has been discussed above (see Immununologic Factors, above). Additional factors have been identified in muscle extracts,[78] and a lack of such a trophic factor might cause a retrograde degeneration of the motor system resulting in motor neuron disease.

There is another group of possible trophic factors that are presently under active study. These are the neuropeptides that can be localized to the spinal cord and may play a role as both neurotransmitters and neurotrophic factors. Analysis of neuropeptides can provide important information regarding neural connections and functions. Furthermore, the study of neuropeptide changes in disease states may lead to a fuller understanding of the pathophysiology and pathogenesis of ALS.

Several neuropeptides have received attention. Choline acetyltransferase activity was reduced in both the anterior and dorsal horns of spinal cords in ALS patients.[81] Further studies of muscarinic receptors revealed profound reductions in Lamina 9 correlating with the degree of motor neuron loss. Glycine receptors were also markedly reduced. Both glycine and muscarinic receptors have a high concentration around motor neurons. Benzodiazepine receptors were only minimally reduced. Such data suggest altered vulnerability of neurons to the ALS process may be based on their neuropeptide receptor components.[47] However, of all neuropeptides, thyrotropin-releasing hormone (TRH) has received the most recent attention. Evidence has now accumulated that there is a distinct TRH neurotransmitter system with specific actions. The majority of TRH is extrahypothalamic.[82] Furthermore, TRH has been immunocytochemically demonstrated in the vicinity of mammalian spinal motor neurons and has been localized to synaptic vesicles using electron microscopy and immunocytochemistry.[82–86] Its activity disappears after cord transection, indicating that TRH-containing fibers are of supraspinal origin.[86] Radioimmunoassay (RIA) studies reveal TRH to be located in the ventral horn throughout the entire spinal cord.[87] Using radioautography techniques, receptors for TRH have been found on motor neurons of Rexed Layer 9 of the anterior horn in human spinal cords.[88] In addition, TRH has a depolarizing effect on neurons in vitro.[89,90] Release of TRH from synaptosomal preparations has been demonstrated.[91] Thus, TRH appears to play a fundamental role in motor system function either as a neurotransmitter or trophic factor. In ALS, the cortical, brainstem, and anterior horn motor neuron dropout parallels the distribution of immunologically identifiable presynaptically located TRH. Such anterior horn neuronal loss may be related to transynaptic loss of a "trophic factor," that is, TRH. The role of TRH as both a neurotransmitter and possible trophic factor in the motor system and spinal cord has stimulated ALS investigators to study TRH and ALS more thoroughly. Examination of spinal cords in ALS patients for TRH-like immunoreactivity has demonstrated a marked reduction of activity in the ventral horn when compared to normal subjects.[92] Studies of TRH in CSF have revealed low levels.[93] These data regarding the role of TRH in the motor system as well as CSF alterations in ALS patients have led to a number of therapeutic trials of TRH in ALS which are reviewed in Therapeutic Trials, below.[93–103]

A TOXIC FACTOR

A toxic factor has long been popular among the possible etiologic mechanisms for sporadic ALS. The toxic factor might include a serum or CSF factor, or perhaps heavy metal intoxication. Several heavy metals, including lead (Pb), mercury (Hg), and selenium (Se) have been associated with a motor neuron syndrome. Additional heavy metals and minerals have also been implicated, including manganese (Mn), aluminum (Al), copper (Cu), and calcium (Ca).[61–71,109–132] These toxins might act directly at the cell body or along the axon of the neuron to cause the pathologic change in ALS and resultant clinical symptomatology. Furthermore, a defect in the motor neuron itself may make the patient more vulnerable to a presumed toxin.

Lead has been associated with motor neuron disease for over one hundred years.[109,113,114] The data regarding Pb toxicity in ALS are controversial.[61,109–114] Some groups have found no difference in either the serum, spinal fluid, red blood cells, or whole blood Pb levels in ALS patients.[110] However, other groups have found an increased Pb level by atomic absorption spectroscopy in both the serum and CSF of patients with ALS.[109,111] Increased fragility of red blood cells exposed to Pb has been reported in ALS patients.[111] Finally, patients may vary in their susceptibility to Pb intoxication because of variations in their Pb absorption metabolism. Lead may be a primary pathogen or it may have secondary effects by its interference with various metabolic pathways.

Other heavy metals have also been implicated. An amyotrophic myelopathy has been reported with Hg.[115–117] Selenium has also been reported to be associated with ALS,[118] but prospective studies of two hundred ALS patients did not find any elevation of urinary excretion of Se.[120] Other trace elements have also been studied with refined analytical techniques. The technique that is selected must offer the best sensitivity and accuracy as well as the best selectivity for the element of interest. Some newer techniques that have been used include atomic absorption spectrophotometry, electron probe x-ray microanalysis, fluorescent spectrometry, and neutron activation analysis.[61] A description of these techniques and their limitations can be found elsewhere.[61] These techniques have been applied to analysis of Mn, Al, Cu, Ca, Se, and other trace metals.[62–71,121–132] Manganese has been analyzed by neutron activation analysis in the spinal cords of seven autopsied ALS patients and six control subjects.[121] There was an elevation of Mn in the anterior and lateral columns in the ALS patients studied. It was postulated that since Mn inhibits neuronal transmission, there may be neuronal degeneration on the basis of local disturbances of Mn metabolism. Additional neutron activation analysis studies of Mn levels in spinal cords from ALS patients from Guam, the Kii Peninsula of Japan, and sporadic ALS patients did not demonstrate any Mn elevation.[16–20] Electron probe microanalysis of Mn levels has also yielded conflicting evidence.[62–64,124] Finally, Mn concentrations in muscle and visceral organs of ALS patients did not differ from control subjects.[125]

Interest in Al as a toxin stems from the similarity between the neurofibrillary pathology of experimental Al toxicity and that of ALS in Chammarro. Neutron activation analysis demonstrated increased Al levels in Chammarro with ALS, Chammarros with parkinsonism–dementia, and sporadic ALS patients in Japan.[62,63,124] Levels were also elevated in Japanese ALS patients in data obtained using electron probe x-ray analysis.[61] Studies using x-ray spectrometry demonstrated an increased Al level in neurons containing neurofibrillary tangles found in Guamanian Chammarro with ALS, parkinsonism–Dementia, or normal subjects.[130] These results may reflect the presence of high levels of Al and low levels of Ca and Mg in the soil and drinking water of Guam as well as other areas of high incidence of ALS (e.g., the Kii Peninsula of Japan, New Guinea).[129,131] These chronic nutritional deficiencies of Ca and Mg coupled with an excess of certain other trace metals; for example, Al, could produce aberrations of mineral metabolism associated with deposition of these metals in the CNS. Furthermore, the constellation of ALS, parkinsonism–dementia, and premature neurofilament formation encountered in the Chammarros of Guam and in Japanese of the Kii Peninsula may indicate that these ALS populations share pathogenetic mechanisms involving environmental factors.

The clinical similarities between ALS and neuromuscular disorders associated with hyperparathyroidism, and the frequently reported skeletal abnormalities and fractures in patients with ALS have implicated alterations of Ca metabolism.[61,65,66] Abnormalities of serum Ca, Ca absorption, and elevated Ca levels in CNS tissue have been reported.[61–69] These investigators have also demonstrated Ca deposition in the spinal cord in both patients with ALS and control subjects.[61] On the other hand, Ca was noted to be reduced in muscle tissue while calmodulin levels were normal.[71] Furthermore, normal serum Ca levels and [45]Ca binding have been observed and lower Ca levels in spinal cord tissues were reported in Chammarro with ALS.[124,128]

Spinal cord Cu levels have also been examined using neutron activation analysis and x-ray fluorescent spectrometry with conflicting results.[64,124] Finally, other trace elements, including sodium, chloride, potassium, chromium, iron, cobalt, zinc, rubidium, silver, cesium, and Se have been measured in the CSF of 20 ALS patients and 14 control subjects with neutron activation analysis.[132] The only abnormality noted was a lowered cobalt concentration.

Thus, the data indicate there are abnormalities of heavy metals and trace minerals in ALS patients, but their role in the pathogenesis of ALS remains unclear.

Heavy metals and trace minerals are not the only source for toxic substances that have been studied. Toxicity of serum and CSF from ALS patients has been evaluated.[20–22,133–136] Wolfgram and Myers were the first to note a toxic effect of sera from ALS patients on cultured anterior horn cell neurons.[21,22] Although others could not reproduce this effect,[133–135] Roisen and colleagues, by duplicating exactly the original experiments, demonstrated cytotoxicity of ALS sera on neurons.[20] However, toxicity to a lesser extent was also seen in family contacts and neurologic control subjects. Cerebrospinal fluid from ALS patients had no effect on morphology or neuron-specific enolase production in cultured mouse neurons.[136] Attempts to transfer ALS with whole plasma from ALS patients injected into mice did not produce any abnormalities after 3 months.[1]

THERAPEUTIC TRIALS

Therapeutic trials are logical extensions of the basic research regarding pathogenetic mechanisms. The modalities that are tested are chosen to modify or alleviate a presumed pathogenetic factor, thus relating the "cure" to the disease mechanism. Many such clinical trials have been carried out in ALS with disappointing results.[35,38,39,88,93–108] Recently, clinical trials have focused on presumed viral mechanisms, immune mechanisms, and the possible lack of an essential trophic factor.

Therapeutic attempts aimed at altering viral infections have utilized interferons[104,106] and antiviral agents such as tilorone.[107] These studies have shown no clinical improvement in ALS patients.

Manipulations aimed at the immune system have included plasmapheresis[35,38,39,105,108] and immunosuppression.[34,37,40] Results of these studies are somewhat more encouraging, with several investigators reporting clinical improvement in a few patients.[34,35,37,40] This was seen especially in patients demonstrating monoclonal gammopathies.[35]

Finally, attempts to replace a possible missing "trophic" factor have spurred a multitude of trials involving the use of TRH.[88-103] Thyrotropin-releasing hormone has been given by multiple routes of administration, including intravenous,[93-97] subcutaneous,[98-100] intramuscular,[102] and intrathecal.[100,102] Slow infusion pumps have also been employed.[103] Although initial reports were enthusiastic,[92] subsequent trials have been disappointing.[96,100,102] While some investigators demonstrate modest clinical improvement,[94,96-98,99] others in placebo-controlled studies have shown no benefit.[100,102] Ongoing studies using TRH analogues are underway as well as additional TRH investigations. At the present time, TRH trials are centered about home administration of individually modified subcutaneous TRH doses. Such studies are aimed at minimizing drug side effects and the "autorefractory" period that has been described.

FUTURE GOALS OF RESEARCH

We have reviewed the most recent research efforts relating to the pathogenesis of ALS and some of the therapeutic trials based on these theories. A chapter on research in ALS would not be complete without some brief comments regarding the future goals of these investigations. It is clear that to understand disease mechanisms in ALS, one must begin by understanding the normal interaction that occurs between nerve and muscle. Thus, further studies of the normal interaction between nerve and muscle are necessary, including anatomy, biochemistry, physiology, and trophism. Such studies are underway both in vivo and in vitro through the extensive use of animal models and tissue culture. Tissue culture provides the added benefit of encompassing an isolated system. In the same way, models for disease must be developed. There now exist several animal models for motor nerve degeneration,[75,138] but more ideal models need to be developed. Such models will allow comparison of neuromuscular interaction in both normal and diseased subjects. Furthermore, such models could provide for testing of proposed therapeutic modalities. Ongoing research in both human ALS and animal disease models must elucidate the immunologic, biochemical, toxic, viral, and trophic disease mechanisms with respect to both their individual and additive roles in the pathogenesis of ALS. As pointed out in Biochemical Factors, above, causative factors need not be mutually exclusive. For instance, neurons may be more susceptible to a particular toxin because of an underlying biochemical alteration. Similarly, latent viral infection within the nervous system may occur because of alterations in the immune system. Finally, the ultimate goal of all disease-related research entails the development of rational and curative therapies based on the delineated disease mechanisms.

REFERENCES

1. Rowland LP: Looking for the cause of amyotrophic lateral sclerosis. N Engl J Med 311:979–981, 1985.
2. Salazar AM, Masters CL, Gajdusek DC, et al.: Syndromes of amyotrophic lateral sclerosis and dementia: Relations to transmissible Creutzfeldt-Jakob disease. Ann Neurol 14:17–26, 1983.
3. Alter M, Kurland LT, Molgaard C: Late progressive muscular atrophy and antecedent poliomyelitis. In Rowland LP (ed): Human Motor Neuron Diseases. Raven Press: New York, 1982, pp. 303–309.
4. Miller JR: Prolonged intracerebral infection with poliovirus in asymptomatic mice. Ann Neurol 9:590–596, 1981.
5. Jubelt B, Meagher JB: Poliovirus infection of cyclophosphamide-treated mice results in persistence and late paralysis. Neurology 34:486–499, 1984.
6. Miller JR, Britton CB, Kormer J: Persistent poliovirus infection in cell culture. Neurology 34:237–238, 1984.
7. Viola MV, Lazarus M, Antel J, et al.: Nucleic acid probes in the study of amyotrophic lateral sclerosis. In Rowland LP (ed): Human Motor Neuron Diseases. Raven Press, New York, 1982, pp. 317–329.
8. Davis LE, Bodean D, Price D, et al.: Chronic progressive poliomyelitis secondary to vaccination of an immunodeficient child. N Engl J Med 297:241–245, 1977.
9. Kurent J, Brooks BR, Madden DL, et al.: CSF viral antibodies. Evaluation in ALS and late onset poliomyelitis progressive atrophy. Arch neurol 36:269–273, 1979.
10. Roos R, Viola M, Wollman R, et al.: Amyotrophic lateral sclerosis with preceding poliomyelitis. Arch Neurol 29:331–333, 1973.
11. Oshero L, Cremer W, Norris FH: Virus-like particles in muscle from a patient with amyotrophic lateral sclerosis. Neurology 26:57–60, 1976.
12. Cremer W, Oshero L, Norris FH: Cultures of tissues from patients with amyotrophic lateral sclerosis. Arch Neurol 29:331–333, 1973.
13. Pena GE: Virus-like particles in amyotrophic lateral sclerosis: Electron microscopic study of a case. Ann Neurol 1:290–297, 1976.
14. Harter DH: Viruses other than poliovirus in human amyotrophic lateral sclerosis. In Rowland LP (ed): Human Motor Neuron Diseases. Raven Press, New York, 1982, pp. 339–342.
15. Brahic M, Cash E, Smith RA, et al.: Detection of picornavirus sequences in CNS tissue of ALS and control patients. Neurology 35:108, 1985.
16. Kascsak RJ, Carp RI, Vilcek JT, et al.: Virological studies in amyotrophic lateral sclerosis. Muscle Nerve 5:93–101, 1982.
17. Miller JR, Guntaka RV, Myers JC: Amyotrophic lateral sclerosis: Search for poliovirus by nucleic acid hybridization. Neurology 30:884–886, 1980.
18. Behan PO, Behan WM, Bell E, et al.: Possible persistent virus in motor neuron diseases (Letter). Lancet 2:1176, 1977.
19. Pertschuk LD, Cook LW, Gupta JK, et al.: Jejunal immunopathology in amyotrophic lateral sclerosis and multiple sclerosis: Identification of viral antigens by immunofluorescence. Lancet 1:1119–1123, 1977.
20. Roisen FJ, Bartfield H, Donnenfeld H, et al.: Neuron specific in vitro cytotoxicity of sera from patients with amyotrophic lateral sclerosis. Muscle Nerve 5:48–53, 1982.
21. Wolfgram F, Myers L: Toxicity of serum from patients with ALS for anterior horn cells in vitro. Trans Am Neurol Assoc 97:19–23, 1972.
22. Wolfgram F, Myers I: Amyotrophic lateral sclerosis: Effect of serum on anterior horn cells in culture. Science 179:579–580, 1973.

23. Antel JP, Noronha ABC, Oger JJF, et al.: Immunology of amyotrophic lateral sclerosis. In Rowland LP (ed): Human Motor Neuron Diseases. Raven Press, New York, 1982, pp. 395–402.
24. Oldstone MBA, Wilson CB, Perrin LH, et al.: Evidence for immune complex formation in patients with ALS. Lancet 2:169–172, 1976.
25. Hauser SL, Henderson CE, Lyon-Caen O, et al.: Analysis of antibodies to muscle protein in amyotrophic lateral sclerosis (ALS). Neurology 35 (Suppl 1):250, 1985.
26. Kletti NB, Marton LS, Antel JP, et al.: Antibodies against neural antigen in sera of patients with amyotrophic lateral sclerosis. Neurology 34 (Suppl 1):S–238, 1984 (Abstr).
27. Brown RH Jr, Ogonowski M, Johnson D, et al.: Antineural antibodies in sera from patients with amyotrophic lateral sclerosis. Neurology 34 (Suppl 1):238, 1984.
28. Gurney ME: Suppression of sprouting at the neuromuscular junction by immunoassay sera. Nature 307:546–548, 1984.
29. Gurney ME, Belton AC, Cashman N, et al: Inhibition of terminal axonal sprouting by serum from patients with amyotrophic lateral sclerosis. N Engl J Med 311:933–939, 1984.
30. Ronnevi LO, Conradi S, Karlsson E: Cytotoxic effects of immunoglobin in amyotrophic lateral sclerosis (ALS). Acta Neurol Scand 69 (Suppl 98):182–183, 1984.
31. Westall FL, Rubin R, Nieder J, et al.: Low percentage of Tμ cells in amyotrophic lateral sclerosis. Immunol Lett 7:139–140, 1983.
32. Behan PO, Behan WM, Bell E, et al.: Possible persistent virus in motor neuron diseases. Lancet 2:1176, 1977.
33. Hoffman PH, Robbins DS, Nolte MT, et al.: Cellular immunity in amyotrophic lateral sclerosis and parkinsonism-dementia. N Engl J Med 299:680–685, 1978.
34. Latov N: Plasma cell dyscrasia in motor neuron disease. In Rowland LP (ed): Human Motor Neuron Diseases. Raven Press, New York, 1982, pp. 273–279.
35. Shy ME, Trojaborg W, Smith T, et al.: Motor neuron disease and plasma cell dyscrasia. Neurology 35 (Suppl 1):107, 1985.
36. Krieger C, Melmed C: Amyotrophic lateral sclerosis and paraproteinemia. Neurology 32:896–898, 1982.
37. Engel WK, Hopkins LC, Rosenberg BJ: Fasciculating progressive muscular atrophy (F-PMA) remarkably responsive to antidysimmune treatment (ADIT)—a possible clue to ALS? Neurology 35 (Suppl 1):72, 1985.
38. Keleman J, Hedlund W, Orlin JB, et al.: Plasmaphoresis with immunosuppression in amyotrophic lateral sclerosis. Arch Neurol 40:752–753, 1983.
39. Olarte MR, Schoenfeldt RS, McKiernan G, et al.: Plasmaphoresis in amyotrophic lateral sclerosis. Ann Neurol 8:644–645, 1980.
40. Pattern MB: ALS of autoimmune origin. Neurology 35 (Suppl):251, 1985.
41. Rowland LP, Defendini R, Sherman W, et al.: Macroglobulinemia with peripheral neuropathy simulating motor neuron disease. Ann Neurol 11:532–536, 1982.
42. Antel JP, Chelmicka-Schorr E, Sprotiello M, et al.: Muscle acid protease activity in amyotrophic lateral sclerosis: Correlation with clinical and pathologic features. Neurology 32:901–903, 1982.
43. Hayashi H, Tsubaki T: Enzymatic analysis of individual anterior horn cells in amyotrophic lateral sclerosis and Duschenne muscular dystrophy. J Neurol Sci 57:133–142, 1982.
44. Belendiuk K, Belendiuk GW, Freedman DX, et al.: Neurotransmitter abnormalities in patients with motor neuron disease. Arch Neurol 38:415–417, 1981.
45. Poloni M, Patrini C, Rocchelli B, et al.: Thiamine monophosphate in the CSF of patients with amyotrophic lateral sclerosis. Arch Neurol 39:507–509, 1982.
46. Bradley WG, Krasin F: A new hypothesis of the etiology of amyotrophic lateral sclerosis. The DNA hypothesis. Arch Neurol 39:667–680, 1982.
47. Whitehouse PJ, Wamsley JK, Zarbin MA, et al.: Amyotrophic lateral sclerosis: Alterations in neurotransmitter receptors. Ann Neurol 14:8–16, 1983.
48. Dale JDD, Engel AG, Rudd NL: Familial hexosaminidase-A deficiency with Kugelberg-Welander phenotype and mental change. Ann Neurol 14:109, 1983.
49. Sliman RJ, Mitsumoto H, Schafer IA, et al.: A study of hexosaminidase-A deficiency

in a patient with atypical amyotrophic lateral sclerosis. Ann Neurol 14:148–149, 1983.
50. Johnson WG: Hexosaminidase deficiency: A cause of recessively inherited motor neuron diseases. In Rowland LP (ed): Human Motor Neuron Diseases. Raven Press, New York, 1982, pp. 159–164.
51. Jellinger K, Anzil AP, Seeman D, et al.: Adult Gm_2 gangliosidosis masquerading as slowly progressive muscular atrophy: Motor neuron disease phenotype. Clin Neuropathol 1:31–44, 1982.
52. Pattern BM, Kurlander HM, Evans B: Free amino acid concentrations in spinal tissue from patients dying of motor neuron disease. Acta Neurol Scand 66:594–599, 1982.
53. Rasool CG, Chad D, Bradley WG, et al.: Acetylocholinesterase and ATPases in motor neuron degenerative diseases. Muscle Nerve 6:430–435, 1983.
54. Tandan R, Robison SH, Munzer JS, et al.: Deficient DNA repair in amyotrophic lateral sclerosis cells. Neurology 35 (Suppl 1):73, 1985.
55. Reyes ET, Perurena OH, Festoff BW, et al.: Insulin resistance in amyotrophic lateral sclerosis. J Neurol Sci 63:317–324, 1984.
56. Harno K, Rissanen HK, Palo J: Glucose tolerance in amyotrophic lateral sclerosis. Acta Neurol Scand 7016:451–455, 1984.
57. Bradley WG, Krasin F: DNA hypothesis of amyotrophic lateral sclerosis. In Rowland LP (ed): Human Motor Neuron Diseases. Raven Press, New York, 1982, pp. 493–500.
58. Johnson WG, Wigger HJ, Karp HR, et al.: Juvenile spinal muscle atrophy: A new hexosaminidase deficiency phenotype. Ann Neurol 11:11–16, 1982.
59. Johnson WG: The clinical spectrum of hexosaminidase deficiency diseases. Neurology 31:1453–1456, 1981.
60. Argov Z, Navon R: Clinical and genetic variations in the syndrome of adult GM_2 gangliosidosis resulting from hexosaminidase-A deficiency. Ann Neurol 16:14–20, 1984.
61. Yanagihara R: Heavy metals and essential minerals in motor neuron disease. In Rowland LP (ed): Human Motor Neuron Diseases. Raven Press, New York, 1982, pp. 233–247.
62. Yoshimasu F, Uebayashi Y, Yase Y, et al.: Studies on amyotrophic sclerosis by neutron activation analysis. Folia Psychiatry Neurol Jpn 30:49–55, 1976.
63. Yoshimasu F, Yasui M, Yase Y, et al.: Studies on amyotrophic lateral sclerosis neutron activation analysis. 2. Comparative study of analytical results on Guam PD, Japanese ALS, and Alzheimer disease cases. Folia Psychiatry Neurol Jpn 34:75–82, 1980.
64. Kurlander HM, Patten BM: Metals in spinal cord tissue of patients dying of motor neuron disease. Ann Neurol 6:21–24, 1979.
65. Patten BM, Mallette LE: Motor neuron disease: Retrospective study of associated abnormalities. Dis Nerv Sys 37:318–321, 1976.
66. Mallette LE, Patten BM, Cook JD, et al.: Calcium metabolism in amyotrophic lateral sclerosis. Dis Nerv Sys 38:457–461, 1977.
67. Yanagihara R, Gajdusek DC, Gibbs CJ Jr, et al.: Search for metabolic and neuroendocrinologic anomalies in Guamanians with amyotrophic lateral sclerosis and parkinsonism-dementia. Tenth International Congress on Tropical Medicine and Malaria, Manila, Philippines, 1980, pp. 383–384 (Abstr 621).
68. Yanagihara R, Garruto RM, Gajdusek DC, et al.: Calcium metabolism in Guamanian Chamorros with amyotrophic lateral sclerosis and parkinsonism-dementia. 12th World Congress of Neurology, Kyoto, Japan, 1981, pp. 375–376 (Abstr PPO296).
69. Yase Y, Yoshimasu F, Uebayashi Y, et al.: Neutron activation analysis of calcium in central nervous system tissues of amyotrophic lateral sclerosis cases. Folia Psychiatry Neurol Jpn 28:371–378, 1974.
70. Yanagihara R, Garruto RM, Gajdusek DC, et al.: Calcium and vitamin D metabolism in Guamanian Chamorros with amyotrophic lateral sclerosis and parkinsonism-dementia. Ann Neurol 15:42–48, 1984.
71. Mishra SK, Kumar S: Muscle calcium, calmodulin levels in amyotrophic lateral sclerosis. Neurology 35:73, 1985.
72. Mann DMA, Yates PO: Motor neurone disease: The nature of the pathogenic mechanism. J Neurol Neurosurg Psychiatry 37:1036–1046, 1974.

73. Davidson TJ, Hartmann HA: RNA content and volume of motor neurons in amyotrophic lateral sclerosis. J Neuropathol Exp Neurol 40:187–192, 1981.

74. Davidson TJ, Hartman HA: Base composition of RNA obtained from motor neurons in amyotrophic lateral sclerosis. J Neuropathol Exp Neurol 40:193–198, 1981.

75. Murakami T, Mastiglia FL, Mann DMA, et al.: Abnormal RNA metabolism in spinal motor neurons in the Wobbler mouse. Muscle Nerve 4:407–412, 1981.

76. Greene LA, Shooter EM: The nerve growth factor: Biochemistry, synthesis and mechanism of action. Annu Rev Neurosci 3:352–402, 1980.

77. Varon S, Adler R: Trophic and specifying factor directed to neuronal cells. Adv Cell Neurobiol 2:115–163, 1981.

78. Smith RG, Appel SH: Extracts of skeletal muscle increase neurite outgrowth and cholinergic activity of fetal rat spinal motor neurons. Science 219:1079–1081, 1983.

79. Varon S, Manthorpe M, Longo FM: Growth factors and motor neurons. In Rowland LP (ed): Human Motor Neuron Diseases. Raven Press, New York, 1982, pp. 453–471.

80. Landmesser L, Pilar G: Interactions between neurons and their targets during in vivo synaptogenesis. Fed Proc 37:2016–2022, 1978.

81. Gillberg PA, Aquilonius S, Eckernan S, et al.: Choline acetyltransferase and substance P-like immunoreactivity in the human spinal cord: Changes in ALS. Brain Res 250:394–397, 1982.

82. Winokur A, Davis R, Utiger RD: Subcellular distribution of thyrotropin-releasing hormone (TRH) in rat brain and hypothalamus. Brain Res 120:423–434, 1977.

83. Hokfelt T, Fuxe K, Johansson O, et al.: Thyrotropin releasing hormone (TRH) containing nerve terminals in certain brain stem nuclei and in the spinal cord. Neurosci Lett 1:133–139, 1975.

84. Hokfelt T, Fuxe K, Johansson O, et al.: Distribution of thyrotropin-releasing hormone (TRH) in the central nervous system as revealed with immunohistochemistry. Br J Pharmacol 34:389–392, 1975.

85. Johansson O, Hokfelt T, Jeffcoate SL et al.: Ultrastructural localization of TRH-like immunoreactivity. Exp Brain Res 38:1–9, 1980.

86. Hokfelt T: In Iversen LL, Nicoll RA, Vale W (eds): Neurobiology of peptides. Neurosci Res Prog Bull 16, 1978.

87. Kardon FC, Winokur A, Utiger RD: Thyrotropin-releasing hormone (TRH) in rat spinal cord. Brain Res 122:578–581, 1977.

88. Manaker S, Winokur A, Rhodes CH, et al.: Autoradiographic localization of thyrotropin-releasing hormone (TRH) receptors in human spinal cord. Neurology 35: 328–332, 1985.

89. Nicoll RA: Excitatory action of TRH on spinal motor neurons. Nature 265:242–243, 1977.

90. Nicoll RA: The action of thyrotropin-releasing hormone, substance P and related peptides on frog spinal motor neurons. J Pharmacol Exp Ther 207:817–824, 1978.

91. Bennett GW, Edwardson JA, Holland D, et al.: Release of immunoreactive luteinizing hormone-releasing hormone and thyrotropin-releasing hormone from hypothalamic synaptosomes. Nature 257:323–329, 1975.

92. Mitsuma T, Nogimori T, Adachi K, et al.: Concentrations of immunoreactive thyrotropin-releasing hormone in spinal cord of patients with amyotrophic lateral sclerosis. Am J Med Sci 287:34–36, 1984.

93. Engel WK, Siddique T, Nicoloff JT: Effect on weakness and spasticity in amyotrophic lateral sclerosis of thyrotropin-releasing hormone. Lancet 2:73–75, 1983.

94. Graco VL, Caligiuri M, Abbs JH, et al.: Placebo controlled computerized dynametric measurements of bulbar and somatic muscle strength increase in patients with amyotrophic lateral sclerosis following intravenous infusion of 10 mg/kg thyrotropin-releasing hormone. Ann Neurol 16:110, 1984.

95. Sufit R, Beaulieu D, Sangua M, et al.: Placebo controlled quantitative measurements of neuromuscular function following intravenous infusion of 10 mg/kg thyrotropin-releasing hormone in 16 male patients with amyotrophic lateral sclerosis. Ann Neurol 16:110–111, 1984.

96. Caroscio JT, Cohen JA, Zawodniak J, et al.: A double-blind placebo-controlled trial of TRH in amyotrophic lateral sclerosis. Neurology 35:106, 1985.
97. Mitsumoto H, Salgado ED, Negroski D, et al.: Double-blind crossover trials with acute intravenous thyrotropin-releasing hormone infusion in patients with amyotrophic lateral sclerosis: Negative studies. Ann Neurol 16:109, 1984.
98. Engel WK, Van der Bergh P, Askanas V: Subcutaneous thyrotropin releasing hormone seems ready for wider trials in treating lower motor neuron-produced weakness and spasticity. Ann Neurol 16:109–110, 1984.
99. Engel WK, Spiel RH: Prolonged at-home treatment of motor neuron disorders with self-administered subcutaneous (sq) high-dose TRH. Neurology 35:106–107, 1985.
100. Mitsumoto H, Salgado ED, Negroski D, et al.: Double-blind crossover trials with chronic, subcutaneous injections of small doses of TRH in patients with ALS. Neurology 35:71, 1985.
101. Munsat TL, Mora JS, Robinson JE, et al.: Intrathecal TRH in amyotrophic lateral sclerosis: Preliminary observations. Neurology 34:239, 1984.
102. Imoto K, Saida K, Iwamura K, et al.: Amyotrophic lateral sclerosis: A double-blind crossover trial of thyrotropin releasing hormone. J Neurol Neurosurg Psychiatry 47:1332–1334, 1984.
103. Taft J, Munsat T, Jackson I, et al.: A constant infusion pump for intrathecal delivery of TRH in ALS. Neurology 35:107, 1985.
104. Farkkila MA, Iivanainen MV, Bergstrom L, et al.: Interferon treatment in amyotrophic lateral sclerosis. Acta Neurol Scand 69:184–185, 1984.
105. Silani V, Scarlato G, Valli G, et al.: Plasma exchange ineffective in amyotrophic lateral sclerosis. Arch Neurol 37:511–513, 1980.
106. Dalakas M, Aksamit A, Madden D, et al.: Recombinant leukocyte alpha-interferon in patients with amyotrophic lateral sclerosis (ALS). Neurology 35:71, 1985.
107. Olson WH, Simons JA, Halaas GW: Therapeutic trial of tilorone in ALS: Lack of benefit in a double-blind, placebo-controlled study. Neurology 28:1293–1295, 1978.
108. Conomy JP, Gerhard G, Goren H, et al.: Plasmaphoresis in the treatment of amyotrophic lateral sclerosis. Neurology 30:356, 1980.
109. Conradi S, Ronnevi LO, Norris FH: Motor neuron disease and toxic metals. In Rowland LP (ed): Human Motor Neuron Diseases. Raven Press, New York, 1982, pp. 201–231.
110. Stober T, Stelte W, Kunze K: Lead concentration in blood, plasma, erythrocytes, and cerebrospinal fluid in amyotrophic lateral sclerosis. J Neurol Sci 61:21–26, 1983.
111. Stockholm LO, Conradi S, Nise G: Further studies on the erythrocyte uptake of lead in vitro in amyotrophic lateral sclerosis (ALS) patients and controls. Abnormal erythrocyte fragility in ALS. J Neurol Sci 57:143–156, 1982.
112. Campbell AMG, Williams ER, Baltrop D: Motor neuron disease and exposure to lead. J Neurol Neurosurg 33:877–885, 1970.
113. Lively B, Sissons CE: Chronic lead intoxication mimicking motor neurone disease. Br Med J 4:387–388, 1968.
114. Simpson JA, Seaton DA, Adams JF: Response to treatment with chelating agents of anaemia, chronic encephalopathy, and myelopathy due to lead poisoning. J Neurol Neurosurg Psychiatry 27:536–541, 1974.
115. Okinaka S, Yoshikawa M, Mozai T, et al.: Encephalomyelopathy due to an organic mercury compound. Neurology 14:69–76, 1964.
116. Kantarjian AD: A syndrome clinically resembling amyotrophic lateral sclerosis following chronic mercurialism. Neurology 11:639–644, 1961.
117. Brown IA: Chronic mercurialism. Arch Neurol 72:674–681, 1954.
118. Adams CR, Ziegler DK, Lin JT: Mercury intoxication simulating amyotrophic lateral sclerosis. JAMA 250:642–643, 1983.
119. Kilness AW, Hochberg FH: Amyotrophic lateral sclerosis in a high selenium environment. JAMA 237:2843–2844, 1977.
120. Norris FH, Kwei Sang U.: Amyotrophic lateral sclerosis and low urinary selenium levels. JAMA 239:404, 1978.
121. Miyata S, Nakamura S, Nagata H, et al.: Increased manganese level in spinal cords

of amyotrophic lateral sclerosis determined by radiochemical neutron activation analysis. J Neurol Sci 61:283–293, 1983.

122. Yoshimasu F, Yasui M, Yase Y, et al.: Studies on amyotrophic lateral sclerosis by neutron activation analysis-3. Systematic analysis of metals on Guamanian ALS and PD cases. Folia Psychiatry Neurol Jpn 36:173–179, 1982.

123. Yase Y, Kumamoto T, Yoshimasu F, et al.: Amyotrophic lateral sclerosis studies using neutron activation analysis. Neurol India 16:46–50, 1968.

124. Yase Y, Yoshimasu F, Yasui M, et al.: Amyotrophic lateral sclerosis—neutron activation analysis on Guamanian ALS and PD cases and their Chamorro controls. Annual Report of the Research Committee of Degenerative Neurologic Diseases. Ministry of Health and Welfare of Japan, 1980, pp. 296–302 (in Japanese).

125. Pierce-Ruhland R, Patten BM: Muscle metals in motor neuron disease. Ann Neurol 8:193–195, 1980.

126. Patten BM, Bilezekian JP, Mallette LE, et al.: Neuromuscular disease in primary hyperparathyroidism. Ann Intern Med 80:182–193, 1974.

127. Mallette LE, Patten BM, Engel WK: Neuromuscular disease in secondary hyperparathyroidism. Ann Intern Med 82:474–483, 1975.

128. Mishra SK, Chandler DB, Desaiah D, et al.: Calmodulin, calcium binding, and calcium adenosine triphosphatase activity of human erythrocytes in amyotrophic lateral sclerosis. Ann Neurol 14:118, 1983.

129. Perl DP, Gadjusek DC, Garruto RM, et al.: Intraneuronal aluminum accumulation in amyotrophic lateral sclerosis and parkinsonism-dementia of Guam. Science 217:1053–1055, 1982.

130. Gajdusek DC, Salazar AM: Amyotrophic lateral sclerosis and parkinsonian syndromes in high incidence among the Auyu and Jakai people of West New Guinea. Neurology 32:107–126, 1982.

131. Yase Y: Amyotrophic lateral sclerosis. Lancet 2:307–318, 1979.

132. Mitchell JD, Harris IA, East BW et al.: Trace elements in cerebrospinal fluid in motor neurone disease. Br Med 288:1791–1792, 1974.

133. Horwich MS, Engel WK, Chauvin PA: Amyotrophic lateral sclerosis sera applied to cultured motor neurons. Arch Neurol 30:332–333, 1974.

134. Lehrich JR, Couture J: Amyotrophic lateral sclerosis sera are not cytotoxic to neuroblastoma cells in tissue culture. Ann Neurol 41:384–385, 1978.

135. Liveson J, Frey H, Bornstein M: The effect of serum from ALS patients on organotypic nerve and muscle tissue cultures. Acta Neuropathol (Berl) 321:127–131, 1975.

136. Askanas V, Marangos PJ, Engel WK: CSF from amyotrophic lateral sclerosis patients applied to motor neurons in culture fails to alter neuron-specific enolase. Neurology 31:1196–1197, 1981.

137. Rowland LP: Peripheral neuropathy, motor neuron disease, or neuronopathy? In: Battistin L, Hashim GA, Lajtha A (eds). Clinical and Biological Aspects of Peripheral Nerve Diseases. Alan R. Liss, New York, 1983, pp. 27–41.

138. den Hartog Jager WA: Experimental amyotrophic lateral sclerosis in the guinea pig. J Neurol Sci 67:133–142, 1985.

CHAPTER EIGHT

ETHICAL ISSUES IN AMYOTROPHIC LATERAL SCLEROSIS

James T. Caroscio, M.D.

Extensive reviews of ethical issues in neurology are available.[1] However, certain issues seem to be stirred up by amyotrophic lateral sclerosis (ALS) and the purpose of this chapter is to touch upon these points.

TELLING PATIENTS THEIR DIAGNOSIS

It seems reasonable to begin a discussion of ethical issues in ALS with the question of whether or not patients should be told their diagnosis.

It is not uncommon for physicians to withhold the diagnosis of ALS from patients, and instead to entrust this information to a family member. At times, such a policy can be defended, especially early on in the disease when the diagnosis is only strongly suspected, or when the physician perceives that the psychological makeup of the patient is such that he is not capable of handling the news at a given point in time.

As time goes by, however, in a disease like ALS whose main symptom, weakness, is readily manifest to the patient, withholding the diagnosis can create an extremely stressful situation. The physician's silence becomes a nonverbal message to the patient that "What you have is so terrible that its name cannot be used in your presence." The family, drawn into "keeping the secret," is perceived by the patient as hiding something (which, indeed, they are) so that psychological stresses are added to physical ones. Additionally, health care workers are handcuffed in providing care because they are faced with the impossible situation of trying to implement a care plan aimed at helping a patient who is ignorant of his disease.

Certainly physicians have moral obligations to their patients to be honest and not to deceive. Physicians can tell patients the truth of their diagnoses, thereby fulfilling their obligation of honesty, without increasing those patients' psychological pain. In fact, personal experience indicates that the opposite is true, and that patients (and family members) are generally visibly relieved at being told the diagnosis. It is comforting to patients that someone knows what they've got and it is a psychological truth that when someone knows what he is confronting he can deal with it. It is fear of the unknown that creates the greatest anxiety.

Our policy has been to tell all patients who are referred to the Mount Sinai Hospital ALS Clinic their diagnosis—of course once we are convinced the diagnosis is correct. Because the Mount Sinai Clinic is a referral center, most of our patients have had symptoms for a long enough time that the news generally comes as a relief. Patients who cannot handle the truth tend not to hear what the physician is saying and thus psychologically defend themselves. In these cases it takes time for patients to come to an acceptance of their diagnosis.

In the individual practice setting, the timing and manner of telling patients their diagnosis requires all of a physician's interpersonal skills. In a disease such as ALS that is relentlessly progressive and has no treatment, a host of negative emotional responses bombard a physician and care has to be taken lest patients pick up on these negative feelings. It is therefore important for the physician to convey the diagnosis to patients in a way that is confident and forthright. It is also possible to be honest and even upbeat with patients, which goes a long way to helping them approach their life with ALS in a positive way. In any disease, no one knows what the course is going to be in any individual patient. The patient is concerned for himself when he goes to a physician seeking a diagnosis, and statistics really need not enter into discussions. The important thing for the patient is what's going to happen to him, and the answer is that no one really knows for sure. This is a source of hope in any serious illness and physicians and patients alike can gain strength from this fact. That is not to say that patients should be deceived or that an unrealistically rosy picture should be painted. This will only undermine the patient's confidence in the physician as time goes by.

The way we handle the problem of telling patients their diagnosis is to present the facts to them as follows:

• We tell patients that they have amyotrophic lateral sclerosis or ALS as it is called for short.

- We stress that we don't know what causes this disease and that at present there is no treatment for it.
- We tell patients that more research is going on than ever before to discover a cure for this disease and certainly there is hope that treatments will be found.
- We stress that generally this disease is progressive (as patients may already know) although some patients do stabilize and recoveries have occurred, though rarely.
- If there is something particularly positive about a patients' course to date, this is emphasized (e.g., slow progression, absence of bulbar symptoms).
- We tell patients' that despite the lack of medication to stop the disease or reverse it, much can be done with symptomatic medications and the input of physical, occupational, and speech therapists to help them with their problems.
- We stress that we are available to help patients and that we want to see them on regular basis.

This approach is honest, and yet instills hope in patients.

One last word on telling patients their diagnosis concerns the tendency of some physicians to quote expected survival times to patients. This practice is to be condemned. As one observer put it, this puts patients in the same league with convicted criminals who are scheduled to be executed. They, after all, are the only ones who actually know when they are going to die.

SHOULD ALS PATIENTS BE TREATED?

The next ethical issue that arises after the diagnosis of ALS has been made is: Should patients be treated? This may seem like a ridiculous question, especially to someone who is reading a volume devoted to the care of the ALS patient, but the medical literature itself contains laments from ALS patients about the unavailability of treatment[2,3] and admissions from physicians on the tendency to abandon patients once the diagnosis of ALS has been made.[4] When the National ALS Foundation made the decision to fund patient care clinics, members of its board of trustees objected, suggesting that there was nothing that could be done for these patients.

That physicians have a responsibility to care for patients with untreatable diseases is as long-standing a cornerstone of the practice of medicine as the code of Maimonides.

Again, the negative emotional responses of avoidance, identification, rejection, inadequacy, frustration, anxiety, feelings of impotence, and loss of control that ALS brings out in physicians have resulted in the common practice of telling patients with ALS, "There is nothing that can be done, go home and prepare to die."

It is the responsibility of the physician, the first link in the chain of caretakers for patients, to become familiar with coping strategies that are helpful in dealing with the negative responses that diseases like ALS bring out. Guidelines for such strategies are available.[5] It is only the physician's open-minded approach to helping patients with symptomatic medications and his readiness to refer patients to nurses, therapists, and social workers that will result in ALS patients receiving every reasonable opportunity to lead as independent and fulfilling a life as possible despite ALS.

Certainly this volume indicates that there is much that can be done to help ALS patients, and that it is ethical and moral to provide care to patients with this disease.

LIFE SUPPORT DECISIONS IN AMYOTROPIC LATERAL SCLEROSIS PATIENTS

The ethical issue of the use of respirators in patients with ALS is often a complicated one. Responsibility in making the decision on the use of a respirator rests with the patient. He alone, not the physician or family, should make the decision and since ALS patients are intact intellectually (in most instances) this takes a great burden from physicians and families.

Responsibility for bringing up the subject lies with the physician, however, and this requires great skill, a sense of timing, and an ability to cope with one's negative responses to this disease. Broaching the subject too early with patients might create undue anxiety, and waiting too long might create a situation where the decision has been postponed until it is too late. Life-or-death decisions like this are best made in rational moments with time to weigh all the consequences. Gert and Culver addressed this issue very well.[6] Either alternative is rationally acceptable (to opt for a life-saving procedure, or to opt for avoiding the discomfort inherent in experiencing the final stages of ALS). The responsibility of the physician is to present the alternatives and their implications as neutrally as possible, so that patients have every opportunity to make their own decision.

Rational decisions are almost impossible in emergency situations. Either there is no opportunity to ask the patient at all or the patient is presented with a choice when he is gasping for breath. In our experience patients tend to opt for life in such situations and if that option is taken without the knowledge of the long-term implications, a truly cruel situation can be created for patients and their families.

Our rule of thumb has been to initiate discussion about life support with patients when they first complain of breathing difficulty. This serves to address their concern over that symptom and yet it is early enough that patients have time to think about their decision. It must be noted that many ALS patients never develop symptomatic breathing difficulty and that oxygenation of the blood remains good even when total disability has occurred. In these individuals discussion of life support should be made, however, since death is usually respiratory.

There has been a tendency in these enlightened times for patients to write living wills. This can be an excellent way of rationally approaching the problem of life support, for it ensures that patient and family have given careful thought to the issue. Caution must be used in making up such wills to stipulate at what point of dysfunction patients would not want life support measures to be employed. The following case provides an example of how living wills can pose problems.

A 42-year-old ambulatory man with ALS had severe dysphagia and dysarthria and moderate arm weakness. He was admitted to the hospital for an elective feeding gastrostomy. He had drawn up a living will requesting that no life support systems be used. One week postop, while still in the hospital, the patient had a respiratory arrest and the nurses called the arrest team. The patient was resuscitated but required a respirator after the incident.

When questioned about the living will, the patient stated he was glad that the nurses had acted as they had because at his level of dysfunction, he certainly was not ready to die.

This case illustrates how living wills must be careful to indicate what the patient feels is the point at which he would forego life support systems. Another point to be made about living wills is that, since they are often drawn up relatively early on in a patient's course, at a time when he has only an abstract idea of what the end-stages of ALS may be like, patients, families, and physicians must keep communication lines open on an ongoing basis over the contents of the will. When the critical moment arrives, patients, faced with the immediate need to opt for life or possible death, may change their minds.

It is the physician's responsibility to be aware of his patient's wishes concerning life support, then, and the extent of this responsibility is underlined by a recent case where a physician has been sued for malpractice for placing an ALS patient on a respirator, when the patient had made it known that he did not want life support measures to be taken.[7]

It must be made clear to patients that once they are placed on respirators, laws are such that as long as there is not a situation of brain death, they cannot be taken off, except under the most extreme circumstances requiring legal intervention and the willing cooperation of physicians and family. The difficulties surrounding this procedure have been detailed recently.[8]

ALTERNATIVE THERAPIES AND AMYOTROPHIC LATERAL SCLEROSIS

Another important issue that confronts physicians caring for patients with progressive incurable diseases such as ALS is how to handle patients' tendencies to seek alternative forms of treatment from faith healers, nutritionists, or even physicians on the fringes of medicine who claim to have something to offer patients (the most prominent example of this was the use of snake venom on ALS patients by physicians in Florida in the 1970s). The tendency when confronted with patients' queries over the unproven therapies might be to say, "Why not try it, I have nothing better to offer." I think this is a dangerous approach for several reasons. First, patients are removed from the mainstream of what medicine does have to offer by way of symptomatic treatment and clinical trials; second, patients are led to physical and financial sacrifice coupled with an inevitable psychological let down. Lastly, great amounts of money and energy are funneled into something that is essentially doomed to failure. No expenditure of energy and money on a treatment is going to yield results unless applied to sound scientific methods.

I think it is the physician's duty to warn patients against seeking out alternate treatment possibilities to prevent waste of financial, physical, and psychological resources. Patients should be encouraged, however, to take part in scientifically controlled clinical trials when feasible. These go a long way toward providing answers as to the efficacy of various treatments in ALS and have the advantage of boosting patients' morale by giving them a sense of contributing to the advancement of medicine.

REFERENCES

1. Bernat JL: Ethical issues in the practice of neurology. Semin Neurol 4:1–116, 1984.
2. Carus R: Motor neurone disease: A demeaning illness. Br Med J 280:455–456, 1980.
3. Anonymous: A man with motor neurone disease. Br Med J 2:40–41, 1971.
4. Fergusson F: Discussion on motor neurone disease. Proc R Soc Med 55:1019–1033, 1961.
5. Gorlin R, Zucker HD: Physicians reactions to patients. N Engl J Med 308:1059–1063, 1983.
6. Gert B, Culver CM: Moral theory in neurologic practice. Semin Neurol 4:9–14, 1984.
7. The New York Times September 18, 1985, p. A-17.
8. The New York Times, December 16, 1984, p. A-1.

CHAPTER NINE

NURSING CARE OF THE PATIENT WITH AMYOTYROPHIC LATERAL SCLEROSIS

Linda Murray, R.N., M.S., and Cynthia F. DeBartolo, R.N., M.S.

This chapter focuses on the care of the ALS patient using the nursing process. Much of the information presented here is the result of the experience of assessing, planning, and coordinating care for hundreds of patients with ALS in an ambulatory care setting. Nursing care in this setting is delivered primarily via teaching, with emphasis on the patient's self-care in an attempt to maintain health and prevent disease.

Amyotrophic lateral sclerosis is a disease that has an insidious onset and fits the criteria for a chronic illness, with problems and complications that are, degenerative, incapacitating, and associated with disuse phenomena. When viewed in this framework, nursing interventions utilized for patients with any chronic disease are both appropriate and necessary for the patient with ALS.

It is not within the scope of this chapter to reiterate basic nursing care principles; instead, we will focus on adaptations of these care plans to patients with ALS. It is hoped that these adaptations may be utilized during changes that may occur as the disease progresses, regardless of whether the care is delivered by the nurse, family members, or others during hospitalization or at home.

ASSESSMENT OF THE AMYOTROPHIC LATERAL SCLEROSIS PATIENT

During the initial visit to the clinic the patient is interviewed and assessed by the nurse for general health status, understanding of ALS, any problems experienced as a result of the ALS (actual and potential), and what is being done to alleviate these problems. These baseline data are used for the initial care plan and later for comparison as the disease progresses. It should be recorded in the chart, in a formalized manner (see Appendix 9–1).

History and Physical Examination

The patient may spent 2 to 3 h during the initial clinic visit being interviewed by members of various disciplines including physical therapy, nursing, occupational therapy (OT), and so forth. This is usually quite tiring for a patient whose presenting symptom is most often weakness. If patients are fatigued and live within a reasonable distance, appointments may need to be rescheduled to allow for evaluations by representatives of all the above disciplines.

A review of the chart for notations by the physician and other medical personnel prior to interview reduces the frustration for the patient caused by repetitive questions. Some of the information needed by the nurse may be obtained if the nurse is present when the neurologist performs a history and physical examination. If the nurse is not present at this time, it is not necessary to repeat the neurologic assessment, since it is essentially used to establish the diagnosis (during the initial visit) or the rate of progression (subsequent visits). Nursing assessments and interventions are most

---

Appendix 9–1. *Amyotrophic Lateral Sclerosis Clinic Nursing Admission Data*

ALL RELEVANT DATA TO BE CIRCLED OR WRITTEN

Date: _____ Doctor: _____ History obtained by: _____ R.N.

From: _____

I. *Physical Assessment*
   Wt.: _____ Ht.: _____ B.P.: _____
   Patient profile: Sex: _____ Age: _____
   Bulbar/spinal Prosthesis/disability: _____

II. *History*
   Reason for admission (cc:) _____
   Past history: Date of onset: _____ Date of dx: _____
   Patient describes ALS as: _____
   Other illnesses: _____
   Allergies: _____
   Clinic/PMD: _____
   Medications: Prescribed: _____

                     OTC: _____

   Substance use/abuse: _____

III. *Activities of Daily Living*
   Self-care deficits: _____
   Sleep pattern: _____

IV. *Social Profile*
   Language: _____ Occupation: _____
   Family/home situation: _____
   Religion: _____

V. Systems Review
   Skin: dry, bruises, abrasions, rash, edema, other: _____
   Chest: pain, palpitations, smoking, cough, sputum,
   last URI: _____, dyspnea on exertion/at rest,
   no. of pillows, resp. aids, exercises, other: _____
   Eyes: glaucoma, cataracts, glasses, contacts, other: _____
   Ears: hearing aid, earache, tinnitus, other: _____
   Nose/throat: difficulty swallowing—liquids/solids,
   gagging, regurgitation, postnasal drip, other: _____
   Mouth: Lips—closure partial/complete, droop R/L side,
   drooling, odor, cracks, dry, other: _____
   Teeth/gums—bleeding, pain, dentures
   Date of last exam: _____ return appt: _____ Other: _____
   Chewing: tires, squirreling, pushes food with finger,
   other: _____
   Tongue: clear, coated, cerrated, weak—R/L, up/down,
   other: _____
   Speech: clear, intelligible, nasal, poor,
   other: _____
   Bowels: no. stools daily: _____, soft/dry, bleeding, hemorrhoids,
   other: _____
   GU: dysuria, frequency, urgency, incontinence, hematuria, nocturia,
   other: _____
   Gyn: Pap smear, date: _____, discharge (describe),
   other: _____

VI. *Nutrition History*
   Appetite: good, fair, poor
   Diet: regular/special

Typical Daily Intake (Please Indicate Exact Amount)*

Meal and Time	Dairy Products	Meat, Fish, Poultry, Eggs	Fruit, Vegetables	Breads, Cereals	Fluids†
Breakfast					
Snack					
Lunch					
Snack					
Dinner					
Snack					
TOTAL					

   *1 teaspoon = 15 cc   Mug = 200 cc
   8-oz (water) glass = 240 cc   Soup bowl = 200 cc
   5-oz (juice) glass = 150 cc   Jello/custard cup = 200 cc
   Cup = 150 cc   Foam cup = 200 cc
   †Fluids include: Jello, custard, ice cream, sherbet, supplements (e.g., Sustacal, Ensure, instant breakfast).

complete when the nurse understands reflex gradings, ratings of cranial nerve function, normal muscle strength, and musculoskeletal range of motion.

Status of the patient's general health may be obtained from standard information. Observations should include height, weight, blood pressure, sex, age, allergies, other illness, and private physicians or clinics attended, including last visits and return appointments. The patient's general appearance, use of prosthetic devices, disabilities, medications, and information on substance abuse are all important data in assessing the patient's patterns of or belief regarding his general health care. It is also important to note whether the patient is able to participate in the interview. Interventions for the patient with ALS vary depending upon the area of involvement. Patients with bulbar involvement, for example, usually require more extensive nursing intervention. This will be discussed in more detail in Intervention, below.

Understanding the Diagnosis

The patient's readiness to learn about the disease is affected by the time of diagnostic confirmation. If diagnosis was made recently, the patient is less likely to be able to absorb information related to the disease. This becomes apparent when the patient is asked to verbalize what the doctor told him about ALS or how he would define ALS. Even if the patient uses the term motor neutron disease, anterior horn cell disease, or Lou Gehrig's disease as the defining statement, the nurse should not assume that the patient actually understands the term, diagnosis, or implications. This may be ascertained if the nurse asks the patient (with the use of a visual aid) to identify the motor neuron or anterior horn cell.

A better indication of the patient's understanding would be a response indicating that the nerves and muscles stop working, die, or degenerate. (Patients may confuse the terminology, symptoms, and treatment of ALS with those of multiple sclerosis.)

At this point in the interview, patients often become uncomfortable and may manifest this by crying, fidgeting in their chairs, avoiding eye contact, tugging at clothing, quoting from their extensive list of reading materials, or simply stating they don't want to discuss the diagnosis. Crying may be related to emotional lability (which is a reflex act of crying or laughing prompted by minimal emotional stimulation. This is a common symptom in patients with bulbar involvement from ALS). It is best at this time to document the patient's reaction and turn to a less provocative subject. When possible during the teaching phase of the intervention, the patient should be offered another opportunity for clarification of the diagnosis. Generally, patients who have some "accurate" information about the disease and its implications appear to accept intervention more readily. Patients appear less anxious by their second or third visit to clinic (3 to 6 months) which suggests that they have sifted through information from previous visits and have selected, accepted, or denied various facts.

Focusing on the chief complaint, self-care deficits or sleep pattern may provide more comfortable topics for discussion while still providing the nurse with the needed information regarding the patient's response to the diagnosis. The above three factors are often interrelated. The availability of help by a family member, home nursing aide, or friend, the frequency of repositioning required, medications used, rest periods, naps, and total numbers of hours slept within 24 h are all areas that must be addressed.

Inquiry as to the patient's occupation is essential because patients who have impaired motor function may have difficulty doing jobs involving use of machinery, climbing, building construction, and so forth. The loss of speech will be problematical for patients with occupations that center around verbal communication.

Spiritual, religious, or philosophical beliefs contribute significantly to the patient's desire for survival. Mitchell states that these "beliefs frequently help give meaning to suffering and illness; they also may be helpful in the acceptance of future incapacities or death. At other times, however, an illness may be interpreted as God's punishment and this feeling increases the patient's discomfort." [1]

Ascertaining what religious denominmation the patient is affiliated with or whether a particular religious preference is followed may allow the patient an opening to verbalize his supports or needs in this area. The nurse may also ask if the patient has shared the diagnosis with clergy or members of his religious group. Members of the patient's religious group are often sources for caregiving during the later stages of the illness.

Since ALS is a progressive disease, it eventually affects almost all muscles and therefore has an effect on many systems of the body—a review of systems will provide the nurse with data that identify areas where problems exist or have the potential to occur.

Patients seen in the early stages of illness with slowly progressive spinal involvement often have few if any complaints. Those with rapid progressive spinal or bulbar involvement may verbalize or exhibit a variety of deficits during the initial interview. It is important to note in each system when no problem is identified.

Skin

The skin should be observed for alterations in integrity even when there is no complaint. Any break in the skin can predispose the patient to additional problems. Patients should be questioned about foot care. Nails of both hands and feet should be inspected. Fissures may develop in joint spaces as hands become contracted. Disorders such as seborrhea, psoriasis, and flaking of the scalp, eyebrows, and lashes as seen in Parkinson's disease may occur. When edema is present, color, pulses, and circumferences of the extremity should be noted as well as degree of pitting. Problems of the skin are associated with other illnesses, immobility, nutrition, and physical care. Information regarding physical activity, range of movement (ROM), fluid intake, frequency of bathing, use of soaps, lotions, history of dermatologic disorders, and therapies should be elicited.

Breathing

The chest history should include information regarding pain, palpitations, smoking, cough, sputum, last upper respiratory infection (URI), frequency of occurrence of URI, dyspnea on exertion or at rest, number of pillows used for sleep, respiratory aids, exercises, or other complaints the patient may express. Patients who have some knowledge of the implications of URI may be reluctant to answer questions related to respiratory function. They may state that they never have any problems with colds or shortness of breath. They may also indicate irritation at this line of questioning. Reassurance is, of course, indicated and is easily handled by reiterating that these are questions asked of every patient.

Sensation

There is no alteration of sensory function in ALS. Any complaints relating to the senses should be documented in the nursing assessment and reported to the physician for further evaluation.

Swallowing

It is particularly important to determine the patient's ability to smell, taste, and touch as part of the dysphagia assessment. Frequency of gagging, choking, regurgitation, and or coughing should be ascertained. Observe and question the patient regarding hyperextension of the head and neck because this increases problems with swallowing. Postnasal drip and drooling are two frequent complaints of dysphagic patients. Medications taken to control this problem can cause excessive mouth dryness and thickened secretions. The combination of weakened facial muscles, drooling thickened secretions, and poor dental hygiene may result in halitosis. Determine measures used to control the problem along with the date of last dental appointment.

Speech

Change in speech may be very subtle. Determine whether the patient has noticed a change in his speech or its volume. If a change was noticed, ask whether this was discussed with the neurologist and if a referral was made for speech therapy. If therapy has been initiated, discuss what it involves as well as the patient's expectations.

Nutrition

Potter states that: "Nutritional assessment, an integral part of patient care, is essential to developing an effective care plan."[2] The nutritional history should include typical daily intake with very specific amounts, for each meal and snack(s) noted. Appetite, special diets, time required to complete a meal, size of portions, fluid intake weight, and other factors affecting nutritional status such as physical limitations, financial situation, and environment must also be evaluated.

Sphincter Control

Amyotrophic lateral sclerosis does not impair bowel and bladder sphincter muscles. Alteration in these systems may occur as a result of immobility and poor dietary intake. Assessment of bowel function should include frequency and character of stool and remedies used. Evaluation of urinary tract function should include assessment of frequency, pain on urination, and inquiries as to the presence of incontinence and nocturia.

Sexuality

Gynecologic assessment should include date of last examination and Pap smear and any current problems.

Questions related to sexual function are less intimidating when they are incorporated as part of the genitourinary assessment. Amyotrophic lateral sclerosis does not impair sexual response. If problems are uncovered, the nurse must determine if they were present prior to the diagnosis of ALS and if treatment was sought from other sources. It is important to consider that "anything that affects strength and general well being can influence sexual interest and activity (e.g., poor nutrition, anemia, insomnia, poor physical conditioning)."[3]

INTERVENTION

Adaptation to the changes and losses in function that accompany ALS is difficult. The nurse must assist the patient and those caring for the patient to identify activities that encourage adjustment to these losses while enabling the patient to maintain a sense of control.

Most patients exhibit at least one and as many as six (or more) problems (actual and/or potential) requiring nursing diagnosis intervention during the initial clinic visit. The nursing diagnoses listed in Table 9–1 are common to patients with ALS. While some are more commonly seen with patients who have bulbar involvement, they can also be present when patients with spinal involvement are severely immobile. The plan and intervention tend to have a different focus depending on the presence of absence of bulbar symptoms.

Standard teaching plans can be utilized but must be individualized for each patient. Consideration must be given to the various principles of adult learning. Readiness to learn is most impaired during the initial clinic visit. The patient may not be able to hear anything other than information

Table 9–1. Nursing Diagnoses Common to Amyotrophic Lateral Sclerosis Patients

Knowledge deficit regarding disease process
Impaired breathing pattern*
Alteration in nutrition*
Impaired communication*
Alteration in elimination*
Inadequate oral hygiene*
Impaired skin integrity
Alteration in comfort: fatigue, pain
Impaired sleep pattern
Ineffective coping
Spiritual distress
Health management deficit
Self-care deficits
Body image disturbance
Impaired sexual function

*Prominent in patients with bulbar involvement.

about the diagnosis. Therefore plans for potential problems are generally not made at that time. Sensitivity on the part of the nurse will pick up cues related to readiness to learn.

While the nurse plans care for patients with bulbar and spinal involvement, priority is most often given to those patients who have bulbar involvement. These patients experience problems that are life threatening (respiratory, nutritional, communication) in nature and they must be prepared to cope with them at home. Patients with spinal involvement, particularly primary lateral sclerosis, experience a slower progression of disease with less-threatening symptoms in the early stages.

Acceptance of intervention is dependent on the patients having a clear understanding of the disease process and its consequences. Resources such as literature handouts and visual aids that illustrate the affected areas of the nervous system help to accomplish this.

Explanation of the roles of clinic staff and the need for return appointments related to further evaluation of disease progression are usually comfortable topics for discussion. In addition, this provides an opportunity for patients to identify what their needs may be and which members of the clinic staff will be able to assist them.

Breathing

Upper respiratory infection is a major cause of hospitalization for patients with ALS. It is usually associated with immobility and/or aspiration of food or secretions. Concerns regarding breathing problems account for over 20% of all telephone calls to clinic that require nursing intervention.

Patients who present with impaired breathing pattern require the following:

1. Measures and techniques to prevent URI
2. Signs and symptoms of URI
3. Use and precautions of oxygen
4. Use and side effects of prescribed medications
5. Consultation for the use of over-the-counter drugs (these may suppress cough reflex)
6. Deep breathing and coughing exercise
7. Counseling regarding use of assistive devices such as intermittent positive-pressure breathing (IPPB) devices, nebulizers, and ventilators, and discussion of tracheostomy

In addition, the nurse must collaborate with other health care services, such as respiratory therapy, physical therapy, psychiatric nursing, social services, visiting nurse service (VNS), equipment vending, and so on.

During the early stages of the disease, deep breathing and coughing may be sufficient to raise secretions to the oral pharyngeal level. When patients are unable to expectorate, suctioning of the oral–pharyngeal area is indicated. The use of the Yankauer suction tip is appropriate and cost effective for suctioning the oral cavity. A soft whistle-tip catheter should always be used to suction the pharyngeal area or trachea.

The use of visual aids and diagrams of the anatomic structures is helpful when teaching patients about airway maintenance and describing physiologic changes necessitating tracheostomy and ventilatory assistance.

Tracheostomy is done when trachial–bronchial secretions become unmanageable causing increased potential for aspiration, or to facilitate ventilation when respiratory failure seems imminent.

The necessity for the use of assistive breathing devices is always regarded as a major loss by the patient. Intervention of the psychiatric nurse clinician and/or social worker becomes crucial at this juncture. Each team member must know what is being discussed with the patient regarding the use of assistive devices and tracheostomy. Patients and family members often ask representatives of various disciplines for advice. Patient and family may become confused and overwhelmed if too many options are presented.

It is suggested that the following be incorporated into the discharge teaching for tracheostomy home care: utilization of the clean technique (nonsterile) with emphasis on handwashing prior to care and keeping equipment clean. Other considerations include:

Participation of the patient and family
Care of the skin around the tube (stoma)
Care of inner cannula
Suction technique
Change of the tracheostomy tube initiated only upon authorization of the physician (some patients with ALS have this done at an ear, nose, and throat (ENT) outpatient facility or by a surgeon)
Humidification
Resuming daily activities
Supplies needed for home care

Families must also be prepared to operate the ventilator and know what action to take should the ventilator fail. Some patients have a standby ventilator at home as well as an ambu-bag should this situation occur.

Nutrition

Approximately 45 to 55% of all telephone calls to the clinic are related to change in appetite, decrease in ability to swallow, related medication, or problems of elimination. A large part of the nurse–patient interaction is spent teaching the patient and family how to manage dysphagia when bulbar involvement is present (Table 9–2). It is important that patients be knowledgeable about the physiology of swallowing and the ana-

Table 9–2. Nutrition Teaching Plan in Amyotrophic Lateral Sclerosis

Goal: To promote optimal nutrition and hydration and prevent aspiration.

Objectives: At the completion of the session the patient and the significant other(s) will:
1. Discuss the prescribed diet identifying the appropriate size of servings/portions.
2. Discuss nerve and muscle activity, stages of normal chewing and swallowing versus ALS impairment relevant to the clients' involvement.
3. Identify considerations for preparation and ingestion of the diet/medications.
4. Identify signs and symptoms of airway obstruction, emergency actions, and need for suctioning.
5. Discuss alternative methods of nutrition.

Diet
1. High-protein (100–200 g), high-calorie (2,000–3,000 calories)
2. Four basic food groups, plus snacks/supplemental feedings
3. 2 quarts of fluids daily
4. Considerations of other medical problems (e.g., diabetes, low-sodium diet, and so on)
5. Temperature—warmer than room or ice-cold
6. Texture—coarse or chunky solids, semisolids, thick liquids
7. Taste—sweet or sour increases saliva, bitter and salty increases desire for fluids

Nerves and muscles
1. Muscles involved in the act of chewing and swallowing include those of the lips, lower jaw, face, tongue, pharynx, larynx, and cricopharyngeal area.
2. These muscles are stimulated by five cranial nerves.
3. When ALS is present:
   a. Lips—incomplete closure causes drooling.
   b. Jaw and face—weakness and stiffness occurs, causing difficulty chewing.
   c. Tongue—weakness and/or atrophy causes inability to move food back into the pharyngeal area.
   d. Pharyngeal constrictors—weakness causes coughing, gagging, nasal regurgitation.
4. Heartburn and/or wet burp may occur when the muscle of the diaphragm is weak.

Meals and medications
1. Equipment—adaptive utensils, use of blenders, and so on.
2. Environment—comfortable, nondistracting, unhurried.
3. Hygiene—clear oral secretions, clean mouth before and after meals. The patient and/or caregiver should observe handwashing techniques before actual feeding begins.
4. Position—45 to 90 degree angle should be maintained.
5. Medications—for example, atropine, should be taken ½ h before meals to decrease saliva and facilitate swallowing.
6. Ingesting—concentrate on the act of swallowing, placement of teeth, tongue, and food, and breath control.
7. Precautions—do not eat alone; do not laugh or talk with food in the mouth; clear the throat before each swallow; do not hyperextend the neck; know the Heimlich maneuver; avoid thin liquids, sticky and starchy foods, chocolate, and nuts; remain upright ½ h after eating.

Table 9–2. **Nutrition Teaching Plan in Amyotrophic Lateral Sclerosis** (*cont.*)

Airway obstruction
1. Complete—occurs if there is an inability to speak, cough, or breathe, when food is stuck in the throat, indicating a need for the Heimlich maneuver.
2. Partial—occurs if there is a weak, ineffective cough, high-pitched or crowing noise while inhaling. Usually this may be alleviated or cleared through the normal cough reflex or change in position.

Suctioning
1. Necessary when there is inability to expel excessive secretions from the mouth and nasopharynx, particularly before meals.
2. Respiratory infections can occur and should be recognized and reported if a change in color, odor, quantity, or thickness of secretions, or fever is present.

Alternative methods of feeding
1. Indications—unable to maintain adequate caloric intake, or meals take inordinate time with frequent choking.
2. Instruct in various surgical procedures, length of hospital stay, and so forth.

tomic structures involved. Positioning, imagery, and concentration techniques are used when the nurse teaches techniques of swallowing. Nurse intervention for dysphagia includes instruction regarding:

Airway maintenance including oral hygiene
Heimlich manuever
Nutritional requirements and recommendations for food preparation
Medications for control of secretions
Use of assistive devices
Maintenance of bowel and bladder function

Counseling regarding alternative methods of feeding begins when moderate involvement becomes severe, choking occurs with each meal, 1 h or more is required per meal, and there is a 10% loss of body weight. The ultimate decision for choosing alternative methods of feeding rests with the patient. Sucking and swallowing are reflexes present in utero. Eating provides us with our earliest form of gratification. It is thus apparent that the need for an alternative method of feeding presents as a major loss. Alternative methods are often refused even though the patient is aware of the risks of aspiration, dehydration, and severe malnutrition. Patients unfortunately may become so debilitated before they consent to surgery that full benefit of such intervention is not always realized. Impending surgery requires extensive preparation and reassurance. Information overload can occur and may result in anxiety. Preoperative teaching should include:

Method of surgical intervention to be performed (i.e., gastrostomy, esophagostomy, jejeunostomy)
Length of hospital stay
Normal postoperative course

Complications associated with surgery
Coughing and deep breathing exercises
If patient expresses an interest, discussion of feeding formulas may also be addressed

The most frequently asked question during counseling is whether eating and drinking can continue after surgery. While some practitioners may allow the patient to continue to take small amounts of food substances orally it must be remembered that aspiration can occur even with very small quantities. Patients may be satisfied by tasting favorite foods or flavors without swallowing. Many patients indicate that they are not hungry or lose their desire for eating after they have stabilized following gastrostomy.

Electrical feeding pumps are sometimes utilized to regulate gastrostomy feeding. Because this requires that the patient remain stationary to complete the feeding and this may result in the complications of immobility, such pumps should be avoided.

Patients may express concern about bathing because of the gastrostomy opening. Submerging for tub baths is prohibited. A hand-controlled shower head may be used, and water should be directed around the stoma but not at the opening. The stoma and tube may be placed in a plastic bag and padded securely to prevent seepage. Care of the skin and stoma must be taught to the patient prior to hospital discharge.

Nutritional intake may also be altered as patients with spinal involvement become increasingly dependent or immobile. Weakness of the head and neck, trunk, shoulders, arms, or hands may prevent patients from preparing foods or feeding themselves. Another concern may be weight gain associated with sedentary activity levels. Decrease in activity level and nutrition can result in problems with bowel and bladder function, skin integrity, and fluid and electrolyte balance. Muscle spascity may affect the patient's ability to chew and perform adequate oral hygiene. Pain associated with spasticity will alter the patient's level of comfort. These problems will be reviewed separately since they impact on the nutritional status of the patient with spinal involvement.

Speech

If communication is impaired the nurse must assure that the patient is evaluated by speech and occupational therapy. The patient and family must be informed that referral is made to maximize remaining speech function and to establish alternate methods of communication and not to restore speech loss. Exercises prescribed by the speech pathologist may be abandoned by the patient as speech deteriorates. The patient should be encouraged to continue these exercises since they facilitate swallowing.

Sphincter Control

Sphincters of the bowel and bladder are not affected in ALS. Dysfunction and successful intervention are dependent upon dietary intake, medications, mobility and the availability of assistance.

Schaupner indicates that, "function of these two systems must be maintained to prevent serious or life threatening complications such as bowel impaction or paralytic ileus, or complications of the urinary tract such as UTI, renal calculi or hydronephrosis which leads to renal damage."[4] While these more serious complications rarely occur in patients with ALS, constipation, impaction, and sympotoms of UTI are common complaints as the disease progresses.

Bowel function takes place by a series of reflex and sphincter actions. It is also dependent upon the response or work of the diaphragm and abdominal muscles that are weakened by ALS. The patient may have a chronic history of bowel dysfunction, usually constipation. Table 9–3 shows the interventions that are effective for alleviating constipation, contrasted with reasons these may not be effective with ALS patients.

Table 9–3. Intervention Usually Recommended to Alleviate Constipation May Not Work for Patients with Amyotrophic Lateral Sclerosis

Usual Interventions	ALS	Altered Treatment for ALS
Rest 6 h/night	Restless—spasms—insomnia	Reduce anxiety Back massage Warm milk Diversional, quiet activity
Exercises	Often sedentary Decreased ambulation—WCB	Passive ROM Suppositories Enemas—Fleet or tap water

8–10 glasses liquid daily
Fiber
	Dysphagia
	Poor appetite
	Medication to reduce
	  secretions, decreased
	  fluid reabsorption
		Thick liquids
		Prune juice
		Chopped or blenderized
		  fruits and vegetables

Fat-containing foods	Mucus producing
	Increasing complaints of
	  dysphagia
		Cooked fats, for example,
		  boiled milk products
		Stewed or blenderized foods
		Colace tablets or liquid

Abbreviations: WCB, Wheel Chair Bound; other abbreviations as in text.

The availability of a caregiver to help with transfer to and from the commode may be a major factor or deterrant in normal bowel function. The urge for stooling may be lost if the rsponse to stimulation is delayed. Bowel evacuation should take place every 2 to 3 days. If a longer time elapses and symptoms of impaction are present, manual disimpaction or high colonic enemas may be necessary. The physician must be consulted before such intervention is undertaken.

Patients should be cautioned about the use of bulk laxatives and mineral oil if dysphagia is a problem because they can be aspirated. Mineral oil also interferes with the absorption of vitamins A, D, E, and K.

The urinary bladder is stimulated to empty when it contains 200 to 500 ml of urine. The patient with ALS may have a decreased urge to urinate as a result of inadequate fluid intake due to dysphagia or self-imposed fluid limitation related to fear of incontinence. Both of the above can result in urinary tract infection (UTI).

The use of Elavil, atropine, and baclofen also contribute to a change in the bladder emptying. Elavil and atropine cause urinary retention. The patient must be taught the Credé maneuver and encouraged to sit longer to encourage bladder emptying. Baclofen causes urinary frequency. Nocturnal frequency can be decreased by eliminating the amount of fluids taken during the evening hours.

Cleanliness is essential to prevent skin irritations in the perineal area. The area should be cleansed twice per day with soap and water and dried thoroughly. Minor irritations can be treated with application of ointments used to treat diaper rash. Exposure of the area to air is also helpful. Females will need more assistance with toileting if hand impairment and immobility are problems. It is recommended that females establish a regimen where by they void every 3 to 4 h to prevent accidental incontinence and UTI. Cleanliness is an important consideration when the external catheter is used for males. The shaft of the penis and the area of the foreskin can become irritated easily and should be checked daily.

Oral Hygiene

Inadequate oral hygine is very frequently a problem for patients with dysphagia. Unfortunately, this is often an area that is given low priority and as a result, infections of the gums, tongue, and tooth decay develop. To prevent problems from occurring, the mouth and teeth should be cleansed after each meal and at bedtime. An electric toothbrush or Water Pik is helpful for patients who tire easily, or have impaired mobility or bleeding gums.

The tongue may be brushed with a soft toothbrush or washcloth soaked in half-strength water and peroxide if crusted or coated with thick mucus. If gagging is a problem, a device called a tongue cleaner can be purchased in most health food stores. It should be dipped in warm water or mouth wash, pressed down lightly on the tongue, and pulled from back to front. This motion scrapes the debris from the tongue surface. Patients who use the device report very little gagging.

The use of mouthwash, lemon glycerin swabs, candy, or chewing gum increases salivation thus reducing dry mouth.

Drooling or sialorrhea is caused by a swallowing deficit. The patient must be instructed to swallow frequently to clear the mouth of secretions. If the patient has difficulty, secretions should be wiped away with a tissue or cloth towel. A bib may be worn but should be changed and washed often since odors develop. Skin areas exposed to secretions should be washed several times a day with soap and water and a protective skin ointment applied. Vaseline or lip gloss may be applied to the lips to prevent or treat fissures.

Halitosis always accompanies inadequate oral hygiene. It can be embarrassing for the patient and offensive to caregivers. Careful oral hygiene, adequate fluid intake, and use of over-the-counter mouth fresheners help to alleviate this problem. In addition, patients should have regularly scheduled dental checkups to clean the teeth and gums and treat problem early.

Skin

Proper care of the skin can prevent skin breakdown. Daily bathing can be very tiring for the ALS patient. A schedule of bathing should be established which meets the basic hygiene needs while not causing over-exhaustion.

The skin of the ALS patient may be quite fragile depending on his age and nutritional status. The following are suggestions for the care of fragile skin:

- Water temperature must be moderate.
- The use of cold cream lotion or oil-based soaps prevents excessive dryness.
- Baby lotion may be substituted for soap to promote friction when bathing.
- Rinsing the skin with clear water removes debris and prevents dryness.
- Massaging with oils or lotions also prevents dryness.
- One hundred percent cotton clothing helps to absorb perspiration.
- Reposition the patient every 2 h and inspect areas for redness.
- Use cotton-covered foam rubber padding generously to prevent pressure over bony prominences.

- Encourage the intake of high-protein, high-calorie foods.
- Itchy rash may be relieved by the application of powder, corn starch, or calamine lotion.

Note: Persistent rash or itching with flaking scales or patches is usually associated with seborrhea or psoriasis and the patient should be referred to a dermatologist for care.

The feet and ankles are particularly vulnerable to skin breakdown due to pressure and dependent edema. Elevation, ROM, use of elastic stockings, and good hygiene can help prevent complications.

Decubiti, once thought to be uncommon is ALS because sensory function remains intact, can occur in patients who have a mobility impairment along with nutrition and speech deficits. Decubiti can be cared for with traditional methods but most importantly, repositioning is essential.

Pain

Painful joints and spastic muscles are the most common pain complaints of ALS patients. Baclofen (Lioresal) and/or Motrin are sometimes prescribed along with heat or cold packs.

Alteration in comfort can also be related to anxiety, depression, body image disturbance, family stress, sleep pattern disturbance, or a variety of other factors. These are most often managed by counseling with the psychiatric nurse clinician or social worker along with medications such as Elavil, Tofranil or Mellaril. Table 9–4 illustrates the commonly prescribed medications and details instructions for their administration.

Sex

The affect of gentle massage or touch can not be overemphasized for the promotion of comfort. The use of gentle touch, cuddling, and stroking is helpful in reducing tension. Patients may associate sexual dysfunction with fatigue, pain, or difficulty with positioning as the disease progresses. Techniques for sexual intercourse taught to patients with chronic obstructive pulmonary disease (COPD), cardiac disease, paralysis, or ostomy may be offered as alternatives. However, problems of sexual dysfunction are quite complex. As in other chronic illnesses, either patient or partner may fear inflicting injury on the patient, and may fail to complete the sexual act or feel repulsion toward a body that has become weak and atrophied. When considering adaptations for sexual intercourse for ostomy patients, Simmons indicates that the sexual act may become ''ex-

Table 9–4. Medications Frequently Used for Amyotrophic Lateral Sclerosis

Drug	Dose and Use	Patient Instructions
Atropine	Reduces saliva 0.4 mg po ½ h before meals and hs	Notify MD Chest pain, palpitations, dizziness, headaches, blurred vision, flushed, dry skin · Dry mouth and thirst alleviated with mouth care and increased fluids · If a dose is forgotten, take the missed dose as soon as it is remembered but don't take a double dose at one time.
Baclofen	Relieves spasticity. Available in 10-mg tablets. 5 mg is given tid and increased Q3days until therapeutic dosage is attained—not to exceed 80 mg daily.	Notify MD Chest pain, palpitations, blurred vision, vomiting · If weakness or increase in mobility occurs as the dosage is increased, go back to previous dosage and continue to take it. · If a dose is forgotten, take the missed dose as soon as it is remembered but don't take a double dose at one time. · Never stop taking baclofen without directions from the doctor. Sudden stoppage can cause hallucinations. · Baclofen can cause drowsiness, confusion, headache, nausea, urinary frequency. · Do not drink moderate to large amounts of alcohol.
Colace	Stool softener Capsule 100 mg (docysate sodium) 1 qd—1 tid Syrup—60 mg	Notify MD Nausea, diarrhea, persistent constipation (more than 5 days)
Peri-Colace	Capsule 100 mg with 300-mg casanthronal capsule Syrup 60 mg with 30 mg/15 ml	
Ducolax	Promote bowel elimination po 10 mg—15 mg in P.M. or before breakfast. Suppository—one 20 min after breakfast.	Notify MD Severe cramps, vomiting, diarrhea · Patient may experience nausea, abdominal cramps, laxative dependency · GI irritations may occur. If tablets are taken as crushed preparation to facilitate swallowing, milk or antacids should not be given. · Medication starts to work 6–12 h after it is taken. · Suppositories start to work 15 m–1 h after administered.
Elavil	Antidepressant Reduces saliva, induces sleep. 25–75 mg po hs or one tablet tid.	Notify MD for Bruises, bleeding, nausea, SOB, palpitations, dizziness, difficulty urinating

Table 9–4. *(cont)*

		• It may take several days or 2 weeks before Elavil works. Continue to take even though you feel you don't need it. • If a dose is forgotten, take the dose as soon as it is remembered but don't take a double dose at one time. If a once-a-day bedtime dose is missed, don't take it in the morning, but do continue the regular bedtime dose. • Do not drink moderate to large amounts of alcohol. • Contraindicated in narrow-angle glaucoma, seizures, CUD, liver disease, if the patient is receiving thyroid medicines.
Pro-Banthine	Reduces secretions 15 mg po ½ h before meals, tid	Notify MD Palpitations, dizziness, nausea, photophobia, impotence • Contraindicated in narrow-angle glaucoma, myasthenia gravis, CUD, hypertension, hiatal hernia, ulcerative colitis. • Vital signs and urinary function should be routinely monitored.
Quinine	Relief of cramps 4–8 oz quinine in water two to three times daily Tablets: 260 mg, one BID	Notify MD Bruises, bleeding, blurred vision, confusion, headaches, nausea • Contraindicated for patients with CVD • Take after meals to decrease GI disturbances.
Tofranil (imipramine)	Antidepressant Reduces saliva 25–75 mg po hs	Notify MD Bruises, bleeding, nausea, loss of appetite, palpitations, dizziness, difficulty urinating • Less likely to cause respiratory distress than other antidepressant drugs. • Same as Elavil.

Source: Wagner M (ed): Drugs—Nurse's Reference Library Series, Nursing 82 Books. Intermed Communications, Springhouse, PA, 1982.
Abbreviations: CVD, cardiovascular disease; GI, gastrointestinal; SOB, shortness of breath.

tra work for an already overburdened spouse.''[5] She also suggests that ''emotional intimacy and closeness are far more important than sexual performance.''[5] Patients with sexual dysfunction should be referred for or encouraged to seek counseling.

Promoting emotional comfort when spiritual distress is identified is a sensitive issue. As health care providers we must be careful not to interject our own bias into the spiritual needs of our patients. Resources should be identified to assist the patient in coping.

EVALUATION AND FOLLOW-UP EVALUATION

Patients are reevaluated by the nurse on each 3-month return visit to clinic or every 6 to 8 weeks in the more advanced stages. Telephone contact is encouraged and utilized by both patient and nurse to clarify questions and alter interventions appropriately.

Patients with ALS may become so engrossed with daily survival that they loose sight of their susceptibility to various health problems that affect the general population. As a result their basic health care can be compromised. Counseling patients to obtain and maintain contact with a medical internist for general checkups is essential to comprehensive care planning. Treatment regimes established for other illnesses that the patient may have should be reviewed by the nurse and reinforced appropriately.

Coordinating care is a major nursing responsibility in the care of the ALS patient. Any given problem may require collaboration with the ALS clinic physician (neurologist, psychiatrist, physiatrist), local medical doctor, psychiatric nurse clinician, social work counselor, therapist (occupational, physical, speech), community health or visiting nurse, equipment supply agency, specialty clinic or physician [dermatologist, genitourinary (GU) specialist, dentist, ophthalmologist, ENT specialist, and so on].

The local VNS is a particularly vital link in the coordination of health care. Visiting nurses provide the essential service of visiting the patient at home for evaluation and monitoring of disease progression as well as giving the patient emotional counseling and support when travel to the clinic becomes difficult. Other services the VNS may be requested to provide include: evaluation of home care in terms of safety, assistance in placement of home health aids, teaching of various regimes, or monitoring the use of oxygen and the patient's respiratory status. In addition, the VNS serves as an excellent resource for placing or referring various therapists and social workers as well as medical internists.

Research drugs are frequently sought after by patients as they offer the hope for survival that standard interventions lack. The nurse is also responsible for coordinating the educational component of the drug research protocols.

Amyotrophic lateral sclerosis patients are generally admitted to the hospital for diagnostic confirmation, acute episodes of URI (in sequence: conservatively treated early stage, then elective tracheostomy, and finally later stage), bowel obstruction, or surgical intervention for alternative methods of feeding. The patient will most likely also have one or more of the problems listed in Assessment of the Amyotrophic Lateral Sclerosis Patient, above. The focus of the hospital care plan is on direct patient care while the clinic care plan prior to admission or after discharge is on teaching or indirect care as seen in Table 9–2.

True discharge planning usually begins as the acute episode subsides and the patient stabilizes. Hickey and McKenna refer to this as the "active coolaborative phase."[6] The team approach will probably produce the most comprehensive discharge plan. This approach must, however, be coordinated by one person. This role has been filled by the nurse (either the staff nurse or home care nurse coordinator) or the social worker. The patient and family must be included in all phases of planning and may be considered members of the team. Other team members include: nurse, physician, therapist, social worker, nutritionist, and community agency representatives (health agencies and equipment suppliers).

A copy of the plan should be given to the patient to serve as written instructions or as a reminder. A copy should also be forwarded to the appropriate community agency involved in follow-up care. It is important to keep in mind that the ultimate goal of discharge planning is continuity of care as the patient makes the transition from the hospital to his home and community.

In summary, we have outlined the management of the ALS patient in the ambulatory care setting, stressing the role played by the nursing process. This approach was selected because ALS patients are primarily cared for in their home and community. While no cure for ALS exists currently, the nursing process provides a framework in which the ALS patient can be cared for holistically.

REFERENCES

1. Mitchell P: Concepts Basic to Nursing. McGraw-Hill, New York, 1977, pp. 201–202.
2. Potter D (ed): Assessment—Nurse's Reference Library Series, Nursing 82 Books. Intermed Communications, Springhouse, PA, 1982, p. 135.
3. Lyons, A, Brockmeir M: Sex and ileostomy and colostomy. Med Aspects Hum Sex 107–108, 1975.
4. Shaupner C: Teaching Neurologically Impaired Individuals Bowel and Bladder Management. In Van Meter M (ed), Neurologic Care: A Guide for Patient Education. Appleton-Century-Crofts, New York, 1982, p. 45.
5. Simmons K, Sexuality and the female ostomate. Am J Nurs 83(3):409–411, 1983.
6. Hickey J, McKenna J: Effective discharge planning and the neurosurgical nurse. J Neurosurg Nurs 16(2):101–107, 1984.

BIBLIOGRAPHY

Blount M, Bratton C, Luttrell N, Management of the patient with ALS. Nurs Clin N Am 14(1):157–171, 1979.
Fish S, Shelly T: Spiritual Care—The Nurse's Role. Inter-Varsity Press, Downers Grove, Ill. 1983.
Gordon M: Manual of Nursing Diagnosis. McGraw-Hill, New York, 1982.

Hickey J, McKenna T: Effective discharge planning and the neurosurgical nurse. J Neurosurg Nurs 16, (2):101–107, 1984.

Lenox A: When motor neurons die. Am J Nurs 81(4):540–546, 1981.

LouStau A, Lee KA: Dealing with the dangers of dysphagia. Nursing 15(2):47–50, 1985.

Lyons R, Brockmeir M: Sex and ileostomy and colostomy. Med Aspects Hum Sex 9:107–108, 1975.

Lyons R, Yuska C: Tracheostomy Care—Home Care Handbook. Shiley.

Mitchell P: Concepts Basic To Nursing. McGrwa-Hill, New York, 1977.

Montague A: Touching: The Human Significance of the Skin. Harper & Row, New York, 1978.

Pallett P, O'Brien M: Textbook of Neurological Nursing. Little, Brown, Boston, 1985.

Potter D (ed): Assessment—Nurse's Reference Library Series, Nursing 82 Books. Intermed Communications, Springhouse, PA, 1982.

Simmons K: Sexuality and the female ostomate. Am J Nurs 83(3):409–411, 1983.

Snyder M, Jackie M: Neurologic Problems—A Critical Care Nursing Focus. Robert J. Brady, Inc., Bowie, MD, 1981.

Van Meter M: Neurologic Care: A Guide for Patient Education. Appleton-Century-Crofts, New York, 1982.

Wagner M (ed): Drugs—Nurse's Reference Library Series, Nursing 82 Books. Intermed Communications, Springhouse, PA, 1982.

CHAPTER TEN

NUTRITIONAL MANAGEMENT OF DYSPHAGIA

Linda A. Slowie, M.S.R.D.

The process of eating involves salivation, chewing, and swallowing. The setting into motion of these activities appears to be organized in the brain stem. The act of swallowing requires many muscles, bones, and cartilages to move in a coordinated manner (Fig. 10–1). The purpose of this chapter is to discuss the nutritional treatment and management of swallowing problems encountered in patients with amyotrophic lateral sclerosis (ALS). Characteristic of this disease is the selective degeneration of motor nerve cells of the central nervous system. Damage to specific cranial nerves causes progressive bulbar dysfunction which results in weakness or paralysis of the muscles controlling swallowing.

Most often, dysphagia, or difficulty in swallowing is described by the patient as a sensation of food sticking somewhere en route to the stomach. The problem may vary widely due to the particular phase of deglutition affected.[24] In order to provide nutritional treatment to patients with dysphagia, an understanding of both normal and diseased pathophysiology of swallowing is required.

PHYSIOLOGY

Deglutition consists of three distinct phases: oral, pharyngeal, and esophageal (Figs. 10–2 through 10–7). These phases are detailed in Table 10–1.[1,2] A swallow is initiated by the tongue and soft palate. A food bolus is directed away from the larynx through coordinated action of the epiglottis, hyoid bone, and suprahyoid musculature function. The superior, middle, and inferior pharyngeal constrictors together with the cricopharyngeus work to progress the movement of the food bolus. The entry of food from the pharynx into the esophagus is controlled by the cricopharyngeus. The progression of the food bolus in the esophagus is controlled by the intrinsic esophageal musculature. As the food bolus

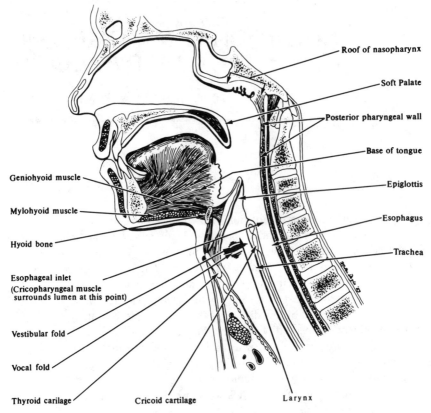

Geniohyoid muscle

Mylohyoid muscle

Hyoid bone

Esophageal inlet
(Cricopharyngeal muscle
surrounds lumen at this point)

Vestibular fold

Vocal fold

Thyroid carilage   Cricoid cartilage   Larynx

Roof of nasopharynx

Soft Palate

Posterior pharyngeal wall

Base of tongue

Epiglottis

Esophagus

Trachea

Figure 10–1. Physiology involved in swallowing (see Table 10–1).

reaches the gastroesophageal junction, the lower esophageal sphincter (LES) relaxes, and the bolus passes into the stomach.[3]

INNERVATION

Innervation of the swallowing mechanism is summarized in Table 10–2. More detailed descriptions can be found elsewhere.[3–5]

Contraction and relaxation, however, both may be controlled by sympathetic innervation to the cricopharyngeus or the vagal branches.[6] The nucleus ambiguous, the primary motor nucleus of vagus, is probably responsible for most of the innervation to the pharyngeal plexus.[7]

Table 10–1. Phases of Deglutition

Oral phase	Jaws close and lips come together. Mastication requires jaw and teeth contact and rotation; tongue lateralization and elevation. Initiation of a swallow requires elevation of tongue tip to alveolar ridge, followed by entire elevation of tongue to hard palate with a slight elevation of larynx.
Pharyngeal phase	A reflex act propels the bolus from the oral cavity into the pharynx. The soft palate moves posteriorly and upwardly to posterior pharyngeal wall. The lateral pharyngeal walls constrict and elevation of tongue effects a tilting of the epiglottis posteriorly toward the laryngeal opening. Simultaneous elevation and forward movement of larynx protects the airway. Laryngeal elevation results in the epiglottis being drawn downward. As a consequence, laryngeal opening closes and food is directed properly. To prevent aspiration, vocal folds close. The cricopharyngeal sphincter relaxes, and the bolus of food is plunged into the esophagus.
Esophageal phase	Contractions of cricopharyngus initiates esophageal peristalsis. The bolus of food is carried to the gastroesophageal junction and the lower esophageal sphincter relaxes.

Source: Dobie RA: Rehabilitation of swallowing disorders. Am Fam Phys 17:5, 1978; Shepherd RS: Human Physiology. Philadelphia, Lippincott, 1971, pp. 412–414.

Table 10–2. Cranial Nerves Involved in Eating Mechanics

Nerve	*Dysfunction*
Trigeminal cranial nerve V	Muscles of mastication
Facial cranial nerve VII	Sensory muscles for taste to front of tongue; sensory to submaxillary and sublingual glands
Glossopharyngeal nerve IX	Swallowing; sensory for taste to cranial posterior one-third of tongue; sensation from soft palate
Vagus cranial nerve X	Soft palate and pharyngeal muscles
Accessory cranial nerve XI	Muscles of soft palate
Hypoglossal cranial nerve XII	Muscles of tongue

Source: Perkins WH: Speech Pathology—An Applied Behavioral Science, Ed 2, Mosby, St. Louis, 1977, pp. 137–139; Warwick R, Williams P: Myology. In Gray's Anatomy. Saunders, Philadelphia, 1973, pp. 506–507.

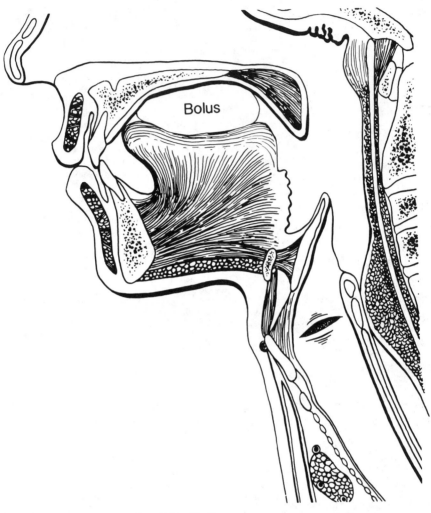

Figure 10–2. Oral phase (see Table 10–1).

PATHOPHYSIOLOGY

Evaluation begins with the patient's description of swallowing ability and difficulty. Assessment of reported symptoms provides clues that suggest impaired stages(s) of swallowing (Table 10–3).[1] These accounts and subsequent examination facilitate identification of muscle weakness or paralysis.

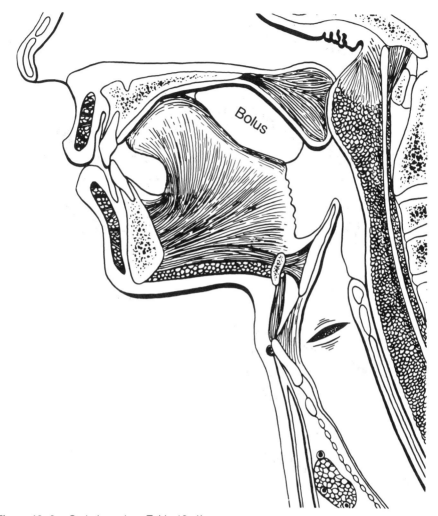

Figure 10–3. Oral phase (see Table 10–1).

Oral stage difficulties include opening and/or closing the mouth, maintaining lip closure, or moving the tongue within the oral cavity. Drooling, oral retention, and leakage of liquids in the mouth are symptoms indicating oral phase disorders. Patient complaints may involve impairment of up-and-down, side-to-side, circular, or front-to-back tongue motions. Loss of liquids through the nose or inability to suck through a straw suggest insufficiency in velopharyngeal closure, associated with

Table 10–3. General Pathophysiology of Dysphagia

Swallowing Phase	Dysfunction	Symptom
Oral	Difficulty opening and closing mouth; difficulty maintaining lip closure and tongue mobility	Movement of food within oral cavity, drooling, oral retention and leakage of liquids
Pharyngeal	Decreased sensitivity or reflex behavior, absence of swallow reflex, premature swallow, poor laryngeal elevation or poor vocal fold closure, hypertonicity of the cricopharyngeal sphincter	Choking, coughing, loss of liquids through the nose or inability to suck through a straw, food lodging in pathway
Esophageal	Insufficient tone and decreased pressure or pressure of the esophageal sphincter and esophagogastric junction	Regurgitation of esophageal contents into pharynx, regurgitation of gastric contents of stomach into esophagus

Source: Dobie RA: Rehabilitation of swallowing disorders. Am Fam Phys 17:5, 1978.

pharyngeal stage involvement. Patients who report choking or coughing episodes usually present with pharyngeal stage disorders as well. Dysfunction during this stage may be secondary to decreased sensitivity or reflex behavior, absence of swallow reflex, premature swallow, poor laryngeal elevation, or poor vocal fold closure. Another deterrent to swallowing is cricopharyngeal hypertonicity, which is described by the patient as an obstruction ("shelf") in the esophagus.[1,2] Esophageal dysfunction may result in regurgitation of contents from the esophagus into the larynx. When the latter occurs, chest pain or heartburn may be a consequence. Esophageal reflex may result because the LES pressure is too low and this interferes with adequate sphincter closure. Various gastrointestinal hormones that are stimulated by certain foods affect the release of these hormones, resulting in either an increase or decrease in LES pressure.[8]

EVALUATION

Ideally, the evaluation of a patient with a swallowing disorder should be conducted by specialists from a number of medical disciplines. Each makes a valuable contribution in terms of diagnostic information, functional assessment, and treatment.

The history should elicit information relative to the onset and duration of the disorder, and solids or liquids that cause the most swallowing difficulty. It is particularly important to learn the consistency of the food bolus best tolerated, that is, the effect solids, semisolids, and liquids have

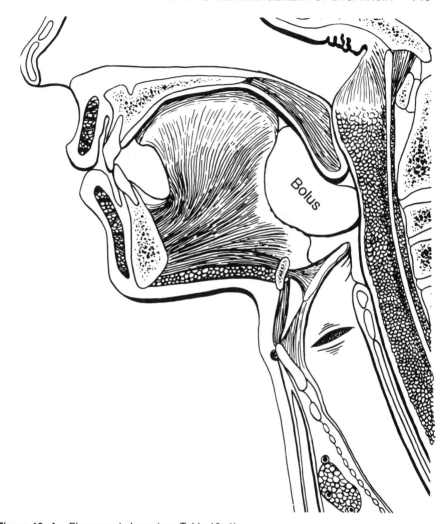

Figure 10–4. Pharyngeal phase (see Table 10–1).

on the difficulty in swallowing. Information should be obtained regarding problems relating to nasal regurgitation, aspiration, and gastroesophageal reflux.

The physical examination should include cranial nerve assessment which is necessary to determine cord mobility. Assessment of the oral mechanism involves observing structure and determining function of muscles of facial expression and mastication [mandible, maxilla, lips, tongue, hard palate, and velum (soft palate)], and the lateral and posterior pharyngeal walls. Color, size, and symmetry relationships are noted. Range,

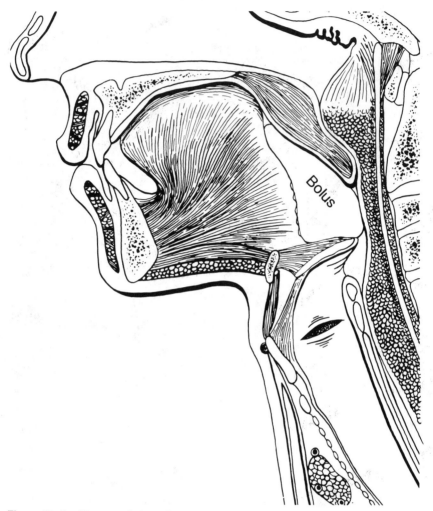

Figure 10–5. Pharyngeal phase (see Table 10–1).

rate, and strength of motion are tested. Oral mucosa and dentition should be inspected and assessed. Laryngeal function is evaluated by asking the patient to cough, clear his throat, hum, and phonate intermittently.[9] Gag and swallowing reflexes are elicited.[24] Observation and evaluation of the patient swallowing liquids and chewing and swallowing foods of varying consistencies should be included. The physical examination should also include anthropometric measurements of height, weight, and upper arm skinfold measurements. In addition to this information, nutritional status of patients is assessed, based on measurement of nutrient intake and bio-

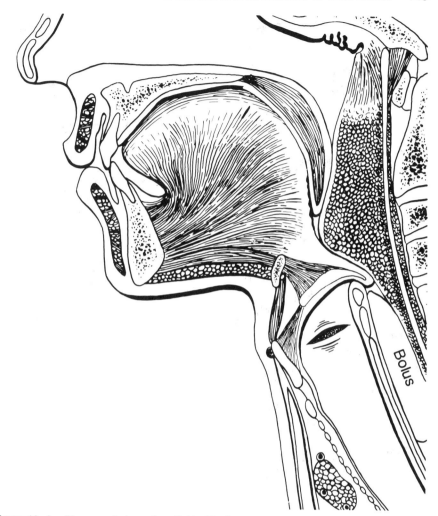

Figure 10–6. Pharyngeal phase (see Table 10–1).

chemical studies (serum albumin, serum levels for total iron, binding capacity, transferrin values, total lymphocyte count, and 24-h urinary creatinine excretion).[10–12] Special attention should be given to the patient's weight, especially in terms of weight loss, as this finding can mark the severity of the swallowing problem and can also serve as an indicator of the progression of the disease. (Though it is also true that in a disease where there is progressive muscle wasting occuring, weight can be lost when presumably an adequate oral intake is maintained.)

Radiologic studies, particularly the videofluoroscopic recording,

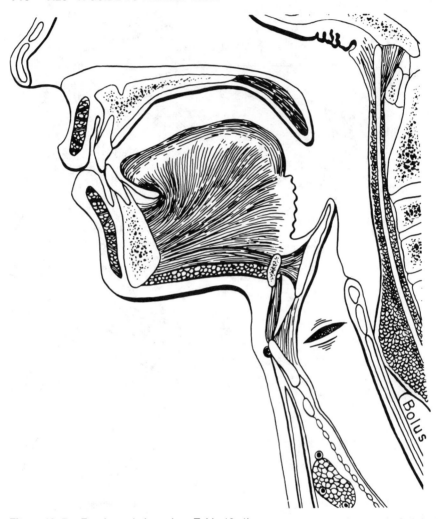

Figure 10–7. Esophageal phase (see Table 10–1).

provide information about all stages of swallowing including pharyngeal and esophageal dysfunction. Oral, pharyngeal, and esophageal transit time and movement can be visualized. In addition, these studies enable diagnosis of cricopharyngeal hypertonicity, stricturing of the lower esophageal sphincter, or presence of tertiary waves. The successful nutritional treatment of patients with a swallowing deficit is dependent on a clear understanding of the functional diagnosis: what swallowing function has been lost and what function remains. With this knowledge, nutritional therapy can be determined in terms of oral intake, and specific foods may be modified in texture, appropriate supplements given, or use of an alternate feeding route instituted.

NUTRITIONAL CONSIDERATIONS

Consideration of the patient's ideal body weight and physical energy requirement is fundamental to planning for optimal nutritional care of the patient. A large number of patients experiencing dysphagia present with significant weight loss. Calorie deprivation occurs secondary to the individual altering food intake out of fear of choking, aspiration, or frustration from the length of time required to eat. Therefore, often the diet needs to provide a level of calories above what is normally required. For many patients a typical high-calorie intake would include one thousand or more supplemental calories.

The major energy-yielding nutrients need to be considered, particularly with respect to the quality and type of protein and carbohydrate as well as fat. A typical high-calorie diet should provide a minimum of 1.5 g protein/kg of body weight; otherwise stated, approximately 20% of the diet should be in the form of protein. The U.S. recommended dietary allowance for protein is 0.8 g/kg.[13] A major concern is that weight loss does not progress to muscle wasting atrophy, hypersensitivity reactions, and altered cell-mediated immune responses. However, protein depletion and its effect on immune response remain somewhat obscure. In formulating high-calorie, high-protein diets, attention needs to be given to the relationship of nonprotein kilocalories and protein nigrogen. A high-calorie, low-protein intake will distort body composition while a high-protein intake requires an increase in nonprotein kilocalories to spare nitrogen waste. A recommended kilocalorie/nitrogen ratio is 150 nonprotein kcal/g nitrogen.[14] It must be remembered that vitamin A and calcium requirements are directly influenced by the protein content of the diet. A high-protein intake increases the demand by the body for vitamin A which may cause the vitamin to be mobilized from the liver, resulting in depleted stores.[15,16] Dietary protein is also known to alter calcium absorption in the gastrointestinal tract which adversely affects calcium balance.[17]

Protein Carbohydrate Fat

Tissue proteins are depleted in advance of changes in serum albumin levels. For this reason the need for a high-calorie, high-protein diet should be considered before changes occur in blood chemistries. A serum albumin level below 3 g/100 ml is indicative of malnutrition and should be corrected by diet.[14]

The source of carbohydrate to incorporate into the diet is of importance because it contributes approximately 45 to 50% of the total kilocalories. Because sucrose is so sweet, glucose and glucose polymers, which are less sweet, may be an acceptable substitute to meet carbohydrate kilocalorie needs.[18]

It is desirable that 30 to 35% of the total kilocalories be in the form of fat.[19] Linoleic acid, the essential fatty acid, must be supplied in the amount of 1 to 2% of total calories.[13] When the diet is high in protein, it is prudent to make appropriate modifications in order to control the cholesterol and saturated fat intake. The cholesterol level of the diet should be equal to or less than 300 mg.[19]

Modifications in the consistency of the diet often result in the limited intake of certain fiber and connective tissue. The average crude fiber intake (nonvegetarian) ranges between 8 and 12 g/day, and the estimated daily adult requirement is 100 mg/kg body weight.[20,21] While bran will increase the bulk of the stool, colonic pressure is increased by fruits and vegetables, either directly by increasing the residue in the colon or by pharmacologic laxative properties.[22]

Although not considered a food, water is a required nutrient. The daily minimum fluid intake must equal the total amount of water lost per day. Water requirement is based on body size and body weight. For adults, that requirement is estimated at 20 to 30 ml/kg body weight. Water requirement may also be estimated according to recommended energy intake. It is suggested that for adults the daily intake be 1 ml of fluid/kcal body weight.[22]

Diet Therapy

The aim of diet therapy is to provide for optimal nutrient and energy intake through proper and specific modifications in food texture and consistency to enable the patient with dysphagia to take nourishment.

Consideration should be given to meal size, time, and frequency. Rather than the customary three large meals each day, generally smaller, more frequent meals served at 2- to 3-h intervals will encourage increased food consumption. In addition, taste preferences and foods disliked by the patient should be taken into consideration.

Modifications in texture range from soft to pureed and any alteration in food consistency should be made concurrently with progression of swallowing dysfunction (Table 10–4).

If jaw movement and tongue mobility are impaired, food becomes

Table 10–4. Recommended Dietary Alterations for Dysphagia

Dysfunction/Symptom	Texture/Consistency
↓ Jaw movement	↓ Tolerance for raw fruits and vegetables; meat cooked tender; food cut or diced into small particle size
↓ Tongue mobility	Soft, cooked, moist foods; small particle size
↓ Mouth and lip closure	Moist foods; mixed and held together; liquids taken separately; placement of food to middle or back of tongue
↓ Sensitivity or ↓ reflex behavior	Pureed and strained foods; ↓ tolerance for liquids
↓ Laryngeal elevation	Ground meat and stewed vegetables well tolerated; head positioned forward and downward to protect airway
↑ Cricopharyngeal tonicity	Small-particle foods avoided; food in bolus form better tolerated
↓ Saliva	↑ Foods of high water content (ice cream, gelatin desserts, puddings); ↑ sour or tart foods and concentrated forms of carbohydrates that will stimulate saliva production; moist food better tolerated, use sauces and gravies
↑ Phlegm/ ↑ mucus	Milk and milk beverages avoided; warm and hot beverages better tolerated; lemon or lime juice concentrated or mixed with water helps break up phlegm
↓ Esophageal sphincter control	↑ Protein, ↓ fat; alcohol and caffeine avoided; ↓ tolerance for citrus fruits
Absence of gag reflex	Alternate feeding route

↑ Increase in
↓ Decrease in

difficult to chew and manipulate in the mouth. Meat, raw vegetables, and fresh fruit are among the foods less well tolerated by patients with even minimal swallowing disorders. Meats prepared by a moist cooking method are better tolerated and can be served with a gravy or sauce which acts as a lubricating agent. Meat or fish may be better tolerated if flaked finely and combined with a sauce, added to egg dishes or pastas, or mixed with a salad dressing and made into a cold salad. The acceptability of vegetables and fruits may be enhanced by cooking them and cutting them into small pieces. Vegetables may be served with cheese or cream sauces or combined with mixed dishes or casseroles. Diced or stewed fruit can be served over cereals or ice cream or mixed with yogurt.

Because bread is so dry it may be better tolerated in the form of milk toast, bread pudding, or bread stuffing. Potatoes, cereals, and pastas are most versatile insomuch as the consistency can be easily altered with the addition of cheese, eggs, meat, and milk.

Certain pastas and grains may be preferred over others on the basis of particle size. Grains, cereals, and rice often fragment in the mouth causing the problem of aspiration. If this is the case, small-particle foods may be better tolerated if held together (combined with cheese, eggs, and sauces) and swallowed in the form of a single bolus.

Milk (one food in which a complete protein is found in liquid form) should be part of the patient's daily diet. If milk is not well tolerated as a beverage, other milk products, such as yogurt, pudding, and custards may be incorporated into the diet.

With minimal swallowing function, it becomes necessary to institute the use of pureed foods. Either homemade blenderized or commercially prepared pureed foods are suitable. Variety and taste appeal of strained meat, fish, and vegetables may be increased when combined with certain foods such as a souffle, mousse, or a chowder.

Intolerance for liquids is most associated with the more extensive deficits in swallowing. Altering the viscosity of a liquid can markedly influence tolerance. The viscosity of coffee and tea may be increased by adding cream, nonfat dry milk solids, honey, or corn syrup. Nectars and various vegetable juices are swallowed easier than most clear juices. To increase the viscosity, strained, fruit, sherbets, and/or unflavored gelatin may be mixed with clear fruit juice beverages. Carbonated drinks are best avoided because of the carbonation often causes spasms in the throat. Ice chips and flavored gelatin desserts are also often poorly tolerated. This is true of any food that decomposes rapidly in consistency (becomes semi-liquid) as it travels from the mouth to the throat.

OTHER CONSIDERATIONS

Saliva

Still another problem interfering with oral feeding is due to either excessive saliva (sialorrhea) or the lack of adequate saliva (xerostomia). To some degree these problems can be managed by controlling the intake of very sour or very sweet foods that cause hypersecretion. To control saliva, it may also be helpful to decrease or increase (as the case may be) foods of high water or fluid content.

Mucus

Another frequent problem associated with dysphagia is the presence of phlegm, which results from weakened muscles involved in respiration. The patient describes this in terms of choking from strangulating mucus.

Often excess mucus production is thought to be caused by the intake of milk, however, this is most unlikely. What may actually happen is that the protein (casein) present in milk binds with salivary secretions to form a tough "ropelike" mucus that is difficult to break up and/or swallow.

Constipation

There may be several diet-related causes of constipation including lack of fiber or bulk in the diet and decreased fluid intake. Despite the fact that major sources of dietary fiber are restricted, specifically raw fruits and vegetables, various other forms of fiber need to be included. Fiber intake can be increased if whole grain pastas are used in casseroles and combination dishes. Fine-cut bran may be added to cooked cereals and casseroles as well. Sometimes the use of prunes and prune juice which contain a natural laxative substance (dihydroxyphenylisatin) may be helpful. It is also most important to meet fluid requirements to assure adequate moisture content of excreta.

If the problem of constipation cannot be managed by diet, it may be necessary to prescribe a bulk laxative.

Formulas and Tube Feedings

Supplemental formulas are indicated when kilocalorie and/or nutrient requirements are unable to be met with food. It is not uncommon for patients to have caloric needs in excess of what they can reasonably eat in any given day. Also if the nutrient intake is deficient, supplemental formulas are a means of providing high-density oral feedings. Palatability and acceptance are key factors when selecting a formula for oral use.

The nature and purpose of the formula will define the type of product desired. If milk is tolerated, homemade blenderized formulas may be used. Composition may be varied with respect to the sources of nutrients and the proportion or ratio of carbohydrate, protein, and fat. Most commercially prepared formulas contain 1 kcal/ml; however, some contain as much as 2 kcal/ml. In addition to these formulas, there are "defined" formula diets commercially prepared for treating patients with problems related to digestion and absorption of solid foods. Patients with an intact functional gastrointestinal tract do not require these special preparations. However, patients with dysphagia who have lactose intolerance may require a nonmilk, lactose-free "defined" formula.

It becomes necessary to use an alternate feeding route in patients with dysphagia when airway protection is compromised and/or when feeding time is prolonged.[23] Common tube feeding sites used for patients with dysphagia include: nasogastric, esophagostomy, gastrostomy, jejunostomy, and pharyngostomy.

In selecting a formula for tube feeding use, special consideration should be given not only to the total calories and composition but also to the rate of administration, volume required, and osmolality. Tube feeding complications may be minimized through careful observation and monitoring of patients' reactions.

CONCLUSIONS

Experience has taught us that a specific form of dysphagia is unique with each patient. Regardless of the etiology, the extent and involvement of the various cranial nerves determine the pathophysiology. An accurate assessment of swallowing function and dysfunction is essential to appropriate therapy, rehabilitation, and nutritional intervention. The nutritional status of the patient is based on assessment of (1) clinical date including medical history, physical examination, and anthropometric measurements, (2) dietary history, and (3) biochemical and radiographic studies.

Most patients with dysphagia are found to be at nutritional risk, with decreased food consumption and restricted protein–calorie intake. Diet therapy consists of prescribing for optimal energy and nutrient intake through modification of food texture and consistency. Most patients with dysphagia who receive appropriate dietary management are able to continue to be nourished via the oral route. As swallowing function diminishes, an alternate feeding route may need to be instituted. In summary, patients with a swallowing disorder require special nutritional and dietary care. Compromised nutritional status may be life threatening if not treated with precise diet therapy.

REFERENCES

1. Dobie RA: Rehabilitation of swallowing disorders. Am Fam Phys 17:5, 1978.
2. Shepherd RS: Human Physiology. Lippincott, Philadelphia, 1971, pp. 412–414.
3. Warwick R, Williams P: Myology. In Gray's Anatomy, Ed. 35. Saunders, Philadelphia, 1973, pp. 506–507.

4. Perkins WH: Speech Pathology—An Applied Behavioral Science, Ed 2. Mosby, St. Louis, 1977, pp. 137–139.
5. Palmer E: Disorders of the cricopharyngeus muscle: A review. Prog Gastroenterol 71:510–519, 1976.
6. Kirchner JA: The motor activity of the cricopharyngeus muscle. Laryngoscope 68:1119–1159, 1958.
7. Lund WS, Ardan GM: The motor nerve supply of the cricopharyngeal sphincter. Ann Otol 73:599–612, 1964.
8. Krause MV, Mahan LK: Food, Nutrition, and Diet Therapy, Ed. 6. Saunders, Philadelphia, 1979, p. 469.
9. Groher ME: Dysphagia: Diagnosis and Management. Butterworths, Boston, 1984, pp. 85–94.
10. Bishop W: Norms for nutritional assessment of American adults by upper arm anthropometry. Am J Clin Nutr 34:2530, 1981.
11. Butterworth CE: The skeleton in the hospital closet. Nutr Today 9:4, 1974.
12. Blackburn GL, Bistrin BR, Maini BS: Nutritional and metabolic assessment of the hospitalized patient. JPEN 1:1122, 1977.
13. Food and Nutrition Board: Recommended Dietary Allowances, Ed. 9. National Academy of Sciences, Washington, DC, 1980.
14. Kinney JM: Calories, Nitrogen, Disease, and Injury Relationships. In White PL, Nagy MD (eds): Total Parenteral Nutrition. Acton, England: Publishing Sciences Group, 1974, p. 90.
15. Arroyane G: Interrelations between protein and Vitamin A and metabolism. Am J Clin Nutr 22:1119, 1969.
16. Roels WA, Lui NST: The vitamins: Vitamin A and carotene. In Goodhart RS, Shils ME (eds): Modern Nutrition in Health Disease, Ed. 6. Lea & Febiger, Philadelphia, 1980, pp. 153–154.
17. Margen D, Chu JY, Kaufmann, NA, et al: Studies in calcium metabolism. I. The calciuretic effect of dietary protein. Am J Clin Nutr 22:584, 1974.
18. American Dietetic Association: Handbook of Clinical Dietetics. Yale University Press, New Haven, CT, 1981, C5.
19. American Heart Association Nutrition Committee: Rationale of the Diet–Heart Statement of the American Heart Association. Arteriosclerosis 2:177, 1982.
20. Hardinge MDG, Chambers AC, Crooks H, et al: Nutritional studies of vegetarians. III. Dietary levels of fiber. Am J Clin Nutr 6:523, 1958.
21. Cowgill GR, Anderson WE: Laxative effects of wheat bran and washed grain in healthy men. A comparative study. JAMA 98:1866, 1932.
22. Nutrition Reviews: Present Knowledge in Nutrition, Ed. 5. Nutrition Foundation, Washington, DC, 1984, pp. 156–71.
23. Shen G: Water and electrolytes. In Howard RB, Herbold WH (eds): Nutrition in Clinical Care. McGraw-Hill, New York, 1978, p. 140.
24. Logemann J: Evaluation and Treatment of Swallowing Disorders. College Hill Press, San Diego, CA, 1984, pp. 129–132.

CHAPTER ELEVEN

SWALLOWING DIFFICULTIES IN AMYOTROPHIC LATERAL SCLEROSIS

Jill Brooks, M.S., C.C.C.-SP

Swallowing difficulty or dysphagia has been associated with many of the degenerative neurologic disorders. When the progressive deterioration of amyotrophic lateral sclerosis (ALS) is confined to the muscles supplied by the spinal cord, dysphagia is not a complication. However, in a significant number of patients, bulbar muscles are involved, resulting in serious difficulties with swallowing. In addition, bilateral corticobulbar tract degeneration can occur, resulting in a pseudobulbar palsy—with characteristic features of swallowing and speech difficulties and emotional liability. A review of the normal physiology of swallowing prior to discussion of swallowing problems associated with ALS is helpful. This can be done by referring to the text and figures in Chapter 10 and by referring to the Glossary of Terms at the end of this chapter.

To review this briefly, the voluntary initiation of the swallow begins with the tongue, followed by the triggering of the swallowing reflex. Next, the bolus of food passes through the pharynx, with the entry of the bolus through the cricopharyngeal sphincter into the cervical esophagus. This completes the pharyngeal stage of the swallow.

PATTERNS OF WEAKNESS OF SWALLOWING MUSCLES IN AMYOTROPHIC LATERAL SCLEROSIS

The ALS patient with bulbar findings can demonstrate both flaccidity and spasticity, and in varying degrees. The muscles of mastication, especially the ptyregoids, can develop weakness, resulting in chewing fatigue. The facial muscles, such as the obicularis oris, may become weak, leading to drooling. The tongue is frequently affected early with fasci-

155

culations, atrophy, and decreased mobility. Thus, the ALS patient may have difficulty controlling material in the oral cavity. Poor control of saliva with subsequent pooling are frequent complaints. Soft palate weakness may result in anterior bulging with food remaining in the oral cavity during chewing. Palatal and pharyngeal weakness are common and nasal regurgitation may be noted. Gag reflexes may range from hyperactive to absent. An intact gag reflex can disappear during the course of the disease. Pharyngeal peristalsis may be decreased, so material remains in the pharynx after the swallow. This material can potentially be aspirated when the patient inhales after the swallow. Usually, at the same time that pharyngeal peritalsis is affected, the swallowing reflex becomes delayed.

The muscles that elevate the larynx may also develop weakness. However, as long as laryngeal function remains adequate to protect the airway, the patient may be able to feed orally. If laryngeal functioning is severely impaired, complete vocal cord adduction during swallowing may not be attained and material may be aspirated. Patients may present with a poor protective cough as a result of respiratory insufficiency and abdominal muscle weakness. Some patients develop cricopharyngeal disorders as a result of discoordination in the entire pharynx. In addition, the cricopharyngeus muscle may fail to relax during swallowing, thus blocking the passage of the bolus into the esophagus.

EVALUATION OF SWALLOWING DIFFICULTY

The major reason for performing a swallowing evaluation is to determine if aspiration actually occurs, and the nature of the swallowing problem leading to aspiration. From this information a treatment plan can then be formulated. In order for material to be aspirated in a person with normal anatomy, it must penetrate all three laryngeal valves (the epiglottic/aryepiglottic folds, the false vocal cords, and the true vocal cords). This may occur under several sets of circumstances. It can occur *before* the swallowing reflex is triggered when the airway has not elevated or closed completely. This may be related to reduced lingual movement or because of a delayed or absent triggering of the swallowing reflex. Aspiration can also occur *during* the swallow, if the laryngeal valves are not functioning adequately, resulting in decreased laryngeal closure. Finally, aspiration can occur *after* the swallow when the larynx lowers and opens for inhalation, resulting in material that has been left in the pyriform sinuses overflowing into the airway.

Evaluation includes clinical examination of the oral musculature and of swallowing, and observation of the patient's symptoms. Obtaining a complete history and description of the problem is necessary. Patients are often quite accurate in their ability to describe and localize their swallowing difficulties. Clinical symptoms can help identify the area of dysfunction (e.g., whether difficulties are present at the oral versus pharyngeal stages of the swallow). This assessment is, however, rather gross and doesn't usually provide enough information to identify specific anatomic or neuromuscular problems.

Swallowing is a dynamic and rapid process, and thus lends itself to study utilizing fluoroscopy. *Cinefluoroscopy* refers to the recording of the fluoroscopic image on movie film. It has the advantage of allowing frame-by-frame analysis of movement patterns. Its disadvantages include greater radiation exposure than other methods and the inability to preserve simultaneous voice recordings. Many hospitals have limited the use of cinefluoroscopy for these reasons.

Another type of fluoroscopy termed *videofluoroscopy* permits simultaneous voice recording with less radiation exposure. It is more difficult to perform than cinefluoroscopy. However, when a tape is numbered and played on a video cassette recorder, frame-by-frame analysis of movement patterns is possible and is similar to analysis of motion picture film.

A procedure known as "the modified barium swallow" can be quite useful in demonstrating swallowing difficulties in ALS patients.

Unlike the traditional barium swallow, the "modified barium swallow" highlights the earlier stages of swallowing. Specifically, the oral, pharyngeal, and cervical esophageal stages are demonstrated as is the physiology. This method of study also differs from the traditional upper gastrointestinal (GI) or barium swallow in other ways, such as the amount and type of contrast material used. In the "modified barium swallow," three consistencies of barium are utilized to evaluate swallowing ability: liquid barium, barium paste, and material requiring mastication (which is coated with a thin layer of paste). Two swallows of each material are given, usually in the following amounts: ⅓ teaspoon each of liquid and paste and ¼ of a small cookie, such as like a Lorna Doone, that has been coated thinly with barium paste.

This method differs significantly from the traditional barium swallow that is designed to diagnose lesions and anatomic deformities. The goal of the traditional barium swallow is to fill the pharynx with material and outline the gross anatomic structures. When this technique is used with dysphagic patients, they tend to aspirate more material than with the modified study.

Other problems detected utilizing the modified barium swallow include abnormal bolus formation, weakness or paralysis, pharyngeal retention, misdirected or asymmetric swallows, and cricopharyngeal sphincter dysfunction. Another benefit of this procedure is that because of the decreased radiation and smaller amounts of barium, treatment strategies can be explored and visualized during the videofluoroscopic study. The inadequacy of subjective impressions *alone* cannot be overstressed. Common difficulties encountered by ALS patients, and illustrated by use of videofluoroscopy and the modified barium swallow are: (1) collections of food can remain on the hard palate due to decreased tongue elevation and mobility; (2) the food bolus spreads from the front of the mouth to the valleculae due to reduced tongue elevation; (3) paste bolus can pool in the valleculae; this occurs in the absence of the triggering of the swallowing reflex; (4) the bolus does not pass through the pyriform sinuses and into the esphohagus when the cricopharyngeous does not relax or opens too early or late; (5) residual material can be found in the valleculae and pyriform sinuses after the swallow due to impaired pharyngeal peristalsis; (6) actual aspiration of food into the trachea may occur.

Another diagnostic procedure utilized in the detection of swallowing problems is the ultrasound evaluation. This study provides information primarily on the anatomy and physiology of the tongue, hyoid, and floor of the mouth without exposure to radiation.

MANAGEMENT OF SWALLOWING DIFFICULTY

Management of dysphagia in ALS patients needs to begin early within the course of the disease process. The patient needs to be instructed to eat in a position that facilitates control during the early stages of the swallow. Recommendations regarding head positioning and placement of food in the oral cavity must be made based on oral musculature involvement. (For example, an upright posture with the neck extended encourages a decrease in the potential vallecular space and may minimize pooling.) Foods that present problems need to be noted so that consistencies within the diet are controlled. In general, patients with poor oral control do best with liquid or foods of thin consistency. Patients with a delayed swallowing reflex do best with food of thicker consistency. Those with reduced pharyngeal peristalsis do best with liquids as do patients with reduced functioning of the cricopharyngeous muscle. Patients with reduced laryngeal closure do best with food of a thicker consistency.

Most blenderized foods act like liquids and fall apart in the mouth and pharynx. Soft foods and custards seem to work quite well. However, sticky foods and substances that combine with saliva to cause thick mucus, such as chocolate or uncooked milk products, should be avoided. Control of saliva may need to be managed medically with drugs such as atrophine, Pro-Banthine, or tricyclics. There have been reports of giving patients meat tenderizer (made from papaya) shortly before meals for the purpose of "liquifying" thick, ropy mucus secretions.

Patients are encouraged to eat in an environment that is free of distractions. Swallowing becomes an activity that requires concentration. The patient may need to be taught a supraglottic swallow in order to protect the airway. This involves holding the breath when swallowing; then coughing, and throat clearing followed by an additional swallow. Good oral hygiene must be stressed. Tooth brushing, mouth rinsing, flossing, and use of a Water Pik after each meal are recommended.

As the disease progresses, management of nutrition by oral feeding may become unsafe. It is the dysphagia specialist's role to recommend procedures that may improve swallowing—such as an oral prosthesis or the exploration of alternate methods of providing nutrition, such as nasogastric feeding, esophagostomy, or gastrostomy.

Cricopharyngeal myotomy has been suggested as a surgical procedure. Release of this muscle allows the bolus to pass more easily into the esophagus. Lebo and co-workers (see Bibliography) reported that 64% of their ALS patients demonstrated improved swallowing following the procedure. Although the benefits may be temporary, the procedure may serve to enhance quality of life in selected patients. Of course, most patients desire to maintain oral intake for as long as possible.

In summary, timing is extremely important when recommending compensatory strategies for decreased functioning or alternatives to swallowing. Because ALS is progressive, the status of the patient's swallowing abilities is continuously changing. It is therefore important to establish baseline functioning, followed by regular assessment, in order to minimize the risk of aspiration and maintain adequate nutritional status.

GLOSSARY OF TERMS

Adduction—movement toward the midline

Aspiration—the inspiratory sucking into the airways of fluid or foreign body

Atrophy—a wasting of tissues, organs, or the entire body

Bolus—a masticated morsel of food ready to be swallowed

Buccal—pertaining to or adjacent to the cheek

Cinefluoroscopy—motion pictures of fluoroscopic views after administration of a contrast medium

Corticobulbar—connecting cortex and motor cranial nuclei in the medulla (part of the brainstem)

Cricopharyngeal—relating to the cricoid cartilage and the pharynx; a part of the inferior constrictor muscle of the pharynx

Deglutition—act of swallowing

Dysphagia—difficulty in swallowing

Fluoroscopy—a procedure for visualizing the shadows of x-rays which, after passing through the body examined, are transmitted through an image intensification tube and projected on a TV monitor.

Labial—relating to the lips

Lingual—relating to the tongue

Mastication—the process of chewing food in preparation for deglutition and digestion

Myotomy—surgical division of a muscle

Peristalsis—a wave of alternate circular contraction and relaxation of the tube by which the contents are propelled onward

Pharynx—the upper expanded portion of the digestive tube, between the esophagus below and the mouth and nasal cavities above and in front

Sulci—(lateral) the grooves or depressions in the oral cavity

Supraglottic—above the glottis or vocal cords and ligament

Valleculae—a crevice or depression between the median and lateral glossoepiglottic folds on either side

Velopharyngeal—pertaining to the soft palate and the posterior nasopharyngeal wall

Velum (palatinum)—pertaining to the soft palate

Videofluoroscopy—video pictures of fluoroscopic views after administration of a contrast medium

BIBLIOGRAPHY

Aronson, A: Clinical Voice Disorders: An Interdisciplinary Approach. Thieme-Stratton, New York, 1980.

Blount M, Bratton C, Luttrell N: Management of the patient with amyotrophic lateral sclerosis. Nurs Clin 14:157–171, 1979.

Carpenter RJ, McDonald TJ, Howard FM: The otolaryngologic presentation of amyotrophic lateral sclerosis. Otolaryngology 86:479–484, 1978.

Delisa JA, Mikulic MA, Miller RM: Amyotrophic lateral sclerosis: Comprehensive management. Am Fam Phys 19:137–142, 1979.

Dworkin, JP, Hartman DE: Progressive speech deterioration and dysphagia in amyotrophic lateral sclerosis: Case report. Arch Phys Med Rehab 60:423–425, 1979.

Farber SD: Neurorehabilitation: A Multisensory Approach. Saunders, Philadelphia, 1982.

Gagic NM: Cricopharyngeal myotomy. Can J Surg 26:47–49, 1983.

Groher ME (ed): Dysphagia: Diagnosis and Management. Butterworths, Boston, 1984.

Lebo CP, Sang UK, Norris FH: Cricopharyngeal myotomy in amyotrophic lateral sclerosis. Trans Pac Coast Otoophthalmol Soc Annu Meet 56:125–133, 1975.

Lebo CP, Sang UK, Norris FH: Cricopharyngeal myotomy in amyotrophic lateral sclerosis. Laryngoscope 86:862–868, 1976.

Linden P, Siebens A: Dysphagia: Predicting laryngeal penetration. Arch Phys Med Re183 64:281–284, 1983.

Logemann J, Evaluation and Treatment of Swallowing Disorders. College Hill Press, San Diego, CA, 1983.

McGuirt WF, Blalock D: The otolaryngologist's role in the diagnosis and treatment of amyotrophic lateral sclerosis. Laryngoscope 90:1496–1501, 1980.

Shawker TH, Sonies BC, Hall TE, Baum BF: Ultrasound analysis of tongue, hyoid and larynx activity during swallowing. Investigative Radiology 19:82–86, 1984.

Shawker TH, Sonies BC, Stone ML: Soft tissue anatomy of the tongue and floor of the mouth: An ultrasound demonstration. Brain and Language 21:335–350, 1984.

Smith RA, Norris FH: Symptomatic care of patients with amyotrophic lateral sclerosis. JAMA 234:715–717, 1975.

CHAPTER TWELVE

REHABILITATION OF PATIENTS WITH AMYOTROPHIC LATERAL SCLEROSIS

Somchat Chiamprasert, M.D.

Since amyotrophic lateral sclerosis (ALS) is a progressive disease, one might ask: How can we help the patient with ALS? Physical and occupational therapy, though not a cure, can be very helpful to both the patient and his family. They must be provided with instruction on proper types of exercises, selection of appliances and equipment, and transfer methods. In addition, they frequently need to be shown how to modify their living environments to accommodate rehabilitation equipment.

Some patients may require active therapy given by the therapist at the hospital, office, or home. This is often necessary to reduce pain and to stretch joints that may be going into contracture which will result in potential difficulty in transfers and hygienic care. Rehabilitative therapy will help the patient to maintain, for as long as possible, his capacity to function, will lessen the deformity or disability, and may indirectly result in improving psychological stability. Patients and families require ongoing psychosocial assistance.[1]

Rehabilitation also includes not only active therapy but also the application of orthoses, braces, or splints to prevent deformity, support weakened limbs, neck, and torso, and thus improve the patient's mobility, balance, and especially his ability to ambulate.

Since there are only a few ALS clinics available to the growing ALS patient population, it is often difficult for the patient and his family to obtain adequate assistance and understanding to enable them to cope with this illness. The members of the rehabilitation team should therefore familiarize themselves with the patient's potential deformities and disabilities. They can then help the patient and his family to prevent, or at least minimize, problems due to these deformities and disabilities.

Any well-informed and well-equipped rehabilitation facility should be able to provide the ALS patient with specific advice and assistance, **163** particularly in physical therapy and occupational therapy. Speech therapy will also be indicated if the patient's ability to communicate verbally is impaired. Although in most of the ALS patient population it is not realistic, vocational rehabilitation may be applicable in the patient with a slowly progressive disease course. For patients who are homebound, homecare services will be needed. These services may include physical therapy, occupational therapy, respiratory therapy, skilled nursing care, and services of a home health attendant. Equipment, appliances, and adaptive devices are provided, as needed, to the patient in order to enhance to the greatest extent possible his comfort and independence. The Muscular Dystrophy Association has given support and financial aid to many patients so that they can utilize the services mentioned above.

Because of the progressive nature of this illness, realistic goals must be set when we consider rehabilitative medicine for the patient with ALS. In some patients the progression of the disease stabilizes for a significant period of time, while in others the deterioration is rapid. Generally speaking, rehabilitation medicine's goals for the ALS patient are: (1) to enable the patient to attain the highest functional level possible. (2) to maintain range of motion (ROM), thereby preventing deformities, (3) to maintain the patient's ability to perform activities of daily living with optimal safety using energy conservation techniques. These goals can be accomplished through closely coordinated efforts of the physical therapist and occupational therapist. Efforts are also made to delay or retard the deterioration process as it affects the patient's overall ability to function. For example, bracing of the lower extremities may enable a patient to remain ambulatory as an alternative to becoming wheelchair-bound. Rehabilitation medicine, in maintaining a patient's physical independence, will also enhance his social adjustment and emotional well-being.

Rehabilitation medicine provides the ALS patient a team with three members: a physiatrist, a physical therapist, and an occupational therapist. The physiatrist evaluates the extent of the disability, the deformity, and gauges the level of functioning. The physiatrist also assesses the residual function capability so that the patient can be taught to maximize his potential for self-care and independence.

On the basis of the physiatrist's evaluation the treatment is planned. As needed, the patient receives physical therapy, occupational therapy, and an activities of daily living (ADL) evaluation. If the patient's physical status warrants them, orthoses and appliances are provided and the patient is taught how to use these devices.

Communication and coordination between the physiatrist and the therapist are essential before orthoses or equipment are ordered. Such orders should be implemented after the patient has been evaluated by all three rehabilitation team members. Exceptions, of course, occur when the device is simple or when the patient's need for equipment is urgent.

Since the patient is seen at our ALS clinic once every 3 months, home programs are emphasized. Counseling should also be provided for the patient, the patient's family, and the patient's companion or attendant so that appropriate management can be carried out at home. The physical therapist evaluates the patient, recommends exercise techniques, and instructs the family regarding assistive devices they can safely give the patient. The occupational therapist assesses the patient's abilities and limitations in terms of ADL. If necessary, the occupational therapist recommends ADL devices, appliances, wheelchairs, and communication aids. The occupational therapist may also evaluate the patient's home environment and recommend possible adaptions or modifications of the home so that wheelchairs and other assistive items can be more easily accommodated. Details on physical therapy and occupational therapy may be found in Chapters 14 and 15 of the present volume.

EXTENT OF DISABILITY, DEFORMITY, AND LEVEL OF FUNCTIONING

In the early clinical phase of the illness, the patient may not have any visible deformity, may be able to ambulate freely, and may also be independent in regard to ADL. Although the patient may not, at this point, need any assistive devices, he may experience fasciculations and fatigue. He should therefore be instructed to limit his activity and to rest frequently; guidelines in this regard should be consistent with the patient's level of endurance.

Some patients may already have moderate or mild limitations in ambulation and activities of daily living when we first evaluate them. In these cases, deformities are visible. The most common deformity is footdrop resulting in gait disturbance. Frequent areas of soft tissue tightness occur beside the gastrocnemius and soleus; affected areas also include the neck flexor, shoulder adductor, elbow flexor, pronator, web space of hand, metacarpal-phalangeal joint extensor, rectus femoris, hip flexor, tensor fascia lata and knee flexor.[2] Patients in this group must be instructed in how to stretch tightened joints; these patients may also need orthotics such as the footdrop correction brace and may possibly require a walking device such as a cane, a wheeled walker, or a walker with a platform attachment if hand weakness interferes with the patient's ability to safely grip a standard wheeled walker. For patients who experience respiratory distress on exertion, breathing exercise and exercise for endurance are needed. Activities of daily life instruction may also be helpful.

The next group of patients are those who are wheelchair-bound and dependent in ADL. Positioning and therapeutic exercise are prescribed to prevent deformities and to facilitate nursing care.[2] The occupational therapist instructs the family on ADL techniques, and teaches the patient's family how to use such devices as wheelchairs.

In the late stage of the disease, the patient is bedridden and in need of total care, including nursing, feeding, which may require a gastrostomy feeding tube, and respiratory care. Tracheostomy and the use of ventilators and suctioning devices can sometimes be necessary for the patient's comfort and survival. Skin care and frequent turning of the patient to prevent decubitus ulcers must be performed by the family, the nurse, or the home health aide. Fortunately, in our experience, very few patients have developed this problem. Although care of patients with impaired speech is discussed in Chapter 17 of this volume, the occupational therapist can—and very often does—provide the patient with nonverbal communication devices. Such devices include application of the computer with appropriate modifications for the individual patient.

ORTHOTIC PRESCRIPTION

The primary purposes of orthotics[3] for the ALS patient are: (1) prevention of deformity, (2) protection of a weakened or painful musculoskeletal segment, (3) improvement of function. Minimal bracing and ambulation aids are helpful for prolonged and safe ambulation. To prolong ambulation efforts the patient should be taught how to fall safely.[2]

The braces provided must be as lightweight as possible while also being efficient. The most commonly prescribed brace is the ankle–foot arthrosis (AFO; Fig. 12–1). When the patient has mild weakness in the ankle dorsiflexor we can order a prefabricated posterior leaf spring (PLS) so the patient need not wait for a custom-made brace. If the patient has weakness of the evertors and/or the invertors of the foot, in addition to weakness of the dorsiflexors, the orthosis must then be custom-made to provide medial and lateral stability. The shoe clasp AFO[4] is sometimes prescribed, but this provides mainly dorsiflexion and slight mediolateral stability. Use of the conventional double metal upright short leg brace is to be avoided with the ALS patient because it is heavy. As the disease progresses, the patient will have increasing weakness not only at the ankle but also at the knee and hip. The leg brace will then act like an anchor,[3] creating even greater difficulty for the patient attempting to lift his leg. The plastic orthosis, in contrast, is light and easy to wear. It is also

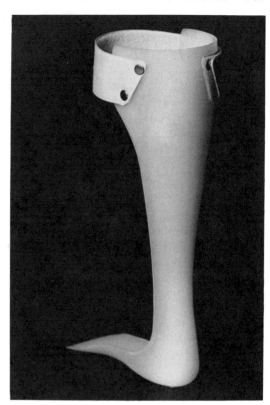

Figure 12–1. Polypropylene ankle–foot orthosis: lightweight, practical, and frequently prescribed for our patients who have ankle weakness. It stabilizes the ankle–foot component and improves the patient's gait and safety on ambulation.

cosmetically advantageous since it is inserted in the shoe and the patient may wear another sock on top of the brace to conceal it. Many patients improve their ability to climb stairs after they begin to use the AFO. Some patients who use bilateral AFOs continue to maintain their ability to ambulate with the assistance of a wheeled walker.

If the patient develops shoulder tightness or subluxation due to weakness, he may suffer from intense shoulder pain that can become so disabling as to interfere with simple activities such as putting on a shirt sleeve. Application of the shoulder elbow orthosis or shoulder abduction assist suspension sling can be made, either attached to the wheelchair or on a stand.[5] We also recommend other supports such as the Bobath sling.

Weakness of the neck musculature creates a major problem. Neck flexion tightness may affect the patient's posture, balance in sitting and standing, mobility and ambulation, feeding and breathing. Development of dermatitis at the neck skinfold areas because of poor aeration and hygienic care can also occur. Therefore, the use of a neck collar (commonly the foam rubber type) is recommended. If the patient is so emaciated that he may not be able to tolerate the pressure of the collar, we consider the use of a headband or modified collar attached to the upper thoracic pads to decrease the size of the neck area under pressure. Details are found in Chapter 14 of this volume.

It should be noted that not all patients benefit from using orthoses. The patient with severe weakness and low endurance may find the use of an orthosis too great an effort for practical use. The patient with quadriparesis, lacking musculature of the trunk and abdomen, and lacking sufficient strength in the upper limbs to utilize crutches or a walker, will not benefit from the lower limb orthosis. If the patient lacks motivation and rejects the orthosis, it is then contraindicated.[3] The patient who has severe back pain and poor strength of the back and abdomen may benefit from using the lumbosacral or the thoracolumbar support. However, if the patient's pulmonary functions are impaired, they may be further compromised by extra force from the support, particularly if it is of the thoracolumbar type.

The patient with mild or moderate weakness of the wrist and hand can be helped to maintain hand function with the fabricated splints given by the occupational therapist. However, when there is rapid muscular atrophy, splints will need frequent readjustment. In these cases, the use of commercially available splints which come in different sizes may be more practical and economical.

SPASTICITY

Spasticity is present in the ALS patients who have upper motor neuron involvement. Patients with severe spasticity may have difficulty in ambulation and may present with spastic dysarthria. There may also be problems regarding personal hygiene. It is true that spasticity of the lower extremities may have a splinting effect and may actually help the patient to walk, even without leg braces.[6] However, spasticity may also cause undesirable effects like plantar flexion or an inverted foot. With the ankle no longer in a neutral position, gait deviation will result. Although we have tried bracing a few patients with spastic ankles, the results have not been satisfactory. Lioresal is usually prescribed for patients with spasticity. Dosages of antispasticity medications should be adjusted so the patient will not develop further weakness and will not experience lowered endurance after the use of these medications.

Factors that are well known for increasing spasticity include the presence of contractures, anxiety, extreme heat or cold, or any ordinarily painful condition such as ingrown toenails, infection, or decubitus ulcers.[7] The use of heat and cold may temporarily reduce spasticity, as has been noted in some stroke patients.[7] Inhibitory techniques carried out by the therapist may also help reduce spasticity. Spasticity can affect the shoulder, causing the scapula to rotate downward and foreward. The angulation of the glenoid fossa, which is dependent upon the position of the scapula on the costal wall, is then impaired, and the glenohumeral joint may subluxate.[8] Subluxation of this joint might also occur in the weak or paralyzed patient. Pain resulting from shoulder subluxation can further disturb the patient. Treatment for this condition includes the use of an appropriate sling, and therapeutic modalities such as hydrocollator pack and ultrasound therapy. Before giving ultrasound therapy, x-ray films should be obtained to determine the severity of osteoporosis since ultrasound can mechanically cause vacuolization of the bones. The application of transcutaneous electrical nerve stimulation (TENS) may also be valuable in pain reduction and can be taught to the patient's family so it can be carried out in the patient's home.

FATIGUE

Fatigue is very common in the ALS patient. It often prevents the patient from doing adequate exercises either at home or under the supervision of the therapist. The patient's exercise program must reflect consideration of his endurance so that overexertion does not occur. Patients should rest as often as they need to during ambulation, exercises, or performance of any ADL. Although a patient may still have fair strength, poor endurance will cause the patient to fatigue easily, thereby increasing the likelihood of the patient becoming disabled relatively early in the course of the disease.

MUSCLE CRAMPS

Muscle cramps and pain are also experienced by ALS patients. Occasionally, even when the quadriceps femoris, biceps, or triceps brachii are first tested, the patients have cramps of such severity as to prevent us from performing a full evaluation of muscle strength. Patients who experience leg cramps at night may benefit from taking quinine sulfate as recommended by the neurologist. Muscle cramps also interfere with the patient's activities or exercises.

TYPES OF EXERCISE

Range of motion exercises, either active or passive, are always needed. However, exercise programs must be appropriate for the ALS patient. Although we usually do not recommend progressive resistive exercise to these patients, those patients with slowly progressive disease will benefit from instruction in mild strengthening exercises for the uninvolved muscles. Isometric[6] and nonstrenuous active exercises are recommended. Details on exercise will be discussed in Chapter 15 of this volume. For the patient who has respiratory impairment we recommend to the patient and his family breathing exercises and postural drainage techniques. An individualized exercise regimen has been found to slow and even prevent development of disuse atrophy and osteoporosis, as well as undesirable side effects such as undue fatigue, muscle strain, and cramping.[6,9]

OBESITY

Obesity is noted in some patients who are not rapidly progressive and have no swallowing problem, but who may be less active or wheelchair-bound with a resultant decrease in energy expenditure. Obesity can cause ADL difficulties and can pose problems for attendants, nurses, or family members who must lift or transfer an obese patient.

ATTITUDES

Trust and cooperation of patients and their families are important components of any rehabilitative program. A realistic and reasonable approach is far more constructive than fostering unrealistic hopes and providing useless recommendations.

CONCLUSION

Although rehabilitation medicine is not a cure for the ALS patient, it has an important role in patient management. Rehabilitation is always essential in assisting the patient and his family to cope with the inevitable deterioration in function caused by this disease. Rehabilitation medicine strives to enable the patient to maintain, to as great an extent as possible, an optimum level of functioning[9] and consequently as much independence as can be realistically accomplished. Indeed, rehabilitation medicine is an integral part of the care and treatment of the ALS patient. Until such time when ALS can be cured, rehabilitation will be needed throughout the duration of the disease.

ACKNOWLEDGMENTS

I gratefully acknowledge the editorial assistance of Ms. Naomi Feld in preparing this chapter.

REFERENCES

1. Rusk HA: Rehabilitation Medicine, Ed. 4. Mosby, St. Louis, 1977, p. 440.
2. Johnson EW, Alexander MA: Management of motor unit diseases In Krusen's Handbook of Physical Medicine and Rehabilitation, Ed. 3. Saunders, Philadelphia, 1982, pp. 679–690.
3 Cary JM, Luskin R, Thomson RG: Prescription principles. In Atlas of Orthotics, Biomechanical Principles and Application. Mosby, St. Louis, 1975, pp. 235–244.
4. Starvos A, deBlanc M: Orthotics components and systems. In Atlas of Orthotics, Biomechanical Principles and Application. Mosby, St. Louis, 1975, pp. 184–234.
5. Guilford A, Perry J: Orthotic components and systems. In Atlas of Orthotics, Biomechanical Principles and Application. Mosby, St. Louis, 1975, pp. 81–104.
6. Sinaki M: Rehabilitation. In Mulder DW (ed): Diagnosis Boston, 1980, pp. 160–193.
7. Anderson TP: Rehabilitation of patients with complete stroke. In Krusen's Handbook of Physical Medicine and Rehabilitation, Ed. 3. Saunders, Philadelphia, 1982, pp. 583–603.
8. Cailliet R: Shoulder Pain, Ed. 2. Davis, Philadelphia, 1981, pp. 140–141.
9. Janiszewski DW, Caroscio JT, Wisham LH: Amyotrophic lateral sclerosis, a comprehensive rehabilitation approach. Arch Phys Med Rehab 64:304–307, 1983.

CHAPTER THIRTEEN

FUNCTIONAL PROFILES BASED ON CLINICAL VARIATIONS IN AMYOTROPHIC LATERAL SCLEROSIS

Janet Zawodniak, B.S. P.T.

A number of functional profiles seen in patients with amyotrophic lateral sclerosis (ALS) and other forms of motor neuron disease will be outlined and discussed in this chapter. These profiles highlight the wide range of problems associated with these diseases that require attention by health care professionals. This chapter is especially directed toward therapists of all disciplines including physical, occupational, speech, respiratory, and psychosocial. To effectively manage these patients, health professionals must be aware of the diversity of problems that may arise. These problems need to be addressed through interdisciplinary management. Interdisciplinary communication is essential because the treatment goals of one specialty may be strongly influenced by critical intervention of another.

The course of ALS and other forms of motor neuron disease is highly variable and health care professionals often face difficulty in planning future care due to uncertainty in predicting the pattern and rate of progression of the illness. Mild to severe stages occurring in patients with a duration of symptoms ranging from 6 months to 8 years will be outlined to demonstrate how varying forms, rates of progression, and patterns of weakness serve as a basis for problem solving. Although it is true that there are shared difficulties among patients, each patient also has problems that are unique to his own case that require individual attention. A single problem or group of problems will be highlighted with each profile. A separate discussion on profiles and problems caused by trunk weakness is also included. Concrete therapeutic management and issues related to patient care based on these profiles are discussed in other chapters throughout this volume.

Table 13–1. Functional Enhancement: Factors To Consider

Preserved	←	PATTERN OF WEAKNESS	→	Involved
Slow	←	RATE OF PROGRESSION MODERATE	→	Rapid
Extent of involvement	←	MUSCLE FATIGUE RATE OF PROGRESSION	→	Daily activity level

FUNCTIONAL ENHANCEMENT

Factors

Table 13–1 lists factors to consider prior to planning therapeutic management. Patterns of weakness are assessed through manual muscle testing and functional evaluations to determine areas of the extremity(ies), trunk, or bulbar musculature that require attention, so that function may be optimally enhanced. The rate of progression is an equally critical factor which is determined through periodic evaluations of strength and function. We at the Mount Sinai Amyotrophic Lateral Sclerosis Clinic recommend that these evaluations be performed at 3-month intervals. We have also found that the approach to management of very slowly progressive patients may markedly differ from those with rapidly progressive disease. Another critical factor is the degree of muscle fatigue patients experience which is influenced by the extent of involvement, rate of progression, and daily activity level of each individual. Psychological factors play a role as well. Consequently, the pattern and rate of progression of the illness as well as muscle fatigue experienced by each individual are interdependent factors when considering therapeutic management.

Therapeutic Considerations

To enhance function, therapeutic considerations include implementing exercise programs, advising patients on compensatory or substitution mechanisms, and applying adaptive (assistive) devices (Table 13–2). One must also be aware of medications that patients may be taking, particularly those that may affect muscle tone.

Exercise

We have found therapeutic exercise to be beneficial to our patients. Exercise programs designed for the extremities, trunk, or speech mecha-

Table 13–2. Functional Enhancement: Therapeutic Considerations

EXERCISE
Extent of weakness
  Rate of progression
  Pattern of weakness
  Activity level   Fatigue
  Occupational
  Recreational

COMPENSATORY MECHANISMS
  Rate of progression
  Pattern of weakness

ADAPTIVE AIDS
  Pattern of weakness
  Rate of progression
  Activity level
  Muscle fatigue
  Patient acceptance
  Family support

nism are intended to maximize neuromuscular function within the context of progressive neuromuscular degeneration. They also serve to prevent contractures and offer psychological support. Muscle fatigue is a common symptom and complaint of ALS patients. Fatigue factors are an integral consideration in exercise program design. Patients with rapidly progressive disease tend to experience higher fatigue than their more slowly progressive counterparts. Critical factors also include the nature of occupational and recreational activities. Contracure prevention is another important consideration. Susceptible areas include the shoulders (extensors, adductors, rotators), hands (digit flexors), hips (extensors, adductors), and ankles (plantar flexors). Details on management of excercise programs in ALS patients are found in Chapter 15 of this volume.

Compensatory Mechanisms

These are commonly referred to as substitution patterns. Compensatory mechanisms are the efficient utilization of unaffected or relatively unaffected muscles in combination with other parts of the body to effectively achieve purposeful function. These are commonly applied in oral speaking, ambulation, and during other activities of daily living (specific examples are discussed later in this chapter). In general, the more slow the rate of progression the more effectively substitution mechanisms are applied. The pattern of weakness dictates the appropriate substitution pattern. Slowly progressive patients have more time to adapt to changes in muscular function and are usually able to more efficiently and safely use compensatory patterns than patients with rapidly progressive disease.

Despite variance in pattern and rate of progression of muscle weakness there are a number of muscle groups that are generally relatively unaffected until later stages of the disease. These include those governing eye movements, cervical spine rotation and lateral flexion, and scapulo-humeral-sternal elevation and depression. Since these movements are generally preserved until later stages they can be counted on in long-range planning for certain critical functions (particularly communication). Other potentially useful movements include elbow and knee extension and ankle and foot plantar flexion.

Adaptive (assistive) Aids

When adaptive aids are appropriate, acceptance by the patient as well as family support may be the most influential consideration in their selection. Chapters 12, 14, 15, and 16 provide information on use of assistive devices in ALS patients.

Functional Problems Due to Trunk Weakness

A highly disabling problem for patients is trunk weakness, particularly in the area of the cervical spine. Most patients experience problems in this area. Cervical extension weakness is most disabling and may cause serious problems in numerous activities during any stage of illness. Often it occurs concurrently with upper extremity or bulbar dysfunction.

Problems During Ambulation

Symptoms of cervical spine weakness often appear during ambulation. Early signs of cervical extensor muscle weakness include muscle cramping or fatigue experienced along the posterior aspect of the neck. The highest demand placed on the posterior neck during ambulation is upon heel strike, where along with the cervical muscles, the thoracolumbar muscles also contract vigorously which induces local muscle fatigue. Initially patients may be asymptomatic during activities performed while sitting.

Biomechanically, when the head is erect the center of gravity falls anterior to the transverse axis of the atlanto-occipital joint for flexion-extension of the neck. If severe cervical extensor muscle weakness is present the head drops forward.[1] Since this posture occurs during ambulation if cervical extensor weakness is moderate, vision is reduced, balance is impaired, and ambulatory function becomes highly precarious. Excess repeated stress is placed on the supporting ligamentous and muscular soft tissues predisposes an individual to develop osteoarthritis and/or spinal subluxation with potential nerve root compression. Safety during ambulation is further endangered if there is significant concurrent upper extremity weakness. In the event of a fall the ability to protect oneself through extension of the arms is lost. A number of patients upon falling have sustained facial and skull lacerations. A few have sustained arm and leg fractures.

If cervical spine weakness progresses into the thoracic area a kyphotic posture during ambulation may occur which may also restrict optimal pulmonary ventilation.

Weakness of the lumbar extensors and abdominal muscles may occur in isolation, but may also occur in combination with upper spine weakness or hip weakness. In isolation a mild lumbar lordosis during ambulation is evident. If lumbar weakness is combined with unsupported cervical extensor weakness, patients attempt to compensate by further increasing postural lumbar lordosis to posteriorally displace their center of gravity to regain or maintain balance and head support. A waddling gait becomes apparent if weakness is present. These patients are predisposed to developing low back pain due to excess stress imposed on the lumbar spine and supporting soft tissue structures.

Problems During Sitting

During activities performed while sitting, if moderate to severe cervical extensor weakness is present, problems may arise during speaking, swallowing, writing, eating, reading, and socializing. When cervical extensor fatigue occurs some patients will posturally compensate through extending the thoracolumbar spine to position the head in extension and thereby enable the cervical flexors take to maintain support. Although this may be practical for short time periods for some patients, it is extremely hazardous for patients with bulbar involvement as it increases risk of choking and aspiration. In patients with added weakness of the thoracolumbar spine, without proper sitting support tremendous physical discomfort may occur, particularly if aggravated by contracture development. Solutions to problems involving trunk weakness are to be found in Chapters 14 and 15 of this volume.

FUNCTIONAL PROFILES

In the following section, ten cases of varying forms of motor neuron disease are described from a functional perspective (Tables 13–3 through 13–5). These include ALS, progressive muscular atrophy (PMA), progressive bulbar palsy (PBP), and primary lateral sclerosis (PLS). Discussion of these cases is intended to convey the diversity of clinical mani-

Table 13-3. Functional Profiles Form: Amyotrophic Lateral Sclerosis (Upper Motor Neuron/Lower Motor Neuron)

Case No.	Age	Sex	DOS	ROP	POW (Extent)	Functional Problems (Common)
1	66	M	6 months	S	RUE Thenar eminence (mild weakness) LMN dominance	Buttoning Writing Manipulating small objects
			12 months	S	RUE Hand intrinsics (mod. weakness) Hand grasp (mild weakness) Forearm supination-pronation (mild weakness)	As above (6 months) Opening jars Turning keys in doors
2	54	M	6 months	M–R	BUEs (symmetrical) Mod. dysfunction proximal and distal UMN dominance (severe spasticity) BLEs (symmetrical) Mild dysfunction proximal and distal UMN dominance (severe spasticity)	Unable to open hands due to severe flexor spasticity causing self-care dependency Barely raises upper arms to horizontal Contracture prone Unable to climb stairs and inclines Difficulty ambulating on uneven terrain Fatigue Depression/anxiety
			12 months	M–R	BUEs (symmetrical) As above (6 months) BLEs (symmetrical) Moderate hip weakness Mild ankle/foot weakness Increased UMN signs (mod. spasticity)	As above (6 months) Contractures: shoulders/hands Increased ambulation difficulty; unable to ambulate on level ground without assistance Assistance necessary during transfers Assistance necessary for bed mobility
3	52	F	6 months	R	All extremities and trunk Mod. diffuse dysfunction UMN dominance	Requires assistance with all self-care (nearly totally dependent) Contracture prone

#	Age	Sex	DOS	ROP	Clinical presentation	Functional status
					(mod.–severe spasticity) Bulbar dysfunction Mod. dysarthria/dysphagia UMN dominance	Requires assistance to ambulate and transfer Requires assistance for bed mobility Communication difficulties: impaired speaking and writing Impaired swallowing Difficulty clearing oral secretions Severe anxiety and fatigue
			12 months		All extremities and trunk Severe diffuse dysfunction Severe UMN signs (severe spasticity) Bulbar dysfunction Anarthric Dysphagic (severe)	Total dependence in self-care Contracture development Wheelchair-bound Unable to communicate: verbally/writing Unable to swallow Difficulty clearing oral secretions Severe depression/anxiety
4	62	F	12 months	S–M	Respiratory Marked diaphragm and intercostal and abdominal muscle weakness BUEs Mild intrinsic hand and shoulder weakness (left greater than right)	Severe dyspnea on exertion causing exhaustive fatigue during daily activities Moderate dyspnea at rest
5	33	F	30 months	M	Cervical spine Severe extensor/flexor weakness Mild lateral flexion and rotation weakness Bulbar dysfunction Anarthric Severe dysphagia BUEs Mod.–severe diffuse weakness	Difficulty ambulating due to poor head control Positioning problems of head while sitting Communication difficulties; unable to speak or write Severe swallowing difficulties Difficulty clearing oral secretions Requires assist with all self-care

Abbreviations: BLE, both lower extremities; BUE, both upper extremities; DOS, duration of symptoms; M, moderate; POW, pattern of weakness; R, rapid; ROP, rate of progression; RUE, right upper extremity; S, slow; other abbreviations as in text.

Table 13–4. Functional Profiles—Form: Progressive Muscular Atrophy (Lower Motor Neuron)

Case No.	Age	Sex	DOS	ROP	POW (Extent)	Functional Problems (Common)
6	52	M	18 months	S	LLE Severe distal weakness ankle and foot (greatest dorsiflexion and eversion) LUE Mild intrinsic hand weakness	Left footdrop causing difficulties during stair climbing (toe catch) and ambulation (toe drag and potential strains/sprains of ankle and foot) Left-handed difficulty manipulating small objects (buttons, coins, and so on)
7	66	M	18 months	S–M	BUEs (symmetrical) Mod.–severe shoulder and elbow weakness Mild hand weakness BLEs Mild ankle and foot weakness	Partial assistance in self-care (feeding, dressing, and the like) Foot slap during ambulation (bilaterally)
8	63	M	18 months	S–M	BUEs Mod.–severe bilateral shoulder and elbow weakness (left greater than right) Mild bilateral hand weakness (left greater than right)	Due to extraordinary use of body compensation mechanisms, independence was sustained in many self-care activities

Abbreviations: LLE, left lower extremity; LUE, left upper extremity; other abbreviations as in Table 13–3.

Table 13–5. Functional Profiles—Forms: Progressive Bulbar Palsy (Amyotrophic Lateral Sclerosis) and PLS (Upper Motor Neuron)

Case No.	Age	Sex	Form	DOS	ROP	POW (Extent)	Functional Problems (Common)

9	66	F	PBP	36 months	S	Bulbar dysfunction
						  Anarthric
						  Dysphagic (severe)
						BUEs:
						  Mild–mod. hand weakness
						    (left greater than right)
						  Mild shoulder weakness
						    (right greater than left)
						Respiratory
						  Mild–mod. impairment
							Communication difficulties;
							  unable to speak and difficulty in
							  writing
							Difficulty swallowing (severe)
							Borderline independence in self-care
							Dyspnea on moderate exertion (ambu-
							  lation greater than 25 yards)
							Difficulty clearing oral and pulmonary
							  secretions
							Two-pillow orthopnea

10	70	M	PLS	96 months	SS	All extremities
						  Mod.–severe diffuse
						    spasticity
						Bulbar dysfunction
						  Severe dysarthria
						  Moderate dysphagia
							Marked increased energy expenditure
							  during daily activities due to spas-
							  ticity
							Severe difficulty speaking
							Moderate difficulty swallowing

Abbreviations: SS, Very slow; other abbreviations as in text or Table 13–3.

festations, on a functional level, that may be presented to therapists of various disciplines. Duration of symptoms in these cases ranged 6 months to 8 years.

The two prime factors or guidelines that serve as a basis for problem solving include the pattern of weakness and rate of progression. In our experience the rate of progression is often the most critical factor. Although there are wide variances in rate of progression among patients, individuals with PMA and PLS have not demonstrated the rapid progression that has been shown in some of our ALS and PBP patients.

Amyotrophic Lateral Sclerosis

Cases 1 through 5 (Table 13–3) outline functional problems characteristic of ALS based on pattern or extent of muscle weakness and rate of progression. Cases 1, 2, and 3 are each compared at 6 and 12 months, case 4 at 12 months, and case 5 at 30 months duration of symptoms.

Case 1 is a 66-year-old man with a fairly slow progression of ALS dominated at this period of his course (6 months duration) by lower motor neuron (LMN) signs of weakness and atrophy in the musculature of the right thenar eminence. Functionally, his problems focused on activities that required thumb opposition. Key factors to consider for independent function in these activities included whether splinting the hand and/or applying assistive devices, or applied use of stronger compensatory muscles to substitute for weakened ones, would be most suitable. The most common substitution pattern for assisting in thumb opposition is thumb interphalangeal flexion through use of the flexor pollicis longus muscle. Muscular fatigue, occupation (this individual was employed as an accountant), and the psychological aspects of accepting splints or devices must all be considered in the decision-making process. Six months later (at 12 months duration of symptoms), clinical weakness had progressed to include mild weakness of the right hand flexors and extensors as well as forearm muscles which caused increased difficulty in opening jars and turning keys in doors. The mild nature of this patient's difficulty at 12 months duration of symptoms makes him a slowly progressive case. Management guidelines for such a patient can be found in Chapter 14 of this volume.

Case 2 is a 54-year-old man who, compared to case 1 at 6 months duration, differs in the disease course in terms of both pattern of weakness and rate of progression. By 6 months all extremities manifested diffuse involvement with upper motor neuron symptoms dominating the clinical course. Consequently, spasticity more than weakness not only resulted in problems performing numerous activities but also caused physical discomfort as well. An increase in rate of progression when spasticity is present results in increased susceptibility to contracture development which further aggravates disability and loss of comfort. Early involvement of hand function (especially if bilateral) is particularly devastating and can result in loss of independence in early stages even if the rate of disease progression is slow. Anxiety and depression are also experienced with such rapid progression of symptoms. By 12 months duration this patient lost independent ambulatory function as well. Without any intervention this individual would be totally dependent in all activities of daily living. The severe physical and emotional strain on the patient's family and/or caretakers often results in their need for as much support as the patient. Chapters 14, 15, and 16 provide advice on physical management of such patients, and Chapters 18 through 20 provide guidance for psychological management.

Case 3, in contrast to cases 1 and 2, is 52-year-old woman whose rate of progression is more rapid. As in case 2, by 6 months duration the patient had diffuse involvement dominated by upper motor neuron (UMN) dysfunction. However, the extent of involvement of the extremities was greater in this patient, and in contrast to cases 1 and 2 she had bulbar involvement impeding communication (oral and written), as well as swallowing difficulties. By 12 months duration of symptoms she was essentially a spastic quadriplegic and anarthric. Not only was she unable to communicate verbally, but her writing ability was also severely impaired as well. Although ALS is physically and psychologically devastating in most forms, this patient had only eye and eyebrow movements, cervical spine:extension, lateral rotation, lateral flexion, and shoulder girdle elevation and depression preserved. Respiratory muscle function was also relatively unimpaired. A critical focus throughout the disease was to sustain her ability to communicate to allow for optimal medical care. Details on how to manage nutritional problems are found in Chapters 6, 9, 10, and 11, and details on treatment of communication difficulties are found in Chapters 14 and 17 of the present volume.

Case 4 describes a 62-year-old woman at 12 months duration whose function was severely restricted due to early progression of ALS into the respiratory musculature. Although she had sufficient motor function within her trunk and extremities to perform independent self-care, her activities became progressively restricted as she rapidly experienced progressive dyspnea, low endurance, and generalized fatigue. This was initially evident upon stair climbing and then eventually at rest. Fear and anxiety levels were high. In this case, the patient's pattern of weakness progressed early on into the respiratory muscles and caused life-threatening symptoms. In terms of total neuromuscular function the rate of progression of her illness was moderately slow. However, due to progression of weakness into respiratory muscles, close medical monitoring of her pulmonary symptoms were critical to prolonging her life. Details of management of breathing difficulty are found in Chapters 4, 5, and 15 and ethical considerations of this most serious symptom are discussed in Chapter 8.

Case 5 is a 33-year-old woman with moderately progressive ALS at 30 months duration. For discussion purposes, description of her functional limitations will focus on those problems arising from trunk weakness. In contrast to the cases discussed previously, in addition to bilateral upper extremity and bulbar dysfunction she had severe cervical spine extensor and flexor weakness. Upper spinal weakness, particularly, caused problems in all areas of function. Despite preservation of lower extremity and thoracolumbar spinal muscles at this stage, ambulation was significantly impaired due to lack of cervical head support. She also had insufficient upper extremity muscle strength bilaterally to support her head during ambulation. Maintaining head support was also difficult while sitting which caused problems in many activities, including eating, communicating, and reading. Postural compensation was only helpful occassionally. Consequently, a critical area of concern was to offer proper head support to sustain safe ambulation and for those activities performed while sitting to ensure comfort and optimal function. Details on how this can be accomplished are found in Chapters 14 and 15.

Progressive Muscular Atrophy

The following three cases have clinical manifestations of LMN signs only (see Table 13–4) and are each outlined and discussed at 18 months duration of symptoms. In our experience (although we have noted wide variances in pattern of weakness) the rate of progression, compared to that experienced by patients with ALS, is generally slower.

Case 6 is a 52-year-old male who at 18 months duration experienced weakness and atrophy distally in both the left upper and left lower extremity. He was considered slowly progressive since his disability was relatively mild. At this time he continued full-time self-employment in the taxi business. A prime consideration was to improve ambulatory function since safety in walking was impeded by a footdrop. To restore a normal heel–toe gait pattern a customized (as opposed to prefabricated) ankle–foot orthosis was considered. In this individual, in addition to psychological acceptance, the rate of progression was the prime determining factor in the selection of the most appropriate orthosis. Advice on orthoses selection for enhancing ambulatory function is to be found in Chapters 12, and 15 of the present volume.

Case 7 is a 66-year-old man with slow to moderately progressive PMA. His pattern presents greater proximal than distal weakness in both upper extremities; however, weakness in both lower extremities is strictly distal. At this time, swallowing was normal as bulbar function was unaffected. However, due to considerable weakness of the upper extremities, he was unable to feed himself. To enhance independence in self-feeding, one may consider selecting a sophisticated assistive feeding device since there would be ample opportunity for such a patient to use this device compared to a patient with rapidly progressive disease. In this patient, not only is the rate of progression a prime determining factor, but also family support in setting up the device. The patient may actually prefer to use compensation or substitution maneuvers. One must be mindful that eating can be a highly repetitive activity (as appetites and nutritional demands do vary among individuals). If a patient must compensate in self-feeding by using alternate muscle groups which may also be somewhat affected by the disease process, the repetitive nature of this activity may lead to fatigue of these compensatory muscles prior to completion of the meal. Management of feeding mechanics is discussed in Chapter 14.

Case 8 is a 63-year-old man with PMA of 18 months duration who was extraordinarily resourceful in using compensation mechanisms to sustain independence in many activities of daily living. Fortunately, within his upper extremities his hands were least affected, and both his trunk and lower extremities were normal. To maintain independence while shaving he hyperextended his trunk to establish forward momentum for arm swing (shoulder and elbow flexion) with gravity ultimately assisting elbow flexion, and by adducting his upper arm against his trunk he could stabilize his arm to shave himself. He remained free of contractures (a strong functional advantage) and through postural compensation with good balance he was able to independently bathe and shower and even carry a 10-pound table across the room.

Progressive Bulbar Palsy

Case 9 (see Table 13–5) is a 66-year-old woman with PBP at 36 months duration. In PBP since the initial symptoms occur in the bulbar musculature resulting in speech and swallowing difficulties, nonvocal communication ineviteably becomes necessary during the course of the illness. Since the extremities generally are not affected until the disease progresses well into the bulbar muscles, we have had patients with PBP who have remained functionally independent for long periods following the initial onset of symptoms. As bulbar manifestations are life threatening close medical monitoring is critical from early onset of symptoms. Although this patient's rate of progression at 36 months is fairly slow, patients with PBP have progressed at a moderate or rapid rate as well. Since the patient lived alone during this stage, a prime focus was to preserve communication through nonvocal means. Some critical concerns included signaling to a neighbor in the event of a fall or choking episode, and to enable her to have long-distance communication with family or friends involved in her care. Chapters 1, 6, 9, 10, 11, 14 and 17 detail ways of managing patients with bulbar problems.

Primary Lateral Sclerosis

Case 10 is a 70-year old man with clinical PLS (UMN signs only) with very slowly progressive disease of 96 months duration. Individuals with PLS can remain functionally independent for some time after the initial onset of symptoms as their rate of progression is generally slow. These patients are most bothered by dysarthria and dysphagia although spasticity causes problems where high energy expenditures are required in striving to remain active. Movement is considerably slowed which adds an appreciable amount of time to performing activities of daily living including self-care. A key focus in this patient was to sustain verbal speech as long as possible and reduce spasticity. Management of patients with spasticity is discussed in Chapters 1, 12, and 15 of the present volume.

It is evident that ALS and its varying forms present highly diverse clinical manifestations. The complexity of problems that arise on a physical and emotional level pose an ongoing challenge to therapists involved in assisting function and offering supportive counseling and care. To best plan for effective management therapists must establish when initial symptoms were manifested to acquire a sense of the rate of progression of the disease and must continually reassess muscle strength changes as the disease progresses. Management varies in slow versus rapidly progressive individuals, and among the varying forms of motor neuron disease, PMA and PLS have not shown the rapid rate of progression that has been demonstrated in some of our patients with ALS and PBP.

Therapists must also be careful not to attempt to service all of the needs of the ALS patient alone as this would be an overwhelming task (Those professionals who treat patients in the patients' homes are most susceptible to such feelings). Consulting with other professionals who are involved or who can potentially be involved in the care of ALS patients is not only rewarding and stimulating but also helps professionals to deliver optimal quality care.

REFERENCES

1. Brunnstrom S: Clinical Kinesiology. Davis, Philadelphia, 1972.

CHAPTER FOURTEEN

SELECTION OF ASSISTIVE DEVICES FOR PATIENTS WITH AMYOTROPHIC LATERAL SCLEROSIS

Valerie L. Takai, B.A., O.T.R.

All patients with amyotrophic lateral sclerosis (ALS) at some point during progression of symptoms in the disease will require assistive devices to maximize function. These aids also serve to promote comfort and to assist the caregiver in caring for the ALS patient. In treating ALS patients, occupational therapists are confronted with an ever-changing disability for which they are called upon to select the most appropriate aids. These may be commercially available, adapted commercial devices, or custom-made aids.

Through experience with a large and diverse ALS population it has been found that by thorough monitoring of self-care needs at 3-month intervals, patients' current equipment and orthotic needs can be met. In addition, anticipated problems and future needs can be dealt with in a timely manner.

In ALS, decisions for selection of these aids can be especially complex. Within the scope of this chapter general guidelines will be presented to assist with problem solving. Their purpose is to make the adjustment to each change in disability as smooth as possible and to avoid the consequences of faulty decisions. Choices for each adaptive aid must be made with the long-term picture in mind with thorough knowledge of individual rate of progression of symptoms and each individual's pattern of weakness. Basic to any consideration is the patient's knowledge and understanding of his disease. Patient and family input are critical for overall satisfaction and acceptance of devices. Any therapist providing or recommending equipment must not only be well informed about each particular aid, but must also be aware of its current availability. Accuracy of information about devices is extremely important. Dashed hopes due to false promises or expectations about a particular device can be devastating to a patient and detrimental to the quality of his life. It is well worth-

189

while to consider the principles outlined in this chapter when selecting the most suitable aids.

EVALUATION

Functional Assessment

Initially one must look at the individual functional profile. This is determined by the results of the current motor assessment. Through manual muscle and functional tests performed in conjunction with the physical therapist the extent of any weakness of the extremities, neck, and trunk may be noted. Other relevant factors include difficulties in speech and swallowing and any respiratory symptoms. Muscle tone and endurance are critical factors as well. In some patients increased tone may be more functionally limiting than weakness. Poor overall endurance may necessitate a wheelchair to conserve energy while ambulating long distances. It may also make the performance of routine self-care activities, such as dressing, too fatiguing and time-consuming (despite use of assistive devices) without the assistance of others.

In cases of severe weakness where only minimal motion is present, one may need to know the specifics of endurance and precision of small discrete movements such as the raising of an eyebrow or the slight turn of the head, if sophisticated technical aids are to be considered.

Second, rate of progression must be examined. When reviewing previous motor assessments, a slow, moderate, or rapid rate of progression can be determined for each individual patient. In cases of slow progression, few devices are needed, as compensatory techniques are often more beneficial. As an example, a patient with over 12 years disease duration exhibits only minimal weakness in the intrinsics of his left hand and a mild footdrop. He still works full-time as an accountant independent in activities of daily living (ADL) using a luggage cart to carry his attache case, a "handicapped person" parking sticker on his car to minimize walking when he visits clients, and a button hook to manage his right cuff button.

In cases of rapid progression many devices are needed within a very short period of time and decisions must be made without delay. One literally cannot afford to wait. For example, in a patient with a course of 4 months duration with total dependence in self-care and very limited ambulation, a bedside commode, hospital bed, patient lift and wheelchair may all be ordered simultaneously.

Determining Activities of Daily Living and Positioning Needs

Once the functional profile is known the occupational therapist must ascertain the needs of the patient in terms of ADL. The ADL evaluation emphasizes feeding, dressing, personal hygiene, management of object manipulation such as turning knobs, handles, and so on, mobility, communication, and leisure activities. Needs for positioning to improve comfort and function must also be determined. Considerations for orthotics and recommendations for support for seating (while keeping in mind appropriate standard furniture as well as wheelchairs) is necessary. Splints must be carefully selected. A splint applied to one part of the extremity to improve function should not compromise function of another part of the same extremity. Take the example of a patient with moderate shoulder and elbow weakness and mild to moderate weakness of wrist extensors and intrinsic hand muscles. Applying a thermoplastic splint to stabilize the thumb in opposition and support the wrist to better enable holding a fork and pen adds considerable weight to the extremity. While the patient should be trying to conserve energy, he or she is actually increasing energy expenditure, and the splint can impede the performance of the activity it was designed to assist. A more reasoned approach would be to adapt the feeding and writing utensils.

Most patients are able to directly state what problems they are having. Those who are familiar with their disease and are followed on a regular basis frequently request devices to perform specific activities. For instance, a patient may state that she has stopped playing bridge with her friends because her hand becomes fatigued when she holds the cards. She adds that she sometimes has difficulty turning the key in the ignition in her car. She asks about card holders and adaptations for keys. Those who are physically uncomfortable generally seek help for improving comfort and may request information on cushions, mattresses, neck supports, and the like.

From the functional profile, the occupational therapist can detect what specific areas of ADL and positioning to concentrate on during the evaluation. By noting the decreased grip strength and the beginning foot and hip weakness, questions may be posed about the patient's ability to open jars and safely get in and out of the tub. Observation is also important. The therapist notices the patient who 6 months ago had only bulbar involvement is now unable to keep his head up when standing for long periods of time due to the presence of neck extensor weakness. With much difficulty he tries to access the keyboard of his communication aid with individual finger movements but the development of finger extension weakness has slowed down his rate of communication. A hand-held typing stick to improve typing speed and a cervical collar to support fatigued neck extensors while standing are considered for trial with the patient prior to final selection.

Long-term ADL and positioning needs must also be assessed. Information about the physical setup of the home including steps, location of the bathroom, chairs, and so forth are needed to assist with long-range planning. In an individual with either slow or moderate progression who may have deterioration in ambulation, home modifications might be an important concern. These could include the conversion of outdoor steps into a ramp, the installation of a stair-glide, and the conversion of a bathroom with a tub into a roll-in shower. These modifications would initially help the patient to maintain independence as long as possible. In the future they would make it easier for others to care for the patient. In a rapidly progressive case such modifications would be inappropriate. Instead plans might have to be made for setting up a bedroom downstairs with an electric hospital bed and a bedside commode as well as arrangements made for spongebathing.

Setting Priorities

To help set priorities when determining assistive device needs, especially when there are time constraints and critical concerns need to be addressed immediately, three special areas of focus are suggested. These include positioning needs, safety, and communication.

With neck and trunk weakness problems may arise in balance for ambulation, discomfort in sitting, compromised respiration with decreased vocal output, and the potential development of spinal deformities. A common positioning problem involves severe proximal upper extremity weakness independent of or coexisting with lower extremity weakness. This can lead to shoulder subluxation, impaired balance in ambulation, and physical discomfort. With a padded clavicle support worn during ambulation many patients are able to ambulate without the discomfort of excess tension in the upper trapezius muscles that occurs when compensating for the weakened shoulder girdle muscles. Neck extensor weakness, if present, is another common positioning problem. A variety of cervical collars can be worn (depending upon the extent of weakness, atrophy, and other factors) to provide proper head support in the car, while ambulating, or sitting in a chair without high back support. An example (Fig. 14–1) shows a common positioning problem illustrated in the functional profile of marked neck extensor weakness and moderate thoracolumbar weakness which severely impeded ambulation. If they are able, patients such as this often use one upper extremity to support the head when

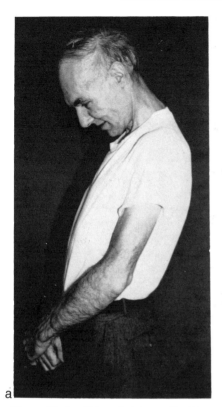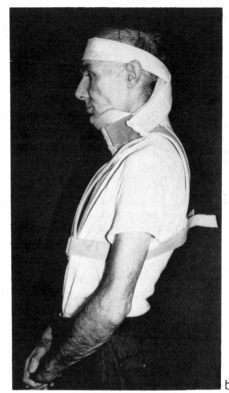

a   b

Figure 14–1. This ambulatory patient has severe neck and trunk weakness which impairs his balance. a. Posture of ALS patient prior to application of cervical orthosis. b. ALS patient wearing Plastazote and Kydex cervical brace with neck and chest straps and the addition of a head strap which enables him to stand erect.

walking. A Philadelphia collar does not provide sufficient support. Instead, a Plastazote cervical support reinforced with Kydex to which an adjustable head strap is added enables independent ambulation with the free use of both upper extremities.

Another positioning problem commonly encountered in ALS concerns trunk and neck weakness while sitting. It should be noted that a highback chair is not sufficient to relieve this fatigue when moderate or severe weakness is present unless the chair can also be reclined. Even in early stages of the disease it is frequently recommended to rest fatigued paraspinal and neck extensor muscles and to conserve energy so as to maximize their strength for activities involving walking and standing.

Safety is another area of special concern. Falls in the bathroom where patients are often unlikely to be wearing lower extremity orthoses in the presence of footdrop, or shoulder or neck supports for neck extensor or

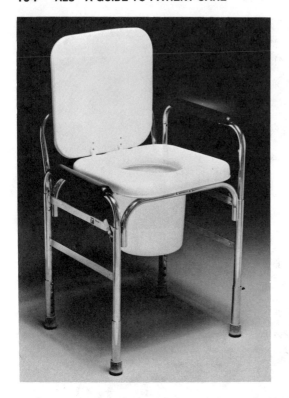

Figure 14–2. Padded drop-arm commode is adjustable in height to accommodate patients with proximal lower extremity weakness who have difficulty getting up from the toilet. (Courtesy of Tenco, Passaic, NJ.)

shoulder girdle weakness, can cause head injuries and fractures. Patients with weakened upper extremities are often unable to protect their heads during a fall and suffer facial injuries. Grab bars strategically placed are often suggested. Adjustable-height padded commodes (Fig. 14–2) are often recommended as they can be used over the toilet in early stages of the disease. Later on they can be used bedside for patients whose bathrooms prove to be inaccessible. Since lower extremity proximal weakness is present in so many ALS patients adjustable height is important for tub seats as well as commodes. Padded seats are important for comfort in those patients for whom atrophy is or may be a consideration in the future.

Communication is a third area of priority. All patients at some point in the course of their disease will encounter communication difficulties due to a variety of causes. These may involve problems of mobility, speech, writing, holding and turning pages of a book, using a telephone, or simply signaling for attention. Ignoring limitations in speech and ability to signal for attention only serves to foster feelings of isolation and abandonment. Total loss of ability to speak coupled with inability to write without any preparation for an alternative system of communication leaves the patient stranded in an unsupportable situation. The occupational therapist working with the speech pathologist can help assure the ALS patient that residual movement can be utilized in a variety of individual ways to help maintain communication. Careful planning is needed in this area to expose patients to augmentative communication aids while the patient is still able to use speech but requires supplementation for it to be intelligible. Small, simple aids such as the lettered cuff in Figure 14–3a, provided on the spot can help alleviate much anxiety and can help to introduce the benefits of augmentative communication.

PATIENT AND FAMILY INVOLVEMENT

From the very beginning, patients and their families are encouraged to engage in active problem solving. The occupational therapist acts as a resource for information concerning aids and solutions for specific problems. Patients and their families are often given simple materials such as cotton stockinette and foam for the fabrication of small cervical pillows, and small pieces of thermoplastics for the adaptations of small knobs on door locks, radios, and so forth. Many patients out of necessity, have designed their own zipper hooks and keyholders. Figure 14–3b shows just one of many unique devices created by ingenious patients. To a pendant with small black beads were added gold stick-on letters. This was designed by a children's librarian to augment her communication during her transition from using vocal to nonvocal communication. When she was not understood by the children seeking her assistance at the reference desk, she pointed to the first letter of the word she was trying to say. The therapeutic value of patients designing their own devices is not to be underestimated.

The acceptance of devices, especially complex technical aids, depends upon the family's acceptance as well as the patient's. In many cases it is the family who must set up the suspension feeder, adjust the placement of the infrared switch (Fig. 14–11a) which operates the electronic communication aid, or disassemble the motorized scooter to place it in the trunk of the car. It is highly recommended that patients have the opportunity to try each device before a final selection is made.

It is important that the patient retain autonomy even in the face of severe disability. In the ALS patient the perception of helplessness may be more devastating than the actual physical disability. With increasing weakness and the concurrent loss of independence there is a need to help

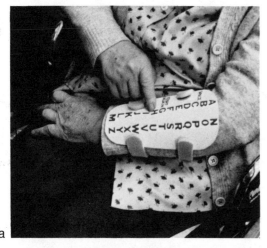

a

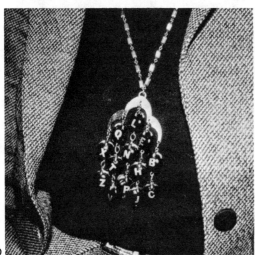

b

Figure 14–3. Communication aids enabling patient to point are often used by patients who are unable to write, but who are able to point with one hand for augmentative communication. a. Lettered cuff worn on forearm. b. Alphabet pendant designed by patient.

the ALS patient adjust to the necessary dependency and to seek help. Also, the family or caregiver need support and guidance. Devices such as patient lifters and electric hospital beds can simplify the family's task.

It has been observed that ALS patients who live alone are often in more desperate need for specific aids even if only of limited or questionable use in order to maintain their independence as long as possible. This is also true for the patient who is home alone during the day while the spouse is at work and will go to all lengths to maintain self-sufficiency so as not to have to hire outside help or force their spouse to stop working. Patients must be confronted when they are placing their health and safety at risk. If weakness progresses to a point where no appropriate device exists that will enable a specific individual to function alone, outside help must be obtained.

ASSISTIVE DEVICE FEATURES

In selecting devices for ALS patients there are several features to keep in mind. For any device that is worn or lifted by the patient, weight is an important concern. This is very true for orthotics, built-up utensils, light-beam head pointers, communication aids mounted on rolling walkerettes, and so on. Light weight is also needed in clothing. Amyotrophic lateral sclerosis patients with marked atrophy along with decreased mobility are especially sensitive to weight and wrinkles in clothing. Thus running suits and quilted jackets are preferred attire for many patients. Any devices that are close to the skin, such as orthotics, cushions, or mattresses, are more comfortable if soft in texture. It has been our experience that patients are generally quite uncomfortable with gel cushions or air mattresses preferring soft foam and synthetic or natural sheepskin.

An additional important feature is the potential for modification to meet future needs. This is especially significant when considering wheelchairs and sophisticated communication aids. A patient whose insurance has already paid for a standard adult wheelchair will probably not be covered if a reclining wheelchair is later needed when neck and trunk weakness become evident. There is no way to convert a standard wheelchair to a reclining one. A portable communication aid with speech output and or a printer without the option for single-switch control will be useless to a patient when he can no longer access the keyboard by direct selection utilizing remaining motor function.

Closely related to this principle of modification is the idea of versatility for a particular device. For example, for many with proximal upper extremity weakness the suspension sling on a locking IV pole is helpful for feeding, grooming, typing, and turning pages. It can be used with either upper extremity while in a regular chair, upholstered recliner, the wheelchair, or a hospital bed. It has often been used for assistive range of motion exercises.

With any devices, not excluding highly sophisticated technical aids, it is important to select systems which the individual is able to use without extensive training. Devices should be relatively simple to set up and easy to maintain. Any device that is burdensome to learn or to set up to the patient and the caregiver does not meet the patient's needs.

ORTHOTICS

Commercial orthotics found to be beneficial to ALS patients include cervical collars, clavicle supports, wrist supports, and suspension slings (Tables 14–1 and 14–3).

With early weakness of hand intrinsics in slowly progressive cases a custom-made short opponens splint may be indicated for activities requiring very fine prehension such as holding a needle. It has been our experience that most patients would prefer a device for a specific task, such as a button hook or a bookholder, to a custom-made splint. Another problem with custom-made orthoses is that progressive atrophy changes the fit and comfort of a contoured splint and necessitates frequent modification or replacement. In slowly progressive cases patients often compensate for weakened intrinsics via stronger compensatory movements and rarely require devices or a splint to improve function. Elastic wrist braces made of soft fabric are comfortable and are used with ALS patients with a weak wrist and hand to better enable holding ambulation aids and various utensils. They are readily available and relatively inexpensive.

Padded clavicle supports are used for the ambulatory patient with severe proximal upper extremity weakness especially when it is bilateral. They are often worn over clothing so that they can be easily put on and removed. In such cases, a larger size than the normal fit is needed. When cosmesis is a critical factor they are worn under regular clothing.

Neck weakness may be initially noticed while sitting in a moving vehicle or ambulating long distances due to increased demand on cervical extensor movements. In cases of moderate extensor weakness open cervical collars can improve balance in ambulation. The wire frame collar is easy to adjust by bending it by hand to get the desired angle of flexion. These collars are suitable for patients with neck weakness who also have

Table 14–1. Commonly Used Commercial Orthoses

Neck	Soft foam collar with back closure
	Philadelphia collar
	Open leather-covered wire frame collar
	Open Kydex frame collar with Plastazote padding
Neck and upper trunk	Plastazote and Kydex cervical brace with neck and chest straps and opening for tracheostomy
Shoulders	Padded clavicle support
Wrist	Elastic wrist brace

Table 14–2. Commonly Used Small Assistive Devices

Feeding	Lightweight built-up handles (to be used with standard or plastic flatware) Plastic Chinese soup spoon Plate guard Rocker knife Universal cuff Flexible and rigid plastic straws Lightweight mugs with easy-grip handles Insulated mug with snorkel lid
Dressing	Button hook Velcro Zipper loops Zipper hook Dressing stick Suspenders Long-handled shoehorn
Personal hygiene	Wash mitt Soap on a rope Lightweight built-up handles (to be used with brush, comb, toothbrush, razor and nail file) Long-handled sponge
Homemaking and meal preparation	Long-lever jar opener with adapted turning knob Adapted paring board Twist-off bottle opener Milk carton holder
Miscellaneous	Doorknob extension lever Light switch extension lever Adapted keyholder Self-opening scissors Lightweight reachers Small pieces of thermoplastics used to adapt small knobs Card holder
Positioning	4-in.-high-density foam cushion Transfer board Wheelchair lap tray Wheelchair bean bag lap desk Head strap (utilized with cervical collars and cervical pillows) Convoluted foam pad for bed/wheelchair Synthetic/natural sheepskin for bed/wheelchair Cervical pillow Foam bed wedge pillow

Table 14–3. Recommended Durable Medical Equipment

Bathroom equipment	Wall-mounted grab bar
	Tub-mounted grab bar
	Raised toilet seat
	Padded height-adjustable drop arm commode
	Padded height-adjustable bath seats and transfer tub benches
	Rolling commode/shower transport chair
	Showerall
Mobility aids	Lightweight manual wheelchair
	Semireclining or fully reclining manual wheelchair
	Add-on power unit for manual wheelchair
	Motorized scooter with height-adjustable seat and adjustable tiller
	Fully reclining powered wheelchair with proportional control
	Wheeled padded recliner
	Glideabout/transport chair
	Mechanical patient lifter with full-body commode sling
Hospital bed	Manual
	Electric
Other	Akros DFD mattress/wheelchair cushion.
	Overbed table with tilting top
	Suspension sling on locking IV pole or on overhead rod for wheelchair
	Electric seat lift recliner

tracheostomies (Fig. 14–4). For patients who are nonambulatory with moderate or severe neck weakness a reclining wheelchair or upholstered recliner are essential (Fig. 14–5). When such patients need to sit upright a head strap, often in conjunction with a cervical collar, can help to maintain good positioning of the head for such activities as reading, watching television, and so forth.

Balanced forearm orthoses, while essentially designed for wheelchair use, are rarely used as they require frequent adjustment due to changing muscle strength and positioning needs. We have found suspension feeders which provide a supinator assist and suspension slings that attach to a locking IV pole to be more beneficial. They are relatively easy to set up, and as mentioned earlier, are very versatile.

Table 14–1 through 14–5 list many of the assistive devices and commercial orthoses that have benefited an ALS population of over eight hundred patients at Mount Sinai Hospital. Their purpose is to offer a starting point for those involved in assisting patients with selecting appropriate aids. Many of the devices in Table 14–2 are provided to patients while

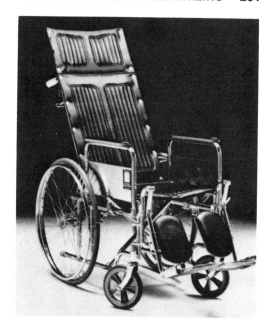

Figure 14–4. This full-reclining wheelchair is the most commonly recommended wheelchair. It has removable full-length armrests and swinging detachable elevating legrests. It allows full support of fatiqued paraspinal and neck extensor muscles and elevation of the lower extremities which is important for alleviating dependent edema.

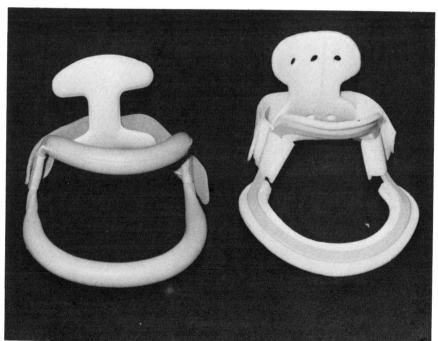

Figure 14–5. Both these collars are lightweight. Open leather-covered wire frame collar (left). Open Kydex frame collar with Plastazote padding (right).

Table 14–4. Examples of Communication Aids

Nonelectronic devices	
Function	
Writing	Triangular pencil grip
	Hand-held typing stick
	Mouthstick for typing
	Headstick for typing
Reading	Bookholder
	Reading table or stand (adjustable height and tilt for bed and recliner)
	Rubber thimble
	Hand-held page turner
	Mouth-held page turner
	Hospital overbed table with tilting top
Telephoning	Shoulder rest for receiver
	Hand-held telephone dialer
Signaling	Classroom bell
	Dinner bell
	Medical emergency bracelet
Conversation (for nonspeakers)	Magic slate
	Assorted letterboards including lettered cuff
	Pointing aids to access displays
	Hand pointers
	Headsticks
	Foot pointers
	Etran and other eye-gaze communication boards
Electronic devices	
Function	
Writing	Voice-activated tape recorders (for speakers)
	Electronic typewriters
	Personal computers (hand-held and desktop)
Reading	Talking books
	Geewa page turner (with scanning option)
Signaling	Portable battery-operated buzzers with option for alternative switches
	Alarms built into augmentative communication aids
	Intercoms
	Emergency alarm systems
Telephoning	Operator headsets
	Speakerphones with automatic dialer
	Hands-free automatic telephone
	TTYs (teletypewriters for nonspeakers)
Augmentative communication*	Texas Instruments (Lubbock, Tx)
	Speak and Spell

Table 14–4. *(cont)*

Electronic devices	
Function	
Augmentative communication*	Adaptive Communication Systems (Pittsburgh, PA)
	ACS Speech Pac/Epson with combo tape
	Prentke Romrich Company
	(Wooster, OH)
	Viewpoint Optical Indicator
	Touch Talker/Light Talker
	Words +, Inc. (Sunnyvale, CA)
	Woods + Living Center III
	Zygo Industries (Portland, OR)
	Scanwriter
	Tetrascan

*Individual device features such as operating technique, language content, communication outputs, portability, and so on are described in Features of Commercially Available Communication Devices, a chart developed by Arlene Kraat and Marsha Sitver-Kogut of the Queens College Augmentative Communication Center in Flushing, New York in February 1985. For the most current information on these devices it is recommended that the reader contact the companies listed.

Table 14–5. Other Commonly Used Assistive Devices

Lightweight electric toothbrush
Water Pik
Lightweight electric razor
Shampoo rinse tray for bed
Bidet with options for foot switch and raised toilet seat
Stairglide
Wheelchair lift
Portable ramp
Van adapted for wheelchair passenger
Upholstered recliner
Highback office chair on wheels
Queen-size and king-size nonhospital electric beds

in the ALS clinic. Most of the durable medical equipment in Table 14–3 is covered by third-party payers. Table 14–5 lists devices that patients have generally obtained on their own without insurance coverage. The orthoses in Table 14–1 are usually fitted in the ALS clinic. Table 14–4 helps to give an idea of the wide range of communication devices.

This section describes the main functional problems in carrying out ADL activities and potential solutions through the use of assistive devices.

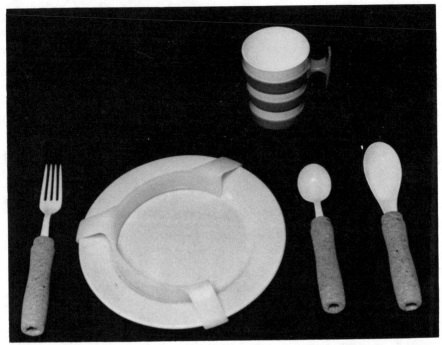

Figure 14-6. Eating equipment adapted to the needs of ALS patients. Lightweight plastic fork and spoon, and Chinese soup spoon have cork fishing rod handles which are often helpful for patients with impaired grasp and pinch. The plate guard is used to assist the patient with getting food onto the utensil. The plastic mug has an easy-grip handle.

DEVICES FOR SPECIFIC ACTIVITIES

Feeding

A common problem in ALS is difficulty holding utensils due to intrinsic hand muscle weakness. Built-up handles are often helpful when compensatory techniques are not possible (Fig. 14–6). Commercial elastic wrist braces are beneficial when the wrist supported in extension improves finger flexion. Proximal weakness may be more limiting than distal weakness preventing the patient from getting hand to mouth. Elevating the plate and forearm used in feeding can facilitate feeding in those with moderate and sometimes severe shoulder abductor weakness as long as sufficient elbow flexion and forearm rotation is present. Suspension feeders with supinator assist and suspension slings also can be of assistance for this problem. Extended plastic straws with large openings and lightweight mugs with easy grip handles are often used. Electronic feeders may be of assistance to those without sufficient upper extremity function and where dysphagia is not a problem. However, these devices are expensive and are not covered by third-party payers.

Dressing

With intrinsic hand muscle weakness come problems with fastening. Zipper loops and button hooks are two of the most utilized devices (Fig. 14–7a). There are many ALS patients who restrict fluid intake while at work to avoid using the bathroom because they are unable to manage a simple zipper. Many have found mass market items with velcro fastenings such as watchbands, wallets, shoes and other clothing to be of assistance to the caregiver as well as the patient. Spasticity is often more of a problem on arising in the morning and can make dressing more difficult than when performed later on in the day. Many times it may be more expedient for the person with ALS who takes an excessively long period of time to get dressed before going to work to have assistance with this task to conserve energy for other tasks.

Personal Hygiene

One of the most humiliating losses in ALS can be the impaired ability to wash, shave, and wipe oneself. Early on this problem should be addressed so that patients can be prepared to accept help when devices are no longer a feasible solution. Built-up handles on toothbrushes and shavers are useful for many with intrinsic muscle weakness. Sitting for grooming and oral hygiene is often recommended to help minimize fatigue in weakened shoulder muscles. Small lightweight electric razors, electric toothbrushes with built-up handles, and a water pik are often beneficial, initially for the patient, and later on for the caregiver.

A patient who is fully ambulatory with very limited function of either upper extremity may appear to the average onlooker to be suffering little disability. For many with such a functional profile a bidet with a foot operated switch has increased their independence in toileting and lessened the psychological discomfort when others must assist in this activity.

Object Manipulation

Difficulty with fine manipulative tasks, such as tuning keys or small lamp switches, television knobs, and so forth is due to intrinsic hand and

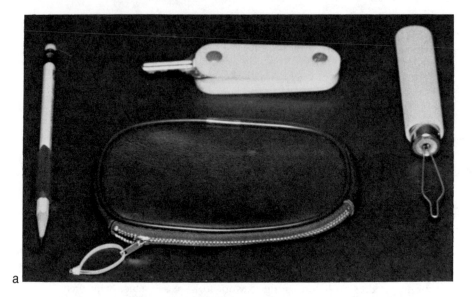

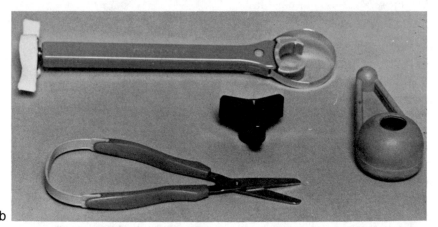

Figure 14–7. a. These small devices assist in activities requiring fine precision. (Left to right) triangular pencil grip, zipper loop, keyholder, button hook. b. These small devices assist with opening jars, turning on lights, opening doors, and cutting for those with impaired grasping and pinching ability. (Left to right) long lever jar opener with adapted turning knob, self-opening scissors, light switch extension lever, rubber doorknob extension lever.

or forearm muscle weakness. In ALS patients with a slow rate of progression, devices for these tasks are rarely needed as patients are able to make use of compensatory techniques. In other patients with mild and moderate intrinsic weakness, special keyholders, adapted knobs and doorknob extenders can be beneficial (Fig. 14–7b).

Mobility

When ambulation is no longer possible for long distances, a wheelchair should be considered. Rate of progression, pattern of weakness, and form of ALS are important factors to consider. As upper extremity weakness and limited endurance often coexist with lower extremity weakness, self-propulsion of manual wheelchairs is often not feasible, or, at best, very limited. In slowly or moderately progressive cases with good upper extremity function and good overall endurance, patients are able to maneuver manual wheelchairs independently. A lightweight wheelchair can assist the caregiver who may frequently be a frail spouse. In moderately progressive cases where neck and trunk weakness are not evident, a standard wheelchair may be considered as a temporary or short-term solution. In rapidly progressive cases a semi-reclining or full-reclining wheelchair is the wheelchair of choice. (Fig. 14–5). In a very slowly progressive case, a reclining wheelchair may not be needed for many years, if at all. Elevating legrests are needed for those who have a tendency to develop dependent edema and who spend most of the day in the wheelchair.

Wheelchairs are not comfortable for many ALS patients. The cushions found to provide the most comfort are high-density foam. The only air-filled cushion we have found to be of assistance to a few patients is the Roho cushion. Most ALS patients cannot tolerate gel, simple air, or water-filled cushions. However, some tolerate well the Akros DFD wheelchair cushion, a combination of foam and gel. Many find that small cushions behind the small of the back add comfort as does a small cervical roll at the nape of the neck.

It has been our experience that even when ALS patients can be accommodated in a narrow adult wheelchair, most prefer a standard adult size that affords increased trunk mobility with more sitting space.

For many patients the wheelchair simply serves as a vehicle to transport them from room to room or to take them places outside the home. Indoors they prefer to spend their time sitting and sometimes sleeping in an upholstered recliner. Others are comfortable in an upholstered reclining geriatric chair. Still others gradually accommodate to the wheelchair after an initial adjustment period. In rapidly progressive cases psychological factors such as anxiety contribute to the poor tolerance for sitting in the wheelchair.

For the patient who is too heavy for the caregiver to transfer alone a mechanical lift can be of assistance for transporting the patient from bed to wheelchair to upholstered recliner, commode, and so forth.

For a select group of ALS patients motorized wheelchairs and scooters have been of assistance, especially at work. Selection of such chairs is highly individualized and depends on the individual pattern of weakness and rate of progression. Safety is an extremely important consideration in selecting a motorized scooter. Scooters have been used most with patients who have less of a problem with neck and trunk weakness and good upper extremity function. A self-regulating height-adjustable seat is a feature to consider for those with proximal hip weakness. An adjustable-angle tiller is another necessary feature to ensure good positioning of arm and forearm, minimizing proximal upper extremity motion.

Add-on power units have become available that are lightweight and joystick-operated with proportional controllers. They fit most manual wheelchairs and some feature special bracketry for reclining wheelchairs. They are simple to install, relatively portable, and can often be rented.

For those who are severely disabled, whose disease is relatively stable, and, who may also be on a ventilator, more customized power wheelchairs should be considered. Chin control, foot control, sip-and-puff as well as joystick control, and a rack to support a ventilator are options to keep in mind.

Many ALS patients and their families have found a van the most practical form of transportation for long trips and well worth the investment to enable the person with ALS to lead an active life outside the home and in the community.

Communication

Assistive devices for communication are notable for their diversity and high degree of individuality. They must meet the broad spectrum of communication needs, namely writing, reading, telephoning, signaling for attention, and conversation. Emergency alarm, computer access, and environmental control may also be included. These devices range from everyday items such as magic slates and classroom bells to highly complex technical aids. Each one should be selected keeping in mind the uniqueness of the individual whose needs are to be met. There is no one device that can meet all these diverse needs. Most likely each individual ALS patient will require several devices.

Table 14–4 lists examples of commercially available aids and custom-made aids that are simple to construct such as letterboards and pointers. Its purpose is to introduce some of the aids that have proved beneficial to a large diverse population of ALS patients.

While some with ALS may lose their ability to rely on oral speech to communicate, there are others who maintain this function. However, they most likely will encounter communication difficulties due to impaired upper extremity function or immobility from lower extremity weakness.

Writing

Writing aids are important for the patient with spoken and or written communication difficulties. In patients with beginning fatigue of hand intrinsics, a triangular plastic pencil grip on a pen or pencil can prolong the ability to write. When writing is no longer feasible with regular writing utensils and their adaptations, typing may be a possibility on light-touch keyboards with typing sticks for the hand, head, or mouth. For those with intelligible speech for whom writing or typing with or without devices is not possible or impractical there are voice-activated tape recorders. These have proved beneficial for writing articles, letters, and memos, and have helped individuals with ALS to continue productive pursuits.

Reading

Reading becomes difficult when it is fatiguing to hold a book and to turn pages. There are wide range of bookholders available for use on regular tables or on stands which can be tilted for the individual reading in bed or in a recliner. When it is not easy to turn pages with a simple device, talking books from the Public Library are a consideration. For those who select an electronic page turner it is important to choose one that can be operated by a single switch, and, if desirable by the user, handle a variety of reading material. Above all it should be reliable, and easy to set up and operate. It should be able to be tilted so that no matter where the patient is sitting or lying the reading material is within the patient's field of vision.

Telephoning

There are a wide selection of mass-market, commercially available telephone products that are beneficial to the individual with impaired ability to dial, hold a receiver, converse, and answer an incoming call. These include automatic dialers, speakerphones, and operator headsets, and even an automatic hands-free telephone (Fig. 14–8) which when set on automatic opens the telephone line after two rings. When the caller hangs up the line automatically closes. Such a feature helps to relieve the anxiety experienced by patients and their caregivers when the patient must be left alone for short periods of time. Thus, the patient's spouse or caregiver can call the patient without the need for the patient to ever touch a button.

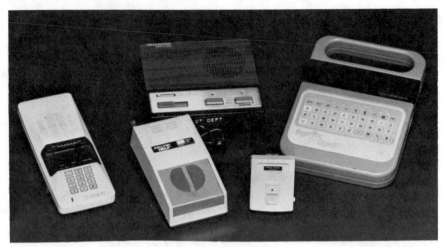

Figure 14–8. There are many electronic communication aids found on the consumer mass market that can be beneficial to ALS patients. Some examples are (left to right) Tranbon automatic automatic hands-free telephone, Call for Help (receiver and signaler), Panasonic speakerphone, and Speak and Spell.

Teletypewriters for the deaf have occasionally been used with ALS patients without intelligible speech who have good hand function. They can communicate regularly with family members who must have the same or comparable device in order to communicate with one another by telephone.

Signaling

For those who due to inability to speak are unable to call out for attention, or due to impaired mobility are not always within earshot, there are several signaling systems available. A medical emergency bracelet is useful for the patient who is unable to effectively communicate by speech or by writing and who goes out of the house alone. It contains important medical information should an emergency arise and the individual with ALS be unable to communicate his special needs. Portable intercoms between individual rooms and portable battery-operated buzzers (Fig. 14–9) enable patients to be left unattended so that those in other parts of the home can be reached by the sound of a voice or the activation of a buzzer. Emergency alarm systems are also available. Some may be used to contact a close neighbor. Others activate a unit attached to the telephone which when a small button worn on the wrist or around the neck is pressed, automatically dials a 24 hr monitoring station to summon help.

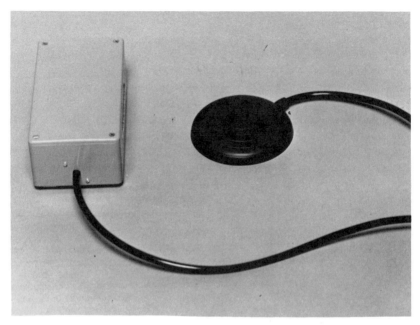

Figure 14–9. Tone caller with flat air cushion switch. This portable buzzer has a variable tone which can be heard over ambient sounds such as those coming from a television or running water. It is very easy to set up and the light touch switch can be activated with minimal pressure from upper and lower extremity and head movements. (Courtesy of Arroyo & Associates, Inc., New York, NY)

Augmentative Communication

Occupational therapists working in conjunction with speech pathologists gradually introduce augmentative communication devices as speech intelligibility deteriorates. By following patients at regular 3-month intervals there is sufficient time to prepare patients and their families for the eventuality of dependence on alternative methods of communication.

As with other assistive devices, patients and their families are encouraged to assist with the selection of suitable communication aids. With help from the patient and guidance from a therapist, many families have been able to make communication boards with supplies provided. Careful motor assessment is needed prior to selection of any communication aid. This involves not only assessment of upper and lower extremity, head, and facial movement, but also eye movement.

Recent experience with ALS patients and reports in the literature indicate that there can be oculomotor abnormalities in ALS, and that these deficits are more common than previously suspected. Most common are deficits in ocular pursuit (the ability to follow a moving target). Clear-cut

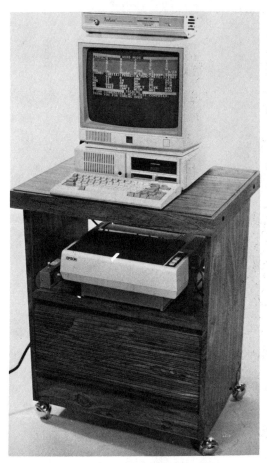

Figure 14–10. Words + Living Center III (IBM-compatible version). This communication system designed for single-switch users utilizes a personal computer with special software, a printer, and a speech synthesizer. It is a multifunctional device with potential for playing games, drawing, controlling appliances, and signaling with an alarm. These functions are in addition to talking through a voice synthesizer and writing on a screen or on a printer. It allows communication by selection from a stored vocabulary and phrase list. Words not in the vocabulary may be stored letter by letter. The user can add or delete vocabulary in the memory which has a capacity for storage of over 1300 words. (Courtesy of Words +, Inc., Sunnyvale, CA)

opthalmoplegia is relatively rare.[1] Thus the characteristics of visual displays are an important concern when selecting sophisticated technical aids.

It has been commonly observed that many patients who must rely on augmentative communication systems have difficulty parting with a motor function that is no longer expedient in permitting communication. For example, ALS patients may insist on writing with much difficulty when another mode of communication, such as pointing to letters, would improve their speed of communication. Patients need to prepare for changes in motor function by gradually employing better preserved and more efficient movements. By introducing other alternatives at the same time, the patient is given the opportunity to gradually part with the residual function that is no longer expedient. For example, in conjunction with a magic

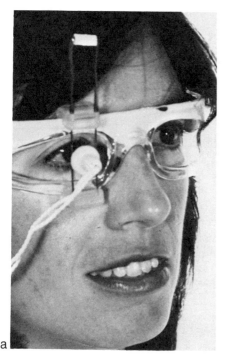
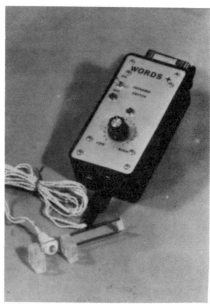

a

b

Figure 14–11. Words + infrared switch is an example of a highly sensitive switch which can employ isolated finger, foot, arm, head, eyelid, or eye movement to operate a communication device. a. Infrared switch mounted on an eyeglasses frame. b. sensitivity of switch may be adjusted to accommodate slight changes in force of movement. (Courtesy of Words +, Inc., Sunnyvale, CA)

slate to which a border of letters and some key conversational phrases such as ''wait,'' ''end of sentence,'' and so on have been added, pointing and writing may be employed using the same transitional aid. There is an intimacy and uniqueness with the simple manual systems that is hard to simulate in the electronic aids. Manual communication systems demand the undivided attention of the communication partner. When examining rate of communication it should be noted that utilizing a manual scanning or manual pointing board is often the fastest way of carrying on a conversation. It allows the message receiver to anticipate and assist the nonvocal individual by constructing words and sentences from the cues received. This feature is not possible with current electronic aids and it is unlikely that the communication rates possible with manual aids can be achieved with electronic devices in the near future.[2]

Today there are several commercially available dedicated and computer-based communication devices with keyboard and single (and multiple) switch input that are suitable for ALS patients. Only 5 years ago, if an ALS patient, whose limited motor capabilities required single-switch input, wished to use a personal computer, custom software had to be designed for a scanning program. Now, besides the visual display and printed output, many devices have synthesized speech output (Fig. 14–10). Some of the dedicated communication devices, such as Scanwriter, Tetrascan, and the Express series have keyboard emulation capability. This enables the single-switch (or multiple-switch) user to bypass the regular keyboard of a second computer which runs regular software (Fig. 14–11). Some of our patients with speech difficulties had been computer users before developing ALS. Having computer access with a communication device can be an important option. To enhance communication rate a variety of strategies have been incorporated into communication aids. The ACS Speech Pac/Epson employs logical letter coding, a form of linguistic prediction. A semantic pictographic code (Minspeak) is utilized in the Light Talker to encode sentences and phrases.

Portability is an especially important consideration for ambulatory patients and for those who wish to take their communication system with them outside the home. This is an area that is rapidly improving with both the dedicated and the computer-based devices.

In selecting any communication aid the patient's daily living routine and 24 hr positioning needs, communication partners and personal messaging needs must all be considered. The motor assessment is performed to determine which movements are most accurate, efficient and least fatiguing. It also helps to determine the type of control and the most suitable location of switches for accurate and efficient interface control. Any sophisticated device should have the potential to meet anticipated deterioration in motor function. Training and customization should be kept to a minimum, and, the system should be ready to use at the time of delivery.[3]

FACTORS OF COST AND AVAILABILITY, SUPPORT SERVICES, AND COMMUNITY RESOURCES

Just as one cannot predict the order of progression of symptoms or duration of disease in an individual patient, it is also impossible to predict the total financial cost of caring for an ALS patient. Underlying every decision about assistive devices is the question of cost and insurance coverage. Third-party payers, including the Muscular Dystrophy Association and the patient's own insurer, cover many assistive devices. However, there is the factor of loss of income for the patient no longer able to work. There may also be a need for the spouse to leave a job to care for the patient as well as expenses for home health aides. All of these factors make it difficult for many to commit funds to pay for specific devices or home modifications which may only be used by the patient for a limited period of time. It is very important that patients be given accurate information about cost and funding so that they can make informed decisions.

We have found that there are many devices in the mass market that can improve function and comfort. Some of these, mentioned earlier are special telephones, upholstered recliners, and personal computers used for communication devices. The fact that they can be shared by other family members may be a consideration in selecting them over devices which are only of use to the patient.

Rental and loan from an equipment pool as well as purchase are options to consider.

It is important for therapists to have accurate knowledge of availability of specific devices to help with the decision-making process. This is especially true for any device that requires customization or a long approval process for payment from the third-party payer. New devices still in the developmental phase are known to have delays in the completion date and may not be ready in time for the individual ALS patient to ever use them.

Patients and their families need to know about individual warranties and servicing. Especially with complex technical aids, they need to know whom to direct their inquiries to when problems arise. If servicing is known to be a problem with a particular aid, perhaps a different device should be selected.

It is strongly recommended that all patients to be registered with the ALS Association and the Muscular Dystrophy Association and to also seek out local resources for the disabled in their own community. We at the Mount Sinai ALS Clinic have been fortunate to work closely with these two organizations as well as Queens College Augmentative Communication Center and Project Open House for meeting the special needs of ALS patients.

SUMMARY AND CONCLUSION

It is important from the initial stages of ALS that patients be seen by an occupational therapist to monitor ADL needs throughout the course of the illness. The goal of assistive devices is to enhance function and quality of life. Another goal is to ease the burden of the caregiver in caring for the patient.

Timing the introduction of specific devices such as bathroom equipment, wheelchairs, and complex technical aids is geared to each individual's pattern of weakness and rate of progression. Also under consideration from past experiences with the patient is that individual's ability to plan and to adapt. Patient and family are treated as a unit and are actively involved in the selection process.

Cost and availability are critical factors, especially with the highly technical aids for which there is rarely insurance coverage. Two very basic issues today regarding assistive devices are getting the appropriate devices to the people who need them, and paying for them.[4] A third issue is getting the devices to those with a progressive disability quickly while they may still make use of them.

It is my personal philosophy that no patient attending an ALS clinic should leave without receiving something, be it a specific device, a source of information, or a suitable solution to a problem.

REFERENCES

1. Cohen B, Caroscio JT: Eye movements in amyotrophic lateral sclerosis. J Neural Transm (Suppl)19:305–315, 1983.
2. Vanderheiden GC: Technology needs of individuals with communication impairments. Semin Speech Lang 5(1):63, 1984.
3. Beukelman DR, Yorkston KM, Dowden PA: Communication Augmentation: A Casebook of Clinical Management. College Hill Press, San Diego, CA, 1984, p. 109.
4. Dixon GL, Enders A: Low cost approaches to technology and disability. In Rehabilitation Research Review, Vol. 19. D:ATA Institute, Catholic University of America, Washington, DC, 1984, p. 3.

BIBLIOGRAPHY

Beukelman DR, Yorkston KM: Computer enhancement of message formulation and presentation for communication augmentation users. Semin Speech Lang 5(1):1–10, 1984.
Braile LE: Support for the dropping head. Am J Occup Ther 35(2):661–662, 1981.
Brammell CA: Assistive devices for patients with neuromuscular diseases: The role of occupational therapy. In Maloney FP, Burks JS, Ringel SP (eds): Interdisciplinary Rehabilitation of Multiple Sclerosis and Neuromuscular Disorders. Lippincott, Philadelphia, 1985, pp. 259–276.
Brammel CA, Maloney FP: Wheelchair prescriptions. In Maloney FP, Burks JS, Ringel SP (eds): Interdisciplinary Rehabilitation of Multiple Sclerosis and Neuromuscular Disorders. Lippincott, Philadelphia, 1985, pp. 364–391.
Charlebois-Marois C: Everybody's Technology: A Sharing of Ideas in Augmentative Communication. Charlecoms, Montreal, Canada, 1985.
Enders A: Questionable devices. In Proceedings of Special Sessions of Second International Conference on Rehabilitation Engineering, Ottawa, Canada, 1984, pp. 271–276

Hayle E (ed): The Source Book for the Disabled. Bantam, New York, 1981.

Sabari J: The roles and functions of occupational therapy services for the severely diasbled. Am J Occup Ther 37(12):811–813, 1983.

Webster JG, Cook AM, Tompkins WJ, et al. (ed): Electronic Devices for Rehabilitation. Wiley, New York, 1985.

Woltosz W: Personal computers as augmentative communication aids. Commun Outlook 5(4):4–7, 1984.

CHAPTER FIFTEEN

EXERCISE, AMBULATION, AND PULMONARY PHYSICAL THERAPY FOR THE AMYOTROPHIC LATERAL SCLEROSIS PATIENT

Janet Zawodniak, B.S. P.T.

The purpose of a physical therapist in an interdisciplinary amyotrophic lateral sclerosis (ALS) team is to help individuals afflicted with ALS to physically function to their maximal neuromuscular capabilities in the presence of progressive neuromuscular degeneration. Since there is no cure for ALS, physical therapists play a critical role in recommending and monitoring therapeutic exercise regimens, optimizing ambulatory function, and assisting in pulmonary management.

The quality of life of the ALS patient can be greatly enhanced, particularly if therapy is instituted soon after the diagnosis is established. Early intervention is most beneficial for optimizing strength, function, and physical comfort.

EXERCISE IN AMYOTROPHIC LATERAL SCLEROSIS

Therapeutic exercise in ALS is beneficial to optimize maximal muscular strength and function within the limitations of the progressive disease process. It also serves to prevent complications such as contractures and disuse weakness.

Commonly asked questions by therapists who are involved in exercising ALS patients include: Is exercise helpful or harmful? What is the appropriate intensity, duration, and frequency of an exercise program? How do I know if I am insufficiently or excessively exercising my patients?

Due to the limited amount of clinical study in ALS, the effects of strengthening exercises were largely unknown and controversial. Consequently, recommended programs were largely empirically based and required cautious judgment. This is understandable since as therapists exercise patients any improvement induced by exercise is usually offset by progressive weakness with the ongoing loss of motor neurons.[1] Prevailing schools of thought have been to advocate activities of daily living alone (unless the disease is slowly progressive),[2] or to advocate frequent participation in active exercise programs as long as overfatigue is avoided.[3,4]

Experience in exercise program design for over eight hundred ALS patients that have attended the Mount Sinai Amyotrophic Lateral Sclerosis Clinic has resulted in the establishment of important parameters to consider when planning exercise programs. These include: the pattern, extent, and rate of progression of muscle weakness, daily activity, and fatigue levels, as well as general physical condition (including coexisting medical problems, if any) and psychological outlook. Due to wide variance in pattern, rate, and individual life-styles, recommended exercise programs are individualized and modified throughout the progression of the disease.

Exercises that may be recommended include general conditioning, isometric, isotonic, isokinetic, postural, and dynamic balancing, and active assistive and passive range of motion (breathing exercises are discussed later in this chapter). Amyotrophic lateral sclerosis patients who tend to show strength gains with exercise are those who are in early or moderate stages of the disease, who have been relatively physically inactive prior to the initiation of the program, and who are among slow versus rapidly progressive individuals. Prior to establishing an exercise program it is critical to know the daily activity level of the individual which includes occupational and/or recreational patterns. Since muscles may undergo activity that may be potentially stressful and fatiguing on a functional level through daily activities, the increased demand imposed on muscle tissue through added "strengthening" exercises must be carefully planned and monitored as the disease progresses.

Systemic or General Conditioning (Endurance Training)

This type of exercise program is designed to optimize systemic strength and includes those activities or exercises that require mild to moderate contractions of multiple muscle groups. Some examples include swimming, bicycling (generally stationary) (Fig. 15–1a), walking or fast walking, and rowing. These activities require relatively low muscular tension and may be sustained over a period of time.[5] Although these may be performed at varying stages of the disease, they are usually recommended during early stages when clinical weakness is minimal and should be performed at submaximal level[6,7] (due to potential choking episodes, swimming is not advised for patients with bulbar involvement).

In support of endurance training is a report of a 36-year-old man with progressive muscular atrophy of 12 months duration who participated in a cardiorespiratory swim training program over an 8-month period.[3] The duration of swimming at the initiation of the program was 30 min which was increased to 90 min over the course of the 8-month period.

In our experience patients seem to respond most favorably to swimming. Swimming has the advantage of allowing a range from very light to fairly high work loads without the risk of injury to muscles, tendons, and joints that are more common in activities such as jogging or heavy weightlifting. The buoyancy of water allows freer movement as energy expenditure during conditioning is reduced. Muscle stretching is facilitated as well, and in patients with a predominance of upper motor neuron signs spasticity is reduced. Water temperature ideally should be warm to reduce the incidence of spasticity, cramping, and premature fatigue. In advanced stages, to ensure safety individuals should be accompanied by a professional who is experienced in swimming therapy for the physically handicapped.

Stationary cycling is also highly recommended and well supported by our patients. Since most cycling apparatus have tension adjustments, work loads can be varied to best suit individual needs. Slowly progressive individuals are usually able to tolerate higher work loads (intensity and/or duration) as compared to those who are rapidly progressive. The advantage attained include promoting muscle and joint flexibility as well as reducing spasticity.

Walking or fast walking is commonly recommended at stages where weakness may be minimal, or, if weakness is more severe, where proper supports (i.e., walking aids such as braces, canes, walkers, cervical collars, manual assist) can ensure safety during this activity. A prime advantage is to maximize the potential for prolonging ambulatory function.

General conditioning offers the benefits of promoting multisystem conditioning, and patients seem to respond most positively to this form of exercise physically as well as psychologically.

Local Muscle Conditioning

Isometric exercises (Fig. 15–1b) are designed to maximize muscle strength in selected muscle groups and reduce spasticity. In lower motor neuron disease they have been shown to increase strength when performed repeatedly at maximal contractions for 6-s interval.[8] One study examined the effects of isometric training on the elbow flexors and exten-

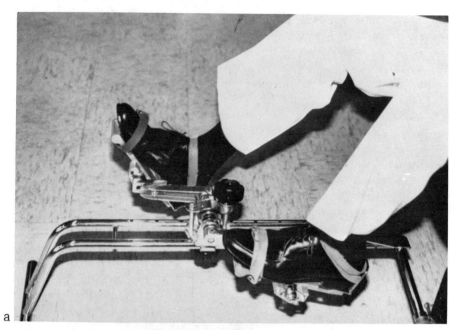

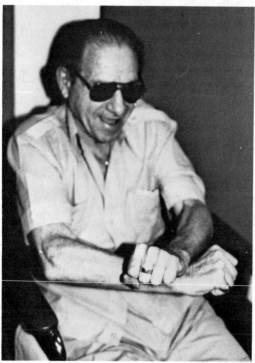

Figure 15–1. a. Example of a cycling exercise apparatus used to perform general (systemic) conditioning exercises. b. Isometric exercises performed to help relieve spasticity and to enhance movement of the upper extremity. c. Isotonic exercise performed against gravity by right upper extremity elbow flexors (local muscle conditioning). d. Isokinetic exercise performance by knee extensors using Cybex exercise apparatus (local muscle conditioning).

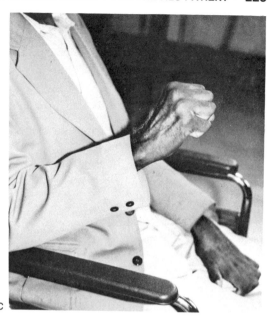

c

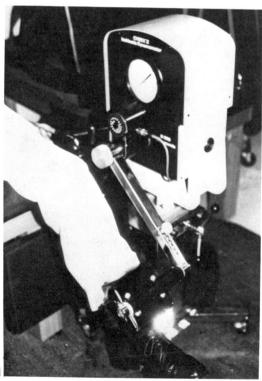

d

sors in six patients with motor neuron disease.[9] Two of the patients were reported to show strength gains in exercised muscles and one had definite functional improvement in bed mobility. However, the occurrence of adverse side effects, the duration of each isometric contraction, frequency of training, and exact number of training sessions are not mentioned in this report.

Isometric exercises in ALS are most suitable when upper motor neuron symptoms (spasticity) cause physical discomfort. Isometrics are useful in temporarily reducing excess muscle tone and facilitate more comfortable stretching of spastic muscles. Maximal isometric contractions should be held for 5- to 10-s intervals (or until the patients experience local muscle fatigue) followed by momentary relaxation and slow stretching of the spastic muscle. Since manual assistance is generally necessary, it is very important that the physical therapist instruct families or attending health personnel in proper technique when performing contract–relax–stretch methods. These patients are usually taking antispastic medication.

In those patients who are not physically bothered by upper motor neuron symptoms or in those with lower motor neuron dominance, isometrics for the purpose of strengthening are not advised. We have found that isometrics often induce local muscle cramping and fatigue which are both uncomfortable and further disabling. Consequently, other forms of exercises discussed in this chapter are preferred.

Isotonic (Fig. 15–1c) and *isokinetic* (Fig. 15–1d) exercises are designed for local muscle strengthening.[5] In ALS patients they may be applied through resistance offered by gravitational forces to added resistance applied either manually or through exercise apparatus.

A recent study supported the effect of manual resistive exercise through training 18 upper extremity muscle groups over a 75-day period.[10] Improvement in static strength as measured by dynamometry occurred in 14 muscle groups. The remaining four groups decreased in strength. Functional enhancement of wheelchair pivoting and sliding board transfer was reported by the patient who did not have prior exercise or functional training. The author concluded that the strength improvement in some but not all muscles may have been influenced by different muscle groups being both variably affected by both exercise and the disease process, and that strengthening exercises are warranted in ALS patients. Although this report supports the application of resistive exercise, we have noted that clinically most ALS patients have complained of significant muscle fatigue either during or following resistive exercise performance of moderate or heavy intensity. This is especially true if the exercises are performed frequently or by a patient who is rapidly progressive. Patients have reported that function of the arm or leg exercised was temporarily diminished as a consequence of heavy exercise. Those who have had involvement of muscles that affect respiratory function have complained of increased shortness of breath and general fatigue either during or immediately following these exercises as well. Although there is lack of evidence as to whether or not moderate or heavy resistive exercise may be detrimental in ALS, if such methods of exercise are applied, close monitoring is essential to avoid overfatigue. Mild resistive exercises seem to be more tolerable.

Patients with slowly progressive disease respond better to resistive exercises than their moderate to rapidly progressive counterparts. Within an individual, extremities with either minimal or no clinical weakness best tolerate resistive exercises. Since areas with moderate or severe weakness are highly prone to excessive cramping or prolonged fatigue, resistive exercises are best avoided in these areas. One must also appreciate the psychological defeat and lowered morale within those patients who experience rapid muscle fatigue following several repetitions or less of heavy resistive exercise.

Balancing and Postural Exercises

Dynamic balancing (Fig. 15–2a) and postural (Fig. 15–2b) exercises are especially helpful to optimize and sustain ambulation as long as possible. These exercises not only condition trunk and extremity muscles to optimize strength and coordination, but also serve to guide patients in safe postural substitution mechanisms as the disease progresses (refer to Ambulation Intervention, below).

Range of Motion Exercise

These exercises be discussed in section Contracture Prevention, below.

EXERCISE PROBLEMS: DISUSE WEAKNESS/OVERWORK

Disuse Weakness (Deconditioning)

The effects of physical inactivity which cause deconditioning and disuse weakness in normal individuals have been well recognized. Reduced physical activity, particularly if prolonged, reduces function of the neuromuscular system in addition to the cardiovascular, skeletal, and other organ systems.[11,12] Normal muscle strength is maintained through muscle

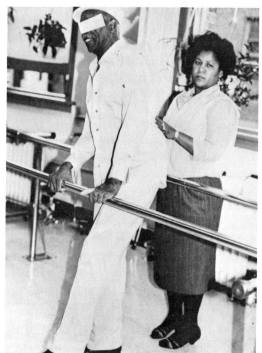

a

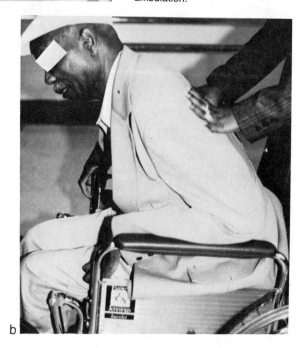

b

Figure 15–2. a. Dynamic balancing exercises performed with assistance of a home health aide to help maximize ambulatory function. b. Patient assisted in upper trunk extension exercises to optimize postural control during ambulation.

contractions that require a certain intensity, frequency, and duration of performance.[5,13] The degree and rate of strength loss through inactivity is dependent upon prior physical conditioning and the degree of reduced activity and stress demand on muscle, which may be endurance and/or power related.[5,12,13] It has been estimated that if the maximum tension a muscle produces is less than 20% of its maximum tension generating capability, the muscle loses strength.[14] Not only does inactivity reduce skeletal muscle function but additionally it may affect optimal cardiovascular adaptations that influence peripheral muscular activity.[5] Strength loss through inactivity and disuse seems to more significantly debilitate individuals with ALS since they are functioning with a diminished motor neuron pool as compared to normal individuals.

A considerable number of our patients have demonstrated disuse weakness sometime during the course of their illness. This has been evident in a number of patients who had been exercising regularly who then temporarily discontinued their programs. These patients subsequently noted a decrease in strength at a rate more rapid than expected when considering the intrinsic rate of progression of their illness. In our experience the rate of progression of the disease process within an individual does not seem to vary throughout the illness (although we have noted stabilization periods).

Most slowly progressive patients upon resuming exercise programs have shown strength gains in temporarily unexercised muscles. A number of moderate and rapidly progressive individuals have demonstrated stabilization in muscle strength for some time after resuming exercise. Some patients also felt their rate of deterioration had slowed. In all patients the balance between strength gains secondary to exercise and the physical daily activity, and strength loss secondary to the inherent rate of progression of the illness along with possible superimposed disuse weakness, must be considered when evaluating exercise response.

Rapidly progressive patients are more prone to disuse weakness. Due to the multiplicity of problems that can develop on a medical and psychological level, time constraints are a factor in the individual's ability to exercise as often as needed. Consequently deconditioning or disuse weakness superimposed on the disease process predisposes these patients to experience more rapid deterioration. Other contributing factors that can adversely affect muscle strength in these patients include malnutrition (particularly in dysphagia) and depression.

As the disease progresses in all patients, those who do not exercise are highly susceptible to developing muscle and joint tightness causing contractures. If severe tightness develops, any potential strength gains in the surrounding area may be lost as movement becomes severely restricted and painful.

Contracture Prevention (Range of Motion Exercises)

As weakness progresses to moderate or severe stages, whether it is generalized or localized to a specific area of the body, even antigravity exercises may be impossible or overfatiguing and muscle and joint tightness may develop. Since increased dropout in the number of motor units within a specific muscle or muscle group places greater stress or demand on remaining muscle fibers, forced compensation through functional activity and added exercise may induce rapid muscle fatigue.[1] Consequently, assistive or even passive range of motion exercises are applied to offer some conditioning and prevent contractures (Fig. 15–3). It is very important for patients' families and/or caretakers to consult with physical therapists for instruction in performing range of motion exercises so that injury and overstress to the musculoskeletal tissues are avoided.

Contracture prevention through daily passive range of motion or stretching exercises is critical to preserve comfort and optimize function by allowing for most efficient use of body substitution methods. Greatest risk of contracture development occurs in those with moderate or severe spasticity where additional exercises as well as antispastic medication may be essential throughout the progression of the illness. If contractures do develop, therapeutic exercise may be supplemented by the application of heat in the form of hot packs, short-wave diathermy, ultrasound, or whirlpool baths. Transcutaneous electrical nerve stimulation has also been of value in relieving pain. The above agents serve to enhance pain relief and promote flexibility of muscles and joints. Massage and joint mobilization may be applied as well. Therapeutic cold agents to relieve pain and inhibit spasticity are avoided, as ALS patients are sensitive to chilling temperatures.

Overwork

The possibility for inducing "overwork" weakness in individuals with ALS through excessive exercise is a common concern among therapists who exercise these patients. Although "overwork" weakness to date has not been scientifically demonstrated in ALS, the advisability for strengthening exercises in ALS and other neuromuscular diseases has been questioned.[6,12] Any reports of deleterious effects of muscle strengthening in other neuromuscular diseases such as muscular dystrophy have been largely anecdotal and unsupported through clinical systematic study. However, it has been stated that "excessive unsupervised overwork certainly can have a detrimental effect on muscle function in neuromuscular disease," and the "active exercise programs must be closely monitored for potential de-

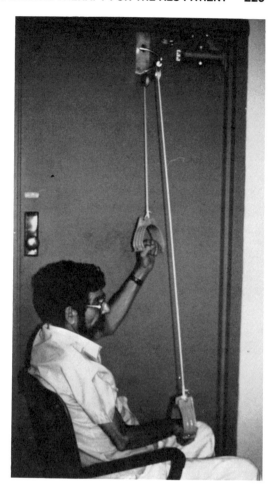

Figure 15–3. Over-the-door pulleys are very useful for conditioning shoulder and other upper extremity musculature and in preserving muscle and joint flexibility and comfort. They are very effective in allowing an individual to perform active-assistive or passive range of motion exercises independently ("holding mitts" are available if hand weakness is severe).

tremental effects on muscle function."[12] However, reports of supervised exercises on ALS and other neuromuscular diseases including isometric, maximal isotonic, or submaximal isokinetic resistive exercises have failed to show deleterious effects on muscle function.[6,9,10,12]

Regarding overwork, not only is there concern over potential adverse effects that may lead to a prolonged reduction in muscle power and endurance, but there is also concern that the immediate transient performance decrement that occurs after moderately heavy work in normals may more significantly impair physical function of the ALS patients.

Since there is a high incidence of muscular fatigue experienced by our ALS patients, we are very careful not to plan vigorous exercise programs for the majority of them. Patients who exercise heavily to the point where excess muscle cramping, aching, and fatigue is experienced either during the exercise, immediately afterward, or on the following day are more susceptible to experience overwork weakness. These patients often report significant temporary functional impairment of the extremity or extremities exercised. This is also evident through muscle testing and observing select activities. Following a period of rest for a few days, recovery seems to occur where function may be performed at preexercise levels until the disease progresses further. Patients who try to maintain a highly active schedule are more susceptible to suffering from overwork weakness. This is usually alleviated somewhat when they reduce their activity level.

Rapidly progressive patients who exercise heavily are more prone to overwork weakness, probably since the rate of motor unit dropout is greater with resultant higher stress placed on remaining motor units which may have also begun active denervation. Slowly progressive patients are less prone to overwork weakness and better tolerate high-intensity or long-duration exercises. This is probably due to the relatively reduced number and rate of motor unit dropout with potential functional compensation through collateral sprouting as compared to patients who are rapidly progressive.[2,6,12] Whether or not there is prolonged weakness as a result of heavy exercise has been difficult to establish because of wide variability in pattern and rate of progression of the disease process among individuals.

There have been limited metabolic studies performed in ALS as well as other motor unit diseases and pyramidal tract disorders.[3,15,16,17,18] One study with ALS and other motor unit diseases using in vivo forearm metabolism methods suggested that abnormalities in oxygen utilization, lactate output, and uptake of glucose and long-chain fatty acids in devervated muscles were consistent with an augmented utilization of blood-borne fuels at rest.[17] During rest and exercise, possible defective autoregulation of skeletal muscle blood flow may have caused the regional muscle ischemia and abnormally high lactate output. It was suggested that blood, oxygen, and nutritive supplies to muscle might be even less during maximal exercise training.[6] Others have commented that in ALS patients with abnormal resting blood flows exercise may improve circulatory efficiency.[3]

Therapeutic exercise is a vital part of management of ALS patients from the onset of the illness and throughout the progression of the disease. All programs must be monitored to avoid side effects such as excess cramping and overfatigue as well as to prevent painful and function-limiting contractures. Despite therapist and patient efforts to maintain muscular strength through therapeutic exercise, patients ultimately weaken. Introduction to other rehabilitative measures including adaptive aids and devices then becomes an integral part of patient management.

AMBULATION INTERVENTION

Ambulation difficulties in ALS are manifested through progressive weakness which is apparent clinically in various patterns: (1) within the lower extremity(ies), (2) within the lower extremity(ies) and trunk, (3) within the upper extremity(ies) and trunk, (4) within the lower and upper extremity(ies) and trunk, or (5) within the trunk (greatest with cervical extensor weakness)

If weakness within one of the above noted areas is mild, postural compensation alone may be sufficient to improve balance and allow for safe ambulation as long as overfatigue does not occur. Dynamic balancing and postural exercises (Fig. 15–2a and 15–2b) are often helpful to enable individuals to maximize strength and coordination, and to most effectively implement substitution mechanisms, or to utilize assistive devices. If ambulation is impaired secondary to spasticity, patients may benefit from antispastic medication and therapeutic exercise to inhibit spasticity if muscle tone is excessive.

Ambulatory Aids

As weakness progresses, ambulation aids and orthotics (splinting or bracing) are recommended. All assistive devices serve to improve function by offering support to weakened muscles and the joints they surround, and to reduce stress on compensatory muscles to conserve energy and minimize local or general muscle fatigue. All aids must be lightweight, but stable to ensure optimal function and safety. The specific aid or device recommended depend upon pattern, extent, and rate of progression of the disease as well as acceptance by patient and family. Knowledge of the time factor to acquire devices and economic constraints are also critical considerations in selection.

Ambulation aids most commonly recommended are listed in Table 15–1. Commonly, weakness of the dorsiflexors of the ankle and foot cause "foot-drop" where the individual is prone to tripping, has difficulty climbing stairs, and is susceptible to ankle strain or sprain. This can be corrected through fitting a customized or prefabricated plastic ankle–foot orthosis (Fig. 15–4a). The selection depends upon the rate of progression of the disease (see Table 15–1). Lightweight shoes or sneakers should be

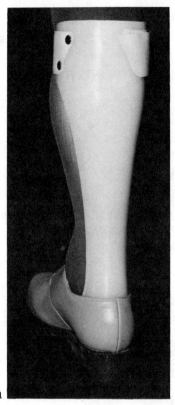
a

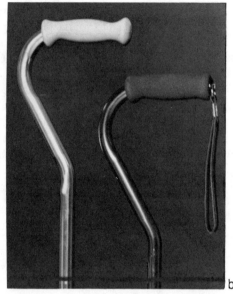
b

Figure 15–4. a. Plastic ankle-foot orthosis used to correct footdrop during ambulation. b. Sample selection of horizontal-grip canes useful for ambulation, particularly in individuals with intrinsic hand weakness. c. Patient descending stairs with aid of forearm crutch. d. Front-wheeled attached walker (most commonly used ambulation aid).

used whether or not bracing is indicated to reduce energy expenditure. At times high-top shoes or sneakers alone may offer adequate support and delay the need for bracing.

With progressive lower extremity dysfunction, if a cane is recommended, horizontal- versus hook-grip canes are used, particularly when there is hand muscle weakness or in moderate or rapidly progressive disease. Horizontal-grip canes minimize hand fatigue, but adequate shoulder strength must be available (Fig. 15–4b) to use them. If weakness progresses and the rate is relatively slow, forearm (Fig. 15–4c) or platform crutches may be used when a cane no longer offers adequate amulatory support. In more rapidly progressive disease, a rolling walker (front-wheeled attachments only) (Fig. 15–4d) may immediately follow use of a cane. Rolling walkers are the most commonly used ambulation aids. Since pro-

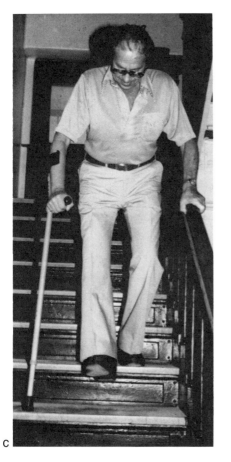

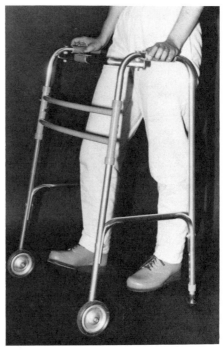

c

d

gressive upper extremity dysfunction makes the lifting required for maneuvering standard walkers (without wheels) difficult, rolling walkers can minimize upper extremity fatigue and reduce overall energy expenditure. If upper extremity weakness progresses to severe stages, platforms may be attached to the walker. If thoracolumbar spinal extension becomes a problem, customized axillary platform attachments may be ultimately necessary.

A 56-year-old white male with slowly progressive bulbar ALS had ceased ambulation after sustaining a fall secondary to progressive diffuse muscular weakness. At that time weakness was moderate to severe proximally and distally in all extremities and cervical spine extensors; however; his strength remained good (4/5) bilaterally in shoulder depressors, thoracic extensors, and knee extensors. Ambulatory function was restored

Table 15–1. Most Commonly Utilized Ambulation Aids

Slow progression
    Compensation manuevers
    Hook- or horizontal-grip canes
    Forearm or platform crutch(es)
    Standard or wheeled walkers
    Platform-attached walker
    Custom-made plastic ankle–foot orthosis(es)

Moderate progression
    Compensation manuevers
    Horizontal grip standard cane(s)
    Wheeled walker
    Custom-made plastic ankle–foot orthosis(es)
    Prefabricated plastic ankle–foot orthosis(es)

Rapid progression
    Compensation maneuvers
    Horizontal-grip cane(s)
    Wheeled walker
    Prefabricated plastic ankle–foot orthosis(es)

Note: Cervical collars are frequently used with varying rates of progression exclusive of or in combination with the above-noted devices. Upper extremity orthosis(es) may also be employed.

through customized adaptation of a walker. Front-castored wheels were attached which enhanced mobility along with a pair of forearm-platform rests with axillary pads which well supported the upper extremities and prevented flexion of the thoracolumbar spine. A pair of lightweight plastic ankle–foot orthoses were applied to the lower extremities to promote optimal foot clearance and ankle stability. The patient advanced the walker using residual lower extremity muscular movements along with upper extremity shoulder girdle depression and protraction.

Within a 3-month period the patient increased his ambulatory distance from 15 ft to 50 yd without overfatigue. During this period his overall endurance and strength in several muscle groups improved. He experienced a positive feeling of psychological well-being and continued to ambulate 30 to 50 yards several days a week for 2 years.

A study of 32 ALS patients that evaluated the effect of physical therapy intervention on ambulatory function revealed that 50 percent of those nonambulatory secondary to progressive weakness became independently ambulatory following physical therapy intervention.[19] The most commonly implemented ambulatory aids were the rolling walker and plastic ankle–foot orthosis.

PULMONARY PHYSICAL THERAPY

Pulmonary physical therapy in the care of the ALS patient assists in maximizing respiratory muscle strength and the efficiency and distribution of ventilation, optimizes the cough mechanism, reduces accumulation as well as facilitating mobilization of bronchial secretions, and enhances general systemic (cardopulmonary) conditioning.[1,3,11] The most commonly used techniques include localized respiratory muscle breathing and coughing exercises, general conditioning exercises, and postural drainage.[11,20]

Respiratory difficulties in ALS mainly occur secondary to degeneration of the upper and lower motor neuron pathways that innervate the respiratory muscles. Problems may occur through spinal or bulbar motor neuron dysfunction. In a given individual bulbar and spinal involvement may occur independent of the other or in varying combination. Since the pattern and rate of ensuing weakness is highly variable, respiratory muscle involvement may occur early or not until later stages of the disease.

Breathing Exercises

Breathing exercises may be performed through local (specific training of respiratory muscles) or general (systemic which include extremity in addition to respiratory musculature) conditioning.[20]Assessment of respiratory muscle function is beneficial during early stages of ALS when respiratory involvement is absent or minimal to best establish normal breathing patterns and initiate conditioning if necessary. Although the training response of respiratory muscles in normal subjects is similar to other skeletal muscles,[20] in restrictive respiratory disorders such as ALS sufficient studies are not available that evaluate the effects of respiratory muscle conditioning (local or systemic) on respiratory muscle strength and pulmonary function. Since respiratory muscles are affected by upper and lower motor neuron dysfunction as are other voluntary muscles, it seems reasonable to parallel concepts of exercise training alluded to earlier to respiratory muscle conditioning. Major goals of breathing exercises then are to maximize ventilatory muscle strength and systemic muscle function, while avoiding overfatigue. Highly active individuals with absent or minimal respiratory muscle dysfunction may not initially require breathing exercises as their muscles are actively conditioned through their daily activities. As the disease progresses specific respiratory muscle conditioning exercises must be instituted. Clinical assessment of respiratory muscle function through clinical inspection, palpation, muscle testing, pulmonary function tests, and screening daily activity levels all serve as a basis for recommending breathing exercise programs.[11,21]

Local Muscle Conditioning

Local muscle conditioning in ALS generally focuses on the primary muscles of inspiration as well as the expiratory muscles.

Inspiratory Muscle Conditioning. The primary muscles of inspiration include the diaphragm and external intercostals.[20] The diaphragm muscle has sternal, costal, and lumbar attachments, all inserted into a central tendon; the diaphragm muscle is frequently affected in ALS patients. Consequently, diaphramatic conditioning should be implemented early in the disease process. These exercises may be performed while the patient is supine, sitting, or during ambulation. Contraction of the diaphragm increases the vertical and transverse thoracic diameter.[20] Ahand placed on the epigastric region during inspiration can offer guidance through tactile feedback when instructing diaphragmatic breathing exercises (Fig. 15–5a). Other methods include expansion against a belt or tape measure circumferentially placed around the lower costal or epigastric region, or through use of a volume incentive spirometer.[11,20,22] Volume incentive spirometers can be very effective in diaphragmatic training (Fig. 15–5b). They encourage the patient to take slow deep breaths which enhances volume and flow of air to the basal lung segments (where atelectasis commonly occurs). A sign of diaphragm fatigue occurs when substitution by accessory muscles is noted.[23]

If sufficient diaphragmatic weakness occurs, the external intercostal and accessory muscles (if intact) become the primary muscles of inspiration and thus sustain ventilation.[11,22] The intercostal muscles interdigitate between ribs and increase the lateral and anteroposterior diameters of the thorax.[22,23] The accessory muscles elevate the sternum and upper ribs and serve as stabilizers for the primary ventilatory muscles.[11,22] The major accessory muscles include the scalene, trapezius, pectoral, and serratus muscles. The external intercostals (Fig. 15–6) and accessory muscles seem to tolerate active exercises during mild to moderate restrictive stages if performed in moderation. In the event of diaphragm and external intercostal paralyses the accessory muscles contract vigorously to sustain ventilation as inspiratory muscle function is severely compromised. As the accessory muscles would be prone to overstress and fatigue at this stage due to functional compensation, active exercises would not be implemented (particularly if external respiratory support is not instituted). However, it would be important to preserve chest cage and shoulder flexibility through passive stretching and mobilization to enhance optimal ventilation and physical comfort.

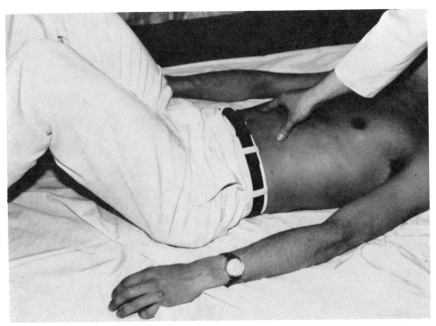

a

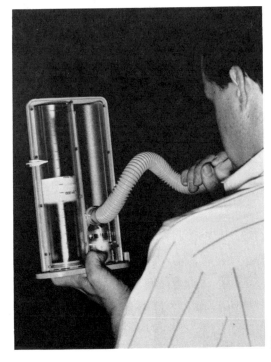

Figure 15–5. a. A method for diaphragmatic muscle training. Patient inspires and exerts outward pressure against hand to enhance epigastric and lower costal expansion. b. Patient using Voldyne volume incentive spirometer which offers visual feedback during diaphragmatic muscle training.

b

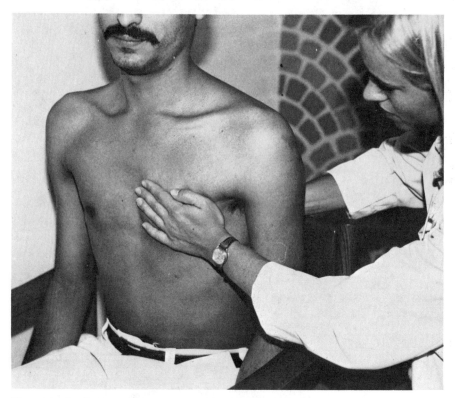

Figure 15–6. Patient conditioning external intercostal muscles for inspiration (mid-costal region) using manual proprioceptive feedback offered by therapist.

Expiratory Muscle Conditioning. Expiration is essentially a passive process at rest. When activity is increased, expiration becomes more active and is performed primarily by the abdominal and internal intercostal muscles.[11,22] The abdominal muscles have attachments to the sternum, ribs (lower two-thirds), pelvis, lumbar fascia, and inguinal ligament. The internal intercostal muscles interdigitate between ribs. Together these muscles generate the high expiratory force and flow rates necessary for an effective cough. Due to motor weakness and excess mucus production in ALS the cough mechanism commonly becomes severely impaired. This impairment results in retained secretions with potential lung infection..

A normal explosive cough occurs in five sequential steps, as follows:[22]

1. Deep breath
2. Inspiratory pause
3. Glottic closure

4. Increased intrathoracic pressure

5. Glottic opening followed by rapid forceful air expulsion

In ALS one or more of the above components may be disrupted. Since expiratory flows are reduced if inspiratory muscle paralyses occurs, inspiratory exercises described earlier must be done to optimize the initial volume of air required for an effective cough (steps 1 and 2). Bulbar dysfunction often causes erratic glottic closure which may impede the intrathoracic pressure buildup and subsequent rapid air expulsion that is optimal for an explosive cough (steps 3, 4, and 5).[3,11,24,25] Patients with bulbar involvement are often unable to volitionally cough so must be instructed in "huffing" to maximize velocity and force of air flow to enhance mobilization of secretions. Just as weak inspiratory muscles affect optimal expiratory muscle function, conversely, weak expiratory muscles affect optimal inspiratory muscle function as well.[20]

Some exercises recommended to maximize expiratory muscle strength include:

• Partial sit-up (to clear scapulae)
• Roll supine to sidelying (both directions) (Fig.15–7a)
• Posterior pelvic tilting
• Neck flexion (lying supine)
• Huffing (bulbar)
• Breathing through a straw (Fig. 15–7b)
• General conditioning exercises
• Cough

If expiratory flows are significantly reduced where the cough becomes weak or nonfunctional, manual assistive compression during expiration over the epigastric (Fig. 15–7c) or lateral costal (particularly with gastrostomy) regions can significantly improve the quality of the cough. If intermittent positive pressure breathing (IPPB) is recommended, during the treatment it increases the patient's tidal volume which augments the potential cough force.[11,22] At this stage the expiratory muscles are often moderate to severely weakened in locations where manual assistive compression when performed in conjunction with IPPB can significantly enhance the force of the cough.

If aggressive pulmonary intervention such as tracheostomy is performed, breathing and assistive coughing exercises are to be continued. This is especially important in patients who suffer an acute pulmonary infection and who required a tracheostomy and mechanical ventilation, who then have the potential for ventilator weaning upon clearing of the infection. Since unaffected respiratory muscles are prone to decondition while on prolonged ventilation, if there is a possibility of partial or complete ventilator weaning, breathing exercises should be implemented as part of the weaning protocol. Another example is patients who have very

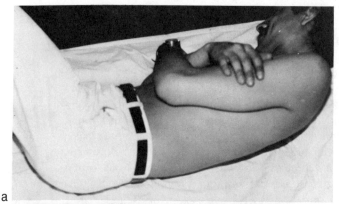

a

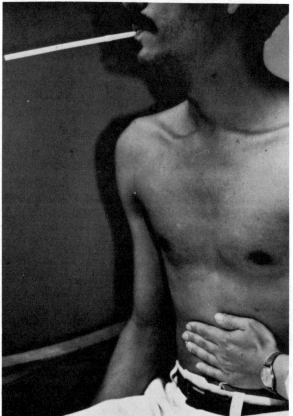

b

Figure 15–7. a. By rolling toward either side (here shown toward the right) weak abdominals are conditioned to optimize bed mobility. b. Patient forcefully exhaling through a straw to maximize expiratory pressure and flow rate. c. Manually assisted compression when synchronized with expiration can significantly improve patient's cough if abdominal muscles are weakened.

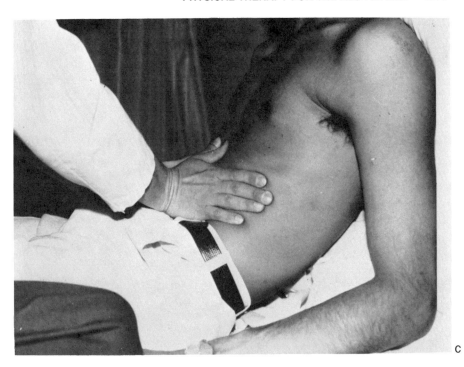

C

slowly progressive disease who then require tracheostomy with assisted mechanical ventilation due to progressive respiratory failure. Due to the slow nature of disease progression, the number of daily hours that assistive ventilation is required can be gradually reduced for a period of time (until the disease further progresses). Again, performance of breathing exercises facilitates attainment of maximal pulmonary efficiency during this process.

Postural Drainage

Since ALS patients (particularly those with bulbar dysfunction) often have difficulty mobilizing secretions, postural drainage may be used adjunctly to maintain pulmonary hygiene. Problems with excess mucus and secretions may occur in early or not until later stages of the disease. Postural drainage includes proper positioning to help drain lung fields susceptible to developing infections or where infection may be active. It also includes percussion (clapping) and vibration (shaking) to mobilize secretions (Fig. 15–8). Vibration is better tolerated than percussion in ALS patients. Breathing and coughing exercises are performed in conjunction

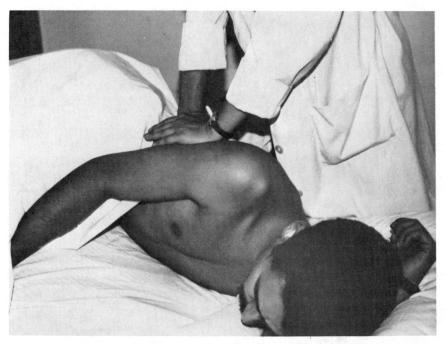

Figure 15–8. Patient receiving postural drainage in Trendelenberg position with vibration to help drain and clear secretions in right lower lobe (lateral basal). Vibration is better tolerated over percussion in ALS, particularly if there is significant atrophy in muscles surrounding the chest wall.

with postural drainage. Patients may concomitantly be receiving antibiotics, humidification, IPPB, intermittent or continuous ventilation, or supplemental oxygen. Physical therapists should instruct patients, families, and caretakers in postural drainage positions to ensure effective drainage of the appropriate lung field(s). There are texts available for reference.[1,11]

To most effectively carry out pulmonary physical therapy in the home, physical therapists should be consulted for instruction in pulmonary physical therapeutic techniques as per individual need. Pulmonary physical therapy should be an integral part of patient management both therapeutically as well as prophylactically in sustaining pulmonary function.

SUMMARY

Physical therapy intervention through exercise program design, optimizing ambulatory function, or implementing pulmonary physical therapy procedures must be monitored by a physical therapist from early to later stages of the disease. Caution must be taken through exercise program design to condition patients' muscles to maximize neuromuscular function while avoiding overfatigue. All programs must consider daily activity levels, pattern of weakness, and the intrinsic rate of progression of the disease. General conditioning exercises are most favored; however; isotonics and isokinetics for local muscle conditioning, and isometrics for reducing spasticity prior to stretching are applied as well. Although slowly progressive individuals tolerate higher work loads as compared to their rapidly progressive counterparts, heavy resistive exercises are generally not recommended as they are fatiguing and may at least temporarily restrict function. Disuse weakness and contractures should be avoided to prevent aggravated disability and physical pain. Exercise additionally offers a psychological boost to enable patients to continously fight against the relentless progression of the disease through maximizing physical strength and function.

Throughout the course of the disease, ongoing education for patients' families and caretakers ensures awareness of changing functional capabilities. This will enable most realistic independent function of the patient and offer guidelines to caretakers for their own physical safety whenever it becomes necessary to physically assist patients in their daily activities.

REFERENCES

1. Maloney FP, Burke JS, Ringle SP: Interdisciplinary rehabilitation of multiple sclerosis and other neuromuscular disorders. Lippincott, Philadelphia, 1985.
2. Sinaki M, Mulder DW: Rehabilitation techniques for patients with amyotrophic lateral sclerosis. Mayo Clin Proc 53:173–178. 1978.
3. Mulder DW: The Diagnoses and Treatment of Amyotrophic Lateral Sclerosis. Houghton Mifflin, Boston, 1980.
4. Norris FH Jr, U KS, Denys EH, et al.: Amyotrophic lateral sclerosis. Mayo Clin Proc 53:544, 1978.
5. McArdle WD, Katch FI, Katch VL: Exercise Physiology. Lea & Febiger, Philadelphia, 1981.
6. Fowler WM Jr, Taylor M: Rehabilitation management of muscular dystrophy and related disorders: I. The role of exercise. II. Comprehensive care. Arch Phys Med Rehab 63:319–328, 1982.
7. Janiszewski DW, Caroscio JT, Wisham L: Amyotrophic lateral sclerosis: A comprehensive rehabilitation approach. Arch Phys Med Rehab 64(7):304–307, 1983.
8. Liberson WT, Asa MM: Further studies of brief isometric exercises. Arch Phys Med Rehab (8):330–336. 1959.
9. Lenman JAR: A clinical and experimental study of the effects of exercise on motor weakness in neurological disease. J Neurol Neurosurg Psychiatry 22:182–194, 1959.
10. Bohannon RW: Results of resistance exercise on a patient with amyotrophic lateral sclerosis. J Am Phys Ther Assoc 63(6):965–968, 1983.
11. Frownfelter DL: Chest physical therapy and pulmonary rehabilitation. Year Book Medical Publishers, Chicago, 1978.

12. Vignos PJ Jr: Physical models of rehabilitation in neuromuscular disease. Muscle Nerve 6:323–338, 1983.
13. Rose SJ, Rothstein JM: Muscle mutability—Part I: General concepts and adaptations to altered patterns of use. Part II: Adaptations to drugs, metabolic factors, and aging. J Am Phys Ther Assoc 62(12):1773–1798, 1982.
14. Kotte FJ: The effects of limitation of activity on the human body. JAMA 196:117–122, 1966.
15. Bar-or O, Inbar O, Spira R: Physiological effects of a sports rehabilitation program on cerebral palsied & post-poliomyelitis adolescents. Med Sci Sports Exerc 8:157–161, 1976.
16. Haller RG, Lewis SF, Cook JD, et al.: Hyperkinetic circulation during exercise in neuromuscular disease. Neurology 33:1283–1287, 1983.
17. Karpati G, Klassen G, Tanser P: The effects of partial denervation on forearm metabolism. Can J Neurol Sci 6(2):105–112, 1979.
18. Moxley RT, Griggs RC, Van Gelder V, et al.: Effects of denervation and wasting on skeletal muscle blood flow in man. Neurology 28:400, 1978.
19. Zawodniak J, Chiamprasert S, Caroscio J: The effect of physical therapy on ambulatory function in amyotrophic lateral sclerosis. (Unpublished data).
20. Shaffer TH, Wolfson MR, Bhutani VK: Respiratory muscle function, assessment, and training. J Am Phys Ther Assoc 61(12):1711–1723.
21. Reinisch ES: Functional approach to chest physical therapy. J Am Phys Ther Assoc 58(8):972–975, 1978.
22. Shapiro BA, Harrison RA, Trout CA: Clinical Application of Respiratory Care. Year Book Medical Publishers, Chicago, 1979.
23. Alvarez SE, Peterson M, Lunsford BR: Respiratory treatment of the adult patient with spinal cord injury. J Am Phys Ther Assoc 61(12):1737–1745, 1981.
24. Fallat RJ, et al: Spirometry in amyotrophic lateral sclerosis. Arch Neuro 36:74–80, 1979.
25. Kigin C: Chest physical therapy for the postoperative or traumatic injury patient. J Am Phys Ther Assoc 61 (12):1724–1736, 1981.

CHAPTER SIXTEEN

HOME CARE OF THE AMYOTROPHIC LATERAL SCLEROSIS PATIENT

Pat Casey Heidkamp, M.S., O.T.R.

Home occupational therapy intervention is required when a patient reports difficulty managing his self-care. Periodic assessment of the patient's functional abilities is made at clinic visits, but as specific problems occur, the recommendation is made for a home visit. However, the home visit is usually not requested until the patient recognizes a certain degree of physical limitation. Limitations usually concern changes in mobility or ability to perform personal hygiene tasks. Successful home occupational therapy intervention requires understanding the patient's adaptive responses to the progression of the disease, assessment of present abilities, and treatment to provide improved function.

HISTORY

The occupational therapist requires the patient's report of onset of symptoms and rate of progression to understand his perceptions about the illness, the importance of specific activities of daily living, and, most importantly, his adaptive ability to the progressive changes that have already occurred. These changes may only be subtle differences in ambulation or hand function, but accommodation to these changes indicates adaptive predisposition. In most instances, a certain amount of adaptation of skills has already occurred with the patient's recognition of the physical limitations. The patient and family report how they have already adapted functioning to this point.

When making the home visit, the therapist observes carefully the family's life-style and apparent priorities concerning general order and living space. This observation is important because as the disease progresses, more equipment may be needed and some changes in uses of space may

247

be required. Openness to the suggestions and willingness to simplify care areas may influence acceptance and uses of assistive equipment.

Sufficient skill in interviewing patients and family caregivers is necessary to develop a level of trust and to ascertain the amount of information they have received about their specific disease process, its rate of progression, and their immediate and long-term priorities. The information they have received from their physician may have been misinterpreted due to fear or anxiety about the prognosis and may have caused misperceptions about some common self-care problems. Careful listening to answers about priorities can direct suggestions to the patient with immediate, concrete solutions that are realistic and within the means of the family to provide. For example, the problem of an inaccessible entrance to the home for a wheelchair may require a ramp instead of an extensive and costly renovation.

ASSESSMENT

The occupational therapist's main function in the initial home visit is to consider the patient's and caregiver's assessment of the home care problems and the solutions they propose, and to supply information about alternative methods or assistive equipment that will provide a workable solution to those problems. An assessment of physical strength, limitations of motion, and present functional abilities must be determined. In addition, the home visit provides the opportunity to assess architectural barriers inside and outside the home, that is, entrances, stairs, hallways, bathroom, and bedroom space, and to observe the patient's and family's abilities and willingness to change methods of performing personal care activities. Assessment is made in the home environment of the patient's ability to assume standing and sitting positions, transfers to and from bed, chair, toilet, tub or shower, and car; mobility in bed; ambulation and ability to negotiate stairs inside and outside the home in addition to ambulation endurance, and ability to drive a car. Other areas of personal care are evaluated either by report or actual demonstration; dressing, showering/bathing, grooming, and eating. Communication, leisure, homemaking, and work activities also are included.

Again, special attention is paid to the person's method of adaptation to the progressive changes of the disease, his needs for maintaining independence in specific areas, and innovative skills in achieving some control in spite of weakness. Matching of these needs with assistive equipment promotes continuation of functional abilities and allows easier transition to the next stage of the illness. Use of specific items of equipment is recommended for specific disabilities rather than "stage" of the disease.

TREATMENT

Recommendations about alternative methods that have been useful to other patients can be made at this time. This method of introducing patient-conceived solutions removes some of the "specialist effect" and allows the patient and family control over solutions. The task of the therapist is to bring alternative solutions to common daily living care problems. This helps to eliminate the frustration of trial and error and the wasting of precious time and energy by all family members. Planting ideas that patients can draw from at certain stages of the illness seems to provide a feeling of control in a seemingly uncontrollable situation and helps reduce anxiety by providing concrete steps to take when problems occur.

The occupational therapist (in conjunction with the physical therapist) spends time in both the clinic and the home setting teaching patients and family members or other caregivers active exercise programs, passive range of motion exercises, positioning of extremities to prevent contractures and reduce edema, correct body mechanics for lifting and transferring, use of ambulation assists, that is, lower extremity plastic orthoses and walkers or canes, and use of patient lifts for transfers or bathing. Other electrical or mechanical assistive equipment are recommended to fit each patient's particular needs. Training may be necessary to use this equipment in the simplest, most efficient way. Use of assistive equipment or a change in self-care routines may be more readily accepted if presented in the home rather than in the clinic setting where physical space and time constraints are better understood by the therapist.

Follow-up home visits are made when progressive weakness warrants more or different assistive equipment, and training to use the equipment or to change routines may be necessary. Indication for training the spouse to use assistive equipment is needed when the patient no longer can walk, stand, or use his hands for personal care. The functional capacity of the spouse (who is likely to be in his fifties or sixties) also must be considered.

Simply providing assistive equipment does not assure the acceptance or use of the equipment or make daily care routines easier. This author has observed that patients and caregivers use the equipment *only* if it makes the personal care routine easier *and* if they cannot continue to perform these tasks in the same manner due to physical constraints. In other words, assuming that the equipment is available to the family, (1) the patient or family must be willing to use the assistive equipment; (2) the present method of activity is no longer working due to physical strain, time, or energy constraints, or limited number of caregivers; and (3) the equipment not only makes the care routine possible, but also makes it easier.

ASSISTIVE EQUIPMENT RECOMMENDATIONS

Recommendations are made for certain items of equipment according to sites of dysfunction, predominance of weakness or stiffness, and rate of progression which differs from patient to patient.

Ambulation With Limited Endurance

Patients who are walking without assistive devices but who are beginning to limit social outings, shopping, or family activities because of limited strength and endurance can consider use of a lightweight, standard or narrow adult width wheelchair with standard footrests, and detachable deskarmrests. These chairs can be placed in a trunk or back seat of a car. Some models have detachable back wheels which make lifting easier in and out of a trunk, especially for a female spouse. An air-filled or foam cushion should *always* be provided with the wheelchair since serious back strain and coccyx and ischial pressure from sitting prolonged periods of time in the sling seat of a wheelchair occur. Some Gel cushions add too much weight both for the patient pushing himself or for the spouse. They also may require extra care to prevent puncture.

Purchase of a motorized cart (i.e., Amigo, Lark, Mobie, and so on) or powered wheelchair is a definite consideration if the overall rate of progression is considered slow, if the amount of stiffness is greater than the amount of weakness, and if the loss of upper extremity and hand function is only slowly progressing. Rental of these items is possible if the rate of progression is considered more rapid. The benefit to patient and family is considerable over the course of the illness, even if use is possible only for a short time. Patients may be less reluctant to give up driving the car if a powered wheelchair of some type is an alternative. The powered carts disassemble to be placed in the car, but the batteries and base are still heavy to lift. Most powered wheelchairs do not disassemble and require a van with a hydraulic lift or van ramp to transport. Both may require a ramp or outside lift to enter a house.

Ambulation Requiring Assistance

When weakness around the ankle causes footdrop, walking on level surfaces and stairclimbing become a problem. Usually a straight cane will be sufficient if only one ankle is involved and the same side hand and wrist are strong. With increased weakness lightweight plastic ankle–foot orthoses (AFOs) are used to stabilize the ankle and prevent foot drop. Recommendation for AFOs are made early to help prevent falling.

Patients whose main complaint is stiffness are plagued by falling and stumbling since increased ankle reflexes thrust them forward. Bracing is not helpful. A straight cane may assist but more likely a folding walker with front casters is useful. This walker does not need to be lifted, so weak or stiff hands need not grasp and release the walker with each step. This only tires and frustrates the patient.

A motorized stair lift may be indicated at this time, especially if the patient lives in a split level home where bathrooms and bedrooms are located on an upper or lower level. Since this is a very expensive item, and some insurance policies do not cover this, other alternatives suitable to the family require investigation.

Trunk and Hip Weakness

Assuming the standing and sitting position is a problem for both patient and spouse when trunk and hip stiffness and weakness occur. Higher seat positioning is required to accommodate the weakened muscles, to improve the safety of transfers, and, to reduce the amount of assistance or lifting by the caregivers.

The powered lift chair affords gradual support to and from the seated position and can be operated by the patient even with weakened hand function. The recliner feature is also an important option since edematous lower extremities can be elevated and trunk and hip position can be changed easily to relieve pressure.

Use of a *full* electric hospital bed provides the same kind of support as the lift chair because it follows the patient while assuming the standing or seated position. Usually a walker placed in front of the patient provides the most security. The bed must be locked in position or butted against the wall for safety. The electric hospital bed also allows the patient or spouse to change positions from lying down to sitting with little effort.

A raised toilet seat is sometimes recommended if the vanity is close and sturdy enough to be used for support while assuming the standing or seated position. The most common alternative is the commode on casters with options that include swing-away armrests, a commode opening with a "C" shape (for easier perineal cleaning), floor brakes (caster locks are considered unsuitable), and padded seat and back. This commode is recommended for several reasons. It can be used for the various stages of the illness—when the patient is ambulatory but requires a raised seat height and armrests over the toilet, when he is not ambulatory and requires toileting and hygiene care in the bathroom, and when he is essentially bedridden but requires the sitting position for improved elimination function. The advantages to the spouse are that it is mobile, it can be easily removed from over the toilet for other family members, it clears most bathroom doors (wheelchairs usually do not), and it eliminates unsafe transfers from chair to toilet in small bathroom spaces.

Difficulty getting in and out of bathtubs is a common problem when either upper or lower extremity function is impaired. Depending upon location of the tub, toilet, and vanity, presence or absence of glass sliding doors, composition of the tub (porcelain, enameled steel, or fiberglass), wall coverings (ceramic or plastic tile or marlite), and amount of turning space, several alternatives can be considered. Grab bars, adjustable height tub benches, and hydraulic or water pressure tub lifts are available. But attention to armrests on tub lifts and placement of controls is imperative. Use of a hand-held shower hose enables a patient to shower or wash hair independently or with assistance while seated on a tub bench without unnecessary mess or inconvenience.

Special support cushions can be used in lift chairs or wheelchairs because weakness in trunk and hip areas cause discomfort when sitting prolonged periods of time. Support of the lower back and pelvis is essential to reduce effects of fatigue, immobility, and gravity. A selection of air-filled or foam cushions that is, Roho, T-foam, provide temporary relief for longer periods of time than other cushions as reported by patients. More than one type of cushion is usually required since no cushion provides relief all of the time.

Neck and Shoulder Weakness

Two types of collars that have been used with more success for neck weakness are soft cervical and lightweight plastizoate Philadelphia-style cervical collars. Some patients prefer the soft cervical collar because it snugly supports the neck muscles. Others prefer the Philadelphia type because it does not compress the cricoid cartilage, but supports the head and neck between the chin and sternum.

Clavicle supports have been used for shoulder weakness with limited success. They do not improve function of the upper extremities but for periods of time relieve muscle pain from strain on the shoulder cuff tendons and neck muscles.

Support for the weak neck and shoulder muscles can be provided by a high-backed and reclined chair, whether it is a recliner wheelchair, a high-back commode, or a recliner lounge or lift chair. Many patients will scoot down in an armchair to provide support to these muscles and rest their heads on the lower back of the chair. This suffices until pressure on the lower back or coccyx becomes apparent.

Upper Extremity Weakness

Most upper extremity devices are used with short-term success due to the progressive nature of the disease. Mobile arm supports provide limited function for eating and typing when shoulder, elbow, and wrist weakness is greater than hand weakness. Usually an added T-bar or a dorsal or volar wrist splint is required to support the wrist. Mobile arm support options include wheelchair or table-mount brackets (for patients who are not in wheelchairs).

Wrist support splints are helpful to some patients but may limit function by restricting substitution motions. Built-up, lightweight handles on eating utensils, toothbrushes, and pens or pencils make continued use of these items possible. A large-handled, lightweight cup is easier to use when all fingers can be placed through the handle. Dressing aids more commonly used include buttonhooks and loops in zippers. Dressing adaptations include pullover dresses or shirts, jogging or leisure clothing with elastic waists or Velcro fastenings, and slip-on shoes. Key holders increase surface area for house and car keys and make turning easier. Turning devices for knobs and handles can also be helpful. Electric toothbrushes and shavers are often too heavy for patients but more convenient for caregivers.

Various electronic switches are available to attach to appliances, such as television, radio, or lights. New styles of telephones requiring light touch or no touch to activate the receiver are also available. Emergency alert systems with easy-touch switches dispatch assistance from hospital emergency centers in some communities.

Upper extremity weakness is a difficult problem with ALS patients since abilities change so quickly. Care in recommending and providing such items is needed. Patients' priorities and long-term concerns, especially in regard to communication and emergency alert, may require more attention than frequent and costly change in adaptive aids that are soon discarded. This area is one in which therapeutic intervention may be particularly helpful since a system of interdependence of patient and caregiver must be developed.

Comfort in Bed

When the patient requires more time supported in bed than in a chair, the value of the full electric hospital bed is apparent. Addition of an overbed table assists with placement of food, writing or communication devices, reading or leisure materials, and hygiene care supplies.

To help prevent skin breakdown and provide comfort, some items have been reported more useful than others. The alternating pressure pad provides an intermittent flow of air to rise and lower parts of the body. The noise of the compressor may interfere with being able to hear the weakened voice of the patient. Foam (eggcrate) mattress pads do relieve pressure but patients cannot move at all once they settle into it. The water mattress is comfortable if an adequate method of heating is available. Sheepskin pads are adequate if perspiration is not a problem for the patient.

The hydraulic patient lift with full-length separating sling is most helpful for caregivers, and patients feel safe being transferred in them. With adequate instruction from the therapist, simple, convenient transfer system can be managed by one caregiver. Toileting can be managed more easily. The aptitude and abilities of the caregiver are the major concern when training with this equipment, although use of it is usually a team effort between patient and caregiver in terms of communication.

Briefly mentioned here are the computer-communication systems which are available and used from the bed by some ALS patients to manage business, leisure, or household tasks.

SUMMARY

Home occupational therapy intervention must augment the patient's and caregiver's adaptive skills to effectively manage this progressive disease. Special care must be taken by therapists to support their independence and present function with alternatives ready when loss of that function occurs. However, care is needed not to overwhelm them with assistive equipment or changed routines or next-stage problems. Adaptation in this disease involves loss of function without loss of dignity or self-worth. The occupational therapist's special task is to facilitate these changes in home caregiving by recommending the appropriate assistive equipment to patient and caregiver.

BIBLIOGRAPHY

Hamilton L: Why Didn't Somebody Tell Me About These Things? Inter Collegiate Press, Shawnee Mission, KS, 1984.

Home Care for the Patient with Amyotrophic Lateral Sclerosis. National Amyotrophic Lateral Sclerosis Foundation, New York, 1977.

Scott A: Amyotrophic lateral sclerosis. In Trombly C (ed): Occupational Therapy for Physical Dysfunction. Williams & Wilkins, Baltimore, MD 1983, pp. 333–335.

Takai V: ADL and adaptive equipment for ALS patients. *AOTA Phys Dis Sp Int Newsletter* 6:1–2, 1983.

CHAPTER SEVENTEEN

COMMUNICATION PROBLEMS IN THE PATIENT WITH AMYOTROPHIC LATERAL SCLEROSIS

Steven H. Blaustein, M.S., M.Ph.

One of the more devastating aspects of amyotrophic lateral sclerosis (ALS) is the progressive loss of the patient's ability to communicate, and it is the role of the speech pathologist working with ALS patients to assist the individual in maintaining some form of functional communication for as long as possible.

It is immediately noted that *communication* is different from speech or "talking." Speech is a complex motor act requiring rapid movements and precise coordination of the respiratory system, laryngeal mechanism, and supralaryngeal articulators, an act that gradually becomes difficult and eventually impossible for many ALS patients. Communication, the expression of thoughts, feelings, or needs, may be delivered via a variety of modalities, such as writing, gesturing, or even blinking. This concept is extremely important and must be discussed with patients as part of the therapy process. Since ALS is a progressive disease, the goal of therapy will eventually be to enable the patient to communicate in any way possible. This must be accepted by the patient and family.

It is recommended that the plan of therapy and options available be discussed with the patient and family at an early point in treatment. Patients are often referred by other professionals to "speech therapy" and the speech pathologist has no idea of what the patient was told or what expectations are. Patients and their families who attend therapy regularly and follow-up at home with practice exercises may expect improvement, or at least stabilization, in the speech disorder. Although temporary improvement in intelligibility is often initially seen through compensatory strategies, the patient's speech eventually continues to deteriorate. Unless the patient is aware of this, he may become disappointed, angry, and frustrated. Patients have been known to discontinue therapy due to un-

Table 17–1.   Common Speech and Related Problems of Amyotrophic Lateral Sclerosis Patients

Dysarthria
Velopharyngeal incompetence
Anarthria
Tracheotomy
Dysphagia

realized expectations or confused goals. It is therefore extremely important that speech pathologists begin the therapeutic relationship with each patient by clearly setting forth realistic expectations concerning treatment.

Experience with numerous ALS patients seen over several years has identified five areas of concern that patients repeatedly and frequently present with and that the speech pathologist must address.

1. Management of dysarthria
2. Management of hypernasality and associated problems secondary to velopharyngeal incompetence
3. Working with the anarthric or unintelligible patient in acquiring and using an augmentative communication system
4. Working with the patient on a respirator or the patient with a tracheostomy
5. Management of swallowing problems (dysphagia)

Table 17–1 summarizes these problems.

Any of these five areas, which often occur singly in other patients, may coexist or occur sequentially in one ALS patient. Thus, it is extremely important to ensure correct timing in managing the patient, deciding when to introduce various therapies and discontinue others, and establishing a correctly focused treatment plan.

DYSARTHRIA

Patients should be referred for a speech and voice evaluation at the first sign of change in voice, resonance, or speech pattern, or repeated chewing or swallowing difficulty. These may be reported by the patients as occurring intermittently. Patients may report reduced intelligibility on awakening or in the evening, difficulty speaking on the telephone, and so on. A complete speech and voice evaluation should be done which should include the following:

1. Oral-peripheral examination to determine structure and function of the articulators

2. Determination of diadochokinetic rates
3. Formal and informal articulation assessment
4. Evaluation of vocal quality, intensity, pitch, and resonance
5. Evaluation of rate and prosodic features
6. Assessment of breath support for speech
7. Investigation into patient's communicative needs and problems
8. Baseline tape recordings

The initial evaluation of the ALS patient with speech involvement at an early stage will differ little from a standard dysarthria evaluation that all speech pathologists are familiar with. Available dysarthria assessment measures and scales are certainly useful and applicable. The oral peripheral examination is extremely important and the speech pathologist should carefully note such things as lingual atrophy and fasciculations, velar involvement, and restrictions in range of movement or weakness in any of the articulators that may affect articulation or the ability to compensate.

If necessary, therapy may be initiated. This consists of compensatory techniques to overcome the dysarthric speech pattern. These include: teaching the patient to overarticulate, heightening self-monitoring skills, reestablishing phrasing patterns to maximize breath support and compensate for slower speech, and helping patients to attain better phonation. In more severe cases, modifying linquistic messages and using supplementary augmentative techniques are considered.

Patients present with varying degrees of dysarthria and varying rates of progression. The amount of intervention is related to the level of involvement. Mildly involved patients may benefit from a few sessions of therapy. Patients with a more marked involvement, and hence less intelligibility, will be seen more frequently. In general, however, patients are seen as long as it takes to attain immediate, realistic goals. Patients have generally not been followed throughout the course of the disease with weekly speech therapy. Rather, they are seen on an as-needed basis, providing intervention to allow for maximum communicative ability based on their current status. Additional care is provided, as needed, based on the progression of the disease. Once immediate goals are met, patients and families are advised to contact the speech pathologist should their level of communication begin to change. In addition, patients are given follow-up visits and are seen regularly at predetermined intervals.

Speech pathologists who work with ALS patients frequently ask about the value of oral motor exercises for their patients. There is little, if any, literature available concerning the efficacy of such exercises. It is therefore the individual pathologist's decision to choose whether to use such "strengthening" or "motor" exercises. It must always be remembered that ALS is a progressive degenerative motor disease and that no matter what is done, the patient's articulation will eventually deteriorate.

It would be helpful for the speech pathologist working with ALS patients to be familiar with the type of dysarthria encountered in this disease. According to the Mayo Clinic schema,[1] the dysarthria found in ALS is classified as a mixed dysarthria. Spastic and flaccid features may both be present. The degeneration may not, however, progress evenly, and spastic or flaccid signs may predominate at any given time. The following speech characteristics were found to be most evident in ALS: distortion of vowels, exceedingly slow speech rate, and shortness of phrases. In addition, imprecision of consonants, marked hypernasality, harsh or strained voice, disrupted prosody, and monotone with excessive intervals between words and phrases were also noted. In the Mayo Clinic study,[1] patients with ALS also attained the highest mean rating for "bizarreness." This category refers to the overall speech pattern being unusual or peculiar.

VELOPHARYNGEAL INCOMPETENCE

Patients with bulbar involvement frequently present with velar weakness causing inability to attain adequate velopharyngeal closure. Loss of velar function has a markedly detrimental effect on speech. The function of the soft palate is to make contact with the posterior pharyngeal wall so as to seal off the oral cavity from the nasal cavity. The effect for speech is to allow for oral resonance and for the establishment of intraoral air pressure which results in effective consonant production and allows for more efficient use of air for speech and phonation. The inability to create a seal at the velopharyngeal port, therefore, creates numerous speech problems for the ALS patient.

An effective way to manage the velar weakness is by providing the patient with a palatal lift. The palatal lift is usually supplied by a dental prosthodontist and is made of acrylic material with wrought wire clasps to attach it to the teeth (Fig. 17–1). In edentulous patients the velar portion of the lift can be attached to the maxillary portion of the patient's denture (Fig. 17–2). In either case, the velar portion of the lift extends posteriorly and serves to elevate the soft palate to attain better closure (Fig. 17–3). In patients where velar movement is present but diminished, the prosthetic elevation may aid closure by helping the soft palate to better approximate the posterior pharyngeal wall. In patients with no functional velar movement at all, the artificially elevated soft palate will at least serve to occlude some of the gap between the posterior pharynegal wall, lateral pharyngeal walls, and flaccid soft palate.

Patients should be considered for a palatal lift if there are any objective or subjective indications of velopharyngeal insufficiency. These may include varying degrees of hypernasality, nasal emission of air, and re-

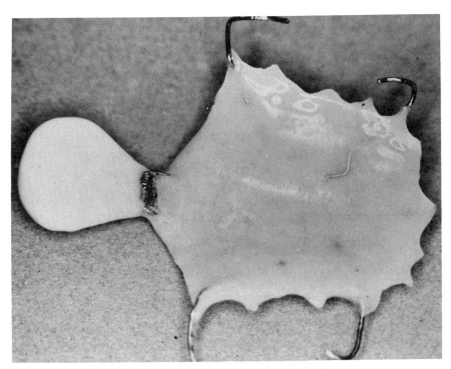

Figure 17–1. Dentulous palatal lift. (Courtesy of Alan Sheiner, DDS.)

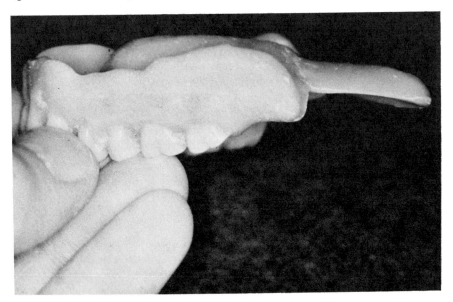

Figure 17–2. Edentulous palatal lift. (Courtesy of Alan Sheiner, DDS.)

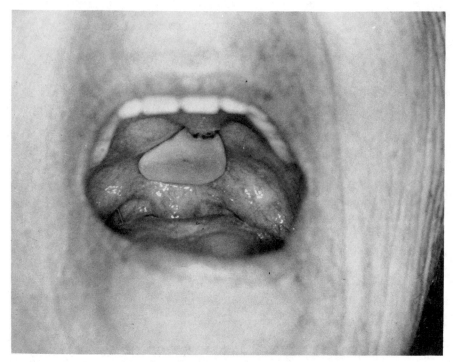

Figure 17–3. Palatal lift in place. (Courtesy of Alan Sheiner, DDS.)

duced intraoral air pressure causing consonant distortions. Patients may complain of "having to push" to speak and "running out of air," especially at the end of phrases. Many patients attempt to increase vocal intensity in an effort to compensate, which actually further distorts speech. Voice therapy is often briefly indicated to reduce hyperfunctional tendencies and to establish maximum vocal use.

A second consideration in recommending a palatal lift is the degree of articulatory control remaining. The patient must maintain sufficient ability to articulate to warrent placement of a lift. For this reason, when indicated, rapid and early provision of a palatal lift is recommended.

ANARTHRIA

Patients with speech involvement will generally progress from mild dysarthria to an anarthric condition. Anarthria means complete loss of functional articulation. Patients at this stage may still be able to phonate, yet, due to the severe progression of the disease, only strained, undifferential vowels may be produced. Once the patient approaches a moderate to severe dysarthria, an augmentative communication system must be considered. An augmentative system is meant to augment, or replace, the patient's no longer functional speech system. It is wise to begin evaluating and training a patient for such a system prior to the time the patient is actually fully dependent on it. This allows time for familiarizing the patient, family, and friends with the system, allowing them to practice with the system, and actually ordering and acquiring the system. Many patients manage the transition from a dysarthric to an anarthric state by using both a residual vocal system and augmentative system to maximize communication.

Advances in personal computers, microelectronics, and communication technology in recent years have tremendously improved options available to patients. The speech pathologist who endeavors to provide augmentative communication systems should be aware of latest developments in this rapidly changing area. If necessary, patients may be referred to a center that specializes in augmentative communication evaluations where systems may be viewed and tried.

In considering an augmentative system for an ALS patient, the needs of the patient must be considered along with his physical limitations. Thus, at this point, it is often beneficial to work with an occupational and physical therapist to select the appropriate system. A large variety of switches are available, including those that operate by blowing, sucking, or wrinkling the forehead. There are systems now available that can operate merely by eye gaze. Available devices may or may not incorporate synthetic speech. There are programmable systems and preprogrammed systems. The decision-making process in choosing an augmentative communication system is complex and must include when to introduce the system, selecting the appropriate system for the needs and ability of the patient, and selecting the type of desired output modality. Finally, the rate and degree of progression of the disease must be weighed. A system should be adaptable enough to be functional for the patient for the maximum amount of time. The augmentative system will provide the patient with a connection to the world and will enhance his quality of life immeasurably.

TRACHEOSTOMY

Some patients with ALS present with pulmonary problems that necessitate a tracheostomy and need for some type of ventilatory support to aid in respiration. Such patients may or may not have speech involvement. It is distressing to see an ALS patient with little or no speech involvement lose his ability to communicate for any amount of time as a result of being "trached." There are many options available to such patients.

The loss of voice in these patients is a direct result of the loss of subglottal pressure at the larynx as the air is diverted through the tracheostomy. This may be a temporary or permanent condition and the speech pathologist must work closely with the pulmonary specialist and otolaryngologist in devising a substitute system. Initially, articulation must be assessed to determine if sufficient articulation is present to warrent continuing to attempt to provide the patient with a manner of "voicing." If the patient is unintelligible, then an augmentative system is considered. If, however, the patient has adequate articulatory control, a variety of options can be considered.

Patients on ventilators may be able to phonate. Factors to be considered include the necessity for a tracheostomy that is "cuffed," the amount of time the cuff must remain inflated, and the size of the tracheostomy tube. The patient's remaining degree of respiratory function is another factor. If the patient is still unable to phonate after all of the above factors have been investigated, commercially available aids such as "Communi-Trach" or "Venti-Voice" may be considered. Finally, many patients do very well with a high-quality electrolarynx.

The ALS patient with a tracheostomy who is dependent on ventilatory support should not be overlooked.

DYSPHAGIA

Progressive swallowing problems are found in patients who present with progressive speech difficulty. The speech pathologist along with the nurse and nutritionist will often be involved in assisting the ALS patient in overcoming these problems. Chapters 9, 10 are devoted to management of this most difficult area.

SUMMARY

Encountering an ALS patient who requires treatment can be an overwhelming and difficult experience for many speech pathologists. Such patients present with numerous, progressive problems that severely hamper communication. Treating such patients requires all of the speech pathologist's skills and repertoire of therapeutic techniques. An open, honest approach with the patient is always best. It must be stressed that what can be accomplished in this difficult disease is limited. What can be offered is appreciated and valued, however. The speech pathologist's role is to keep patients communicating and when this is accomplished it is a most rewarding experience.

REFERENCE

1. Darley F, Aronson A, Brown J: Motor Speech Disorders. Saunders, Philadelphia, 1975.

BIBLIOGRAPHY

Beukelman D, Yorkston K, Dowden P: Communication Augmentation—A Casebook of Clinical Management. College Hill Press, San Diego, CA, 1985.
Darley F, Aronson A, Brown J: Motor Speech Disorders. Saunders, Philadelphia, 1975.
Groher M: Dysphagia Diagnosis and Management. Butterworths, Boston, 1984.
Logeman J: Evaluation and Treatment of Swallowing Disorders. College Hill Press, San Diego, CA, 1983.
Musselwhite C, St. Louis: Communication Programming for the Severely Handicapped: Vocal and Non-Vocal Strategies. College Hill Press, San Diego, CA, 1982.

CHAPTER EIGHTEEN

REACTIONS OF PATIENTS, FAMILY, AND STAFF IN DEALING WITH AMYOTROPHIC LATERAL SCLEROSIS

Philip B. Luloff, M.D.

It is apparent from the foregoing chapters that the nervous system of a person with amyotrophic lateral sclerosis (ALS) degenerates. What is not so apparent, however, is that other systems that tie the life of a person together degenerate as well.

The psychological system of an individual is obviously affected, as is his family system. What is less apparent is how the connections between the patient and the health professional often degenerate and become disrupted.

Although this chapter does not permit an exhaustive discussion of the various dynamics and mechanisms underlying the reactions of patients, their family, and staff in dealing with ALS, an attempt will be made to elucidate major areas of concern based upon observations made in dealing with large numbers of ALS patients over several years.

In working with patients, their families, and staff one notices an interesting and often consistent reaction, a parallel process, if you will. Much of what has been observed as a reaction of patients is also mirrored in the reaction of family and medical staff in a more attenuated form.

In the face of the stresses of ALS, the patient often regresses to less mature forms of behavior. The degree of regression depends upon the nature and severity of the disease, the patient's early life experiences, and the quality of the interrelationships between the patient, family, and health care professional team.

In general, certain immature character patterns which are reasonably well attenuated during periods of health, may emerge with particular clarity when the disease strikes. For example, profound regression may be manifested by the withdrawn, uncommunicative behavior of one patient, or another's guarded suspicion.

267

Other behavior patterns may be similarly interpreted as indicative of regression to earlier levels of psychosexual development. The patient may plead for care, attention, and love or may demand it aggressively. Other patients may show behavior which ranges from extreme self-control, obedience, and cooperativeness to rebellion and outbursts of temper, while still others may manifest fears of being hurt physically or a wish to compete with and to take over the medical care professional's job.

Whatever form the patient's behavior takes, its regressive components are often evident, motivated by the wish to have the health professional take over a role of a confident, authoritative, omnipotent, protective parent who will safeguard him during his illness.[1]

This often leads to conflict when staff tries to fulfill this need only to be defeated by the vicissitudes of the disease. Often family members, too, are subject to regressive behavior and are seen as saboteurs of the therapy plan by staff or patient. The regression of family members is often matched by staff who manifest emotions such as anger, avoidance, fear, denial, guilt, depression, hopelessness, and helplessness and who attempt to find a powerful, all-knowing figure to make things right.

Another way of viewing the behavior of individuals in relation to ALS is from an adaptational frame of reference. Loss of resources—physical, psychological, social, and economic—evokes grief and depression. As the patient anticipates or experiences failures in mastering the problems and challenges of everyday life, he develops feelings of helplessness. For most people such feelings are unpleasant and frustrating. Helplessness and failure, real or anticipated, lead to decrease of self-esteem, sense of worth, dignity, and confidence. Anger becomes mixed with fear and is accentuated by limitations in ability to master everyday problems, in achieving relief from tensions, and in providing oneself with gratifying experiences. Anger is often directed against oneself for being damaged, helpless, worthless, and a failure, which further decreases self-esteem and confidence. Anger is also directed against persons, and at natural processes which appear to be increasingly harsh and threatening as the individual becomes progressively impaired and weaker.

At other times, anger adds to feelings of strength and permits patients to mobilize their remaining resources, but experiences of anger usually lead to increased fear due to guilt, with the associated conviction that one should be punished.[2]

In this setting of increasing fear, anger, and helplessness, the patient's need for others becomes accentuated. In attempting to get support and aid, the patient often is susceptible to charlatans who promise help at first, but ultimately leave the patient feeling more devastated.

In the face of a disease process in which realistic expectations are less ambitious than immediate cure, staff understandably has difficulty dealing with the reactions of those they are trying to help. This is especially true when their help is not seen as good enough, or unrealistic expectations of patients and families are shared by staff.

Family members often have similar reactions to patients, and feel guilty, helpless, and ambivalent in dealing with the change in status of the patient from provider to dependent individual.

For the couple, marital boundaries and issues of power and control provide a springboard for degeneration of the family system. Old family problems and battles may reemerge with family members being subject to outbursts of anger or even physical abuse.

Health professionals with the desire to help and a fair amount of omnipotent feelings are often devastated by the disease. Its relentless course, the discouragement of patients, and their anger and pain are often overwhelming to staff. Staff will complain about working conditions and lack of time, engage in interdisciplinary arguments and territorial disputes, and generally act in nonconstructive ways. Displacing their feelings of being overwhelmed by the disease, staff will manifest behavior ranging from displays of anger to sabotage, passive noncompliance, and open rebellion.

It is clear that having a team of similarly committed health care professionals which meets regularly is very helpful. Even then, problems occur. For a sole practitioner it is much more difficult to deal with the disease, which explains why so many patients have felt abandoned by their doctors after a diagnosis of ALS. We have found that an open atmosphere where people can share their feelings in a nonjudgmental way has been helpful to all health care professionals. For staff, regular meetings to clarify feelings are especially important. When they have not occurred the result has always been an increase in intrastaff conflicts and anxiety with a concomitant decrease in morale. So, too, in families in which people can talk to one another and share their feelings in a reassuring emotional atmosphere, the effect is to decrease intrafamily conflict. This is also true for the individual patient who has an ongoing relationship with a health care professional who is consistently supportive.

USE OF PSYCHOTROPIC MEDICATIONS

An approach to use of psychotropic medications must be individualized for each patient. Although anxiolytic agents such as the benzodiazepines have been widely used to decrease tension, experience has clearly indicated that these should be avoided in ALS patients because of their effect on accentuating muscle weakness. It has been shown that in low doses (50 to 75 mg daily) the tricyclic antidepressants, such as amitriptyline, have been effective in reducing anxiety, with the beneficial side effects of decreasing the emotional lability associated with pseudobulbar palsy and decreasing the amount of oral secretions. In patients with more significant anxiety, and agitation mixed with depression, it has been found that thioridazine in doses of 10 to 25 mg four times a day has been effective. This drug has the beneficial anticholinergic side effect of drying up secretions.

The incidence of major affective disease, schizophrenia, or other psychosis seems to be no greater than that found in the general population.

Sleep problems frequently occur in ALS patients. In evaluating this situation one must keep in mind the possibility of respiratory depression and increased muscle weakness that are associated with such medications and cause special problems for certain ALS patients. Benzodiazepine derivatives and barbiturates are avoided in favor of antihistamines or tricyclics with strong soporific side effects (amitriptyline).

Depression in ALS must be viewed in light of the whole disease process. Reactive, not endogenous, depressions are frequently encountered. Viewed as a reaction to the disease the depression does not necessarily require treatment with medication. Rather, a consistently compassionate approach which views this response as a normal reaction to the situation is what is necessary. It is frequently a stage that patients (as well as family and staff) pass through.

Only an approach that takes into account a multiplicity of determinants from several frames of reference will ultimately explain the different individual reactions to this disease and provide an understanding to the hidden meanings of the communication and behavior of patients, family, and staff in dealing with ALS. It is to be hoped that this individualized approach will help health professionals to be more compassionate in dealing with fellow human beings who are suffering from ALS.

REFERENCES

1. Kaplan SM: Psychiatry and medicine. In Freedman AM, Kaplan HI (eds): Comprehensive Textbook of Psychiatry. Williams & Wilkins, Baltimore, 1967, pp. 1124–1130.
2. Goldfarb AI: Psychotherapy of the aged: The use and value of an adaptational frame of reference. Psychoanal Rev 43:68, 1956.

BIBLIOGRAPHY

Gorlin R, Zucker HD: Physicians' reactions to patients. N Engl J Med 308:1059–1063, 1983.

Kübler-Ross E: On Death and Dying. Macmillan, New York, 1969.

CHAPTER NINETEEN

LIVING AND COPING WITH AMYOTROPHIC LATERAL SCLEROSIS: THE PSYCHOSOCIAL IMPACT

Nurit Ginsberg, C.S.W.

Amyotrophic lateral sclerosis (ALS) is a progressive, degenerative motor neuron disease which affects the body while preserving personality and intellect. After experiencing early symptoms of extremity weakness or bulbar involvement, the patient begins the urgent search for an explanation, often seeing several physicians before a diagnosis of ALS is made and often not comprehending its implications until it is redefined as "Lou Gehrig's disease." At this point his life gets turned upside down. He learns that physical deterioration is inevitable and that he has no control over what will be progressive deterioration of muscle function. The fact that there is no cure for this disease provokes strong feelings of helplessness and vulnerability in patients. The question of how patients and families will cope in the face of this ravaging illness becomes more urgent. As health care professionals we are charged with assisting the patient to cope as well as he can and to help his family support him as well as they can. How do we do this? How do we help the patient maintain his feelings of self-worth? How do we support the family as they cope with inevitable, persistent, and continuous crises?

The psychosocial impact of ALS is as devastating as its physical assaults. They are inseparable and intertwined. Just as in all aspects of life some individuals cope and function better than others, so too with ALS patients. While adaptation is difficult for all, some manage better than others. Although we cannot generalize how to help patients since they differ greatly, some basic principles of behavior can be identified. When these are understood, they help us tune in to the patient's struggle to adjust and this helps us to assist him more effectively.

273

USE OF DENIAL

Denial is a defense used by most newly diagnosed ALS patients. The patient cannot believe or admit to himself that this is happening to him. The use of denial can be beneficial, as it helps the patients to function and cope. As described by Brian Gould, partial denial is maintained throughout a patient's course of illness in a healthy fashion: "Reality was not denied as much as redefined. The most distressing, immutable aspects of the disease were not part of ordinary conscious functioning, and hope was maintained" (Gould, 1980, p. 159). Health care professionals can distinguish when denial is helping the patient and when it is jeopardizing his safety.

In the case of Mr. A., denial allowed him to continue working, which included driving to and from work. The family and staff were aware of the great loss he would sustain if he was prohibited from driving. Yet, it was dangerous for him to continue to drive. This was discussed sensitively with the patient who was able to acknowledge the danger only after his family admitted to him that they felt unsafe as passengers in his car.

DEPRESSION ACCOMPANYING PROGRESSION OF DISEASE

For this patient, facing the fact that he could no longer drive a car began the process of the breakdown of the denial defense. This caused depression, as it forced the patient to look at his reality. Depression occurs in all patients as their symptoms progress. There is a mourning process with each functional loss. Patients struggle to maintain a given level of functioning by compensating in one way or another for muscle dysfunction. They cannot tolerate the awareness that with further deterioration, in the months, weeks, or even days ahead, further loss will occur. And when it does occur, the frustration is intense and the depression severe. How do we help the patient cope with crises within chronicity? How do we help them adjust to a disability that steadily gets worse?

Anxiety is high in all newly diagnosed patients. This may lessen when the progression is slower, enabling them to adjust and find ways of coping.

STRUGGLING WITH DEPENDENCY

It is important that we understand how difficult it is for the patient to lose his independence and self-sufficiency. This is an ongoing struggle that will continue throughout the remainder of his life. Most patients, having been active and independent throughout their lives, experience anger and frustration at needing to rely on others for help in the activities of daily living. This anger and frustration often leads to demanding and regressed behavior, which in turn may provoke resentment in family members caring for the patient. The family feels powerless to meet his needs. This may cause guilt and results in overprotection by the family, in their attempts to do too much. The family's anger and resentment build up and are manifested in various ways, such as fantasies of escape or displacement of feelings on other family members or other health care professionals.

This was illustrated in my work with the B. family. The patient, a 59-year-old married man, became ill and deteriorated at a steady pace. Initially, he fought the disease, resenting the limitations it placed on him and his transformation from "provider" and head of the household to one dependent on his wife. There was a clear role reversal as the wife moved swiftly from her background position in the family to that of decision maker and head of the household. The family continued to function but as the patient became further disabled, the wife exhibited increasing guilt and resentment at being a prisoner in her own home and burdened with the care of her husband. She did a great deal for her husband but was very angry at the situation. Her anger was displaced on her children and friends whom she felt did not understand her. This couple was able to bring their feelings of frustration, resentment, anger, and guilt to session, and by sharing them found ways of coping and going on.

As the patient's physical deterioration increases, he begins to fear he is becoming too difficult for the family to handle. This leads to fears that he will be abandoned by them. He is in conflict. He does need his family's help but is angry at being in this position. He hesitates to express his anger or to make too many demands, which might alienate the family and provoke them to abandon him.

In the case of Mrs. C., a 63-year-old woman, symptoms included weakness in all four extremities as well as bulbar involvement. She exhibited much anger on receiving the diagnosis. This anger, in addition to difficulty adjusting to her limitations, caused her to reject all attempts of staff to provide services and assist her. The patience and support of staff, as well as their not abandoning her as she continued to act out her rage, enabled her to form a trusting relationship and begin to accept the interventions of members of various disciplines. She struggled to maintain as much control as possible. As she became more disabled, dependent on others, and unable to maintain the active, independent life-style she was accustomed to, Mrs. C.'s demands on her husband increased and her behavior at home became very disruptive. As the demands increased, her husband withdrew from her, fulfilling her prophecy of abandonment and thus exacerbating this behavior. Crisis conjoint therapy began as patient and spouse alternately requested that she be placed in an institution. Therapy sessions provided both spouses with an opportunity to verbalize feelings of anger, frustration, resentment, and helplessness at the situation. Having acknowledged these feelings and having them legitimized in conjoint therapy, both husband and wife were able to recognize they did not want to seek placement for the wife. However, because both were feeling overwhelmed, the request for placement had functioned as a cry for help. Ongoing therapy provided them with a safe environment to deal with stressful situations and feelings as they occurred rather than allowing them to build up and become unmanageable.

THOUGHTS OF SUICIDE AND REACTIONS OF DESPAIR

It is draining for health care professionals to work with depressed patients. However, we need to recognize that depression is normal in ALS patients. We must resist our inclination to sidestep or avoid it. Depression ranges from minor reactive to more serious levels of major depression.

Patients may express thoughts about suicide directly but more often we hear these expressed through questions about whether there is any reason to go on living. Although the incidence of suicide is surprisingly rare in this population, all expressions of suicide intent should be taken seriously and carefully explored. Psychiatric consultations should be sought when the health care team evaluates the risk as high. It is common to find that the patient's talk about suicide is his way of expressing his feelings of despair.

LEGITIMIZING FEELINGS

It is important to legitimize the patient's and family's various strong, negative but normal feelings. The patient has a right to feel enraged at this devastating illness. It has already begun to affect his and his family's lives, and future drastic changes are inevitable. Loss of job, diminishing financial security, decreasing social and sexual gratification, changes in appearance and loss of self-esteem, all create profound feelings of loss, provoke intense anxiety, and produce depression.

Some patients and their families are able to acknowledge their feelings about the illness. Others find these issues too painful to deal with directly and will focus on less threatening and more tangible issues. Talking about equipment, help at home, moving to a new location, and so on channels their anxiety away from these difficult feelings. Help with these daily life issues is important in its own right but solutions to these practical issues will not lessen the anxiety the patient and family are experiencing.

FUNCTION OF SUPPORT GROUPS

Many patients feel strongly that only others who are experiencing the same illness and difficulties can really understand and appreciate what they are going through. It is for that reason that we organized the support group consisting of ALS patients.

The group is a forum providing mutual support. It is where patients discuss with each other the fears, difficulties, and concerns they cannot express with their families. The group members are open in sharing feelings and facts about their physical deterioration. Fantasies of death are explored indirectly. The theme of death emerges from time to time yet is dealt with primarily through intellectualization and rationalization. Suicide is explored but reinterpreted by the group as giving up. By setting limits to how far they are willing to go in painful discussion, they cling to a sense of mastery over their feelings, even though they have no control over the disease itself.

A separate group provides family members and others involved in the patient's care a similar forum for them to talk together about their caregiving tasks and their apprehensions of the future. They share, express, and explore the mixed feelings they have.

ROLE OF THE SOCIAL WORKER

Because of the lack of cure of ALS, the focus and interventions of health care professionals with the patient and family take the form of supportive care. This caring activity involves many professional judgments.

Initial psychosocial assessment involves determining the patient's and family's understanding of the illness and its implications. The social worker sees all patients on the basic premise that every ALS patient and his family will have multiple adjustment problems. In getting to know the patient and family, one learns about both their present and past coping abilities. This understanding gives the mental health practitioner an indication of how best to intervene. Timing is important as one must be cautious not to intervene prematurely and upset the equilibrium of a patient struggling to maintain control and independence. It is also important not to assume that the patient is managing well as this can leave him feeling frustrated, ashamed, and helpless because he is not.

Some patients can be helped to get in touch with their feelings. When patients give clear messages of their desire not to deal with painful issues, these should be respected.

Much discussion revolves around the benefits of a patient exploring fears and feelings about illness and death, yet some patients choose not to deal with these areas. Based on her work with cancer patients, Ruth Adams points out that some patients desire to talk about illness and death and will do so readily, whereas others choose not to. Often it is persons involved with caring for patients—whether family, caretakers, or health care professionals—who raise these issues, rather than patients (Adams, 1974, p. 77).

As they act to support one another, patients and their families need guidance and assistance in communicating. Feelings may be frightening to both parties and therefore not easily talked about. Husband and wife may be concerned that they will upset each other by raising difficult feelings and issues. Gradual exploration combined with legitimizing and supporting the feelings that are raised may enable the patient and family to feel safer discussing them. Careful monitoring of emotional states of the patient and family is needed as changes occur in his medical condition.

In some cases, it is best to work with the patient and other family members individually, while joint therapy is preferable in other instances. Family sessions are essential where communication has broken down, feelings are displaced onto others, and the stress and tensions building up at home interfere with the family's ability to adequately care for the patient. Sometimes a patient's behavior provokes the family. This situation needs to be explored to avert buildup of resentments which might disrupt patient care.

Families stressed by the physical and emotional needs of the patient often need an advocate to help them obtain and use community resources, such as home care, Medicaid, and chronic care facilities. They also need an advocate when patients are hospitalized for medical procedures. By using community resources and support of the ALS team, patients are maintained at home throughout the course of the illness and placement in various institutions and chronic care facilities are rare.

The following case illustrates a couple's struggle in adjusting and coping with ALS. Mrs. D., 69, was diagnosed with ALS 2 years ago. She was first relieved at being given a diagnosis, since it ruled out a psychiatric base to her physical symptoms. Relief quickly dissolved to shock as she learned of the implications of the disease. Her good muscle functioning helped her emotionally deny her illness but it also caused her to reject services offered by members of various team disciplines.

Mrs. D. began to feel very anxious when bulbar involvement made her speech difficult to understand. She was frustrated when peers in her senior center began avoiding her. As she could no longer participate in activities, she began withdrawing socially. Her husband lamented the deterioration of their golden years together. He was angry and frightened about her illness. The guilt he experienced over his anger manifested itself in his determination to do whatever he could for his wife. He set up unrealistic expectations for himself about what he could do for her, which inevitably led to failure.

As the disease spread to her extremities, she became increasingly dependent on him and the tensions between them were exacerbated. Individual and joint therapy was initiated to help them deal with their reactions. Mrs. D. joined the patient support group which provided social stimulation as well as helping her to share her experiences with others with whom she could identify. It was frightening for her to see other patients more disabled than she. Group members were supportive and helped her with her fears and distress. Mr. D's engagement with the caregivers group was short-lived as he could not accept comfort, solace, or legitimization of his feelings from the group.

Gastrostomy and tracheostomy were performed to alleviate swallowing and respiratory distress. This caused depression as the patient viewed her respirator dependence as a life sentence.

During hospitalization the patient's behavior and the husband's anxiety was interpreted for the house staff. The floor staff were able to be more patient, supportive, and empathetic as they better understood where her demanding and regressed behavior came from. They recognized, too, that Mr. D's anxiety came from his anger at not being able to help his wife.

Mr. and Mrs. D.'s difficulty in dealing with each other's feelings immobilized them to the point of setting up for failure several plans to discharge the patient home. The patient was eventually transferred to a long-term care facility. She experienced further depression on leaving Mount Sinai Hospital, since it took away her one goal, to return home, and she was now facing the reality that she would remain in the new facility for the rest of her life.

Although this case is unusual because few ALS patients require institutionalization, it does illustrate how issues of helplessness and hopelessness dominate the lives of ALS patients and their families. There is a natural tendency for the human being to turn away from others in pain, who manifest helplessness and hopelessness. Health care professionals working with ALS patients will often feel a similar kind of helplessness in the face of the incurable, progressive nature of the illness. However, they do not turn away and this is their important way of helping. Health care professionals stay with the patient and family and provide understanding, empathy, and patience which makes patient and family feel less alone and less isolated. This is not a one-time infusion of support, but rather a long-term commitment to work along with the patient and family as they struggle day by day with the difficult tasks and demands of adapting to life with ALS.

BIBLIOGRAPHY

Adams R: Not Alone with Cancer. Thomas, Springfield, IL, 1974.

Gould Brian S: "Psychiatric Aspects" in Diagnosis vs Treatment of Amyotrophic Lateral Sclerosis. DW Mulder (ed), Houghton Mifflin, Boston, MA, 1980.

Masser I, Caroscio JT, Luloff P, et al.: The team approach to the care of patients with amyotrophic lateral sclerosis (ALS): A psycho-social perspective. In Psychosocial Aspects of Muscular Dystrophy and Allied Diseases. Thomas, Springfield, IL, 1983.

CHAPTER TWENTY

EMOTIONAL RESPONSE TO AMYOTROPHIC LATERAL SCLEROSIS AND ITS IMPACT ON MANAGEMENT OF PATIENT CARE

Eliana Horta, M.S., R.N.

Peter is 44 years old. He laboriously emerged from painful poverty, having worked since childhood. He worked his way through medical school and became a respected surgeon, yet he never forgot the lessons of his life experience. He has lived with generosity, kindness, and compassion for his fellow man. Now, here he is—agonizingly aware of his illness and its imposed deterioration—becoming more and more imprisoned by his own body.

Carlos is 49 years old. He grew up amidst devastating violence in Colombia. Overcoming poverty and lack of education, he immigrated to the United States and went on to become a successful welder. Now he is being invaded by a disease that he barely understands, and is unable to use the hands that gave him a sense of self-worth and a power to master his life.

Mary was 65. She died 9 months after the diagnosis of amyotrophic lateral sclerosis (ALS).

Christine was 36 years old. She lived 3 years after the diagnosis of ALS.

We could continue this list. In each ALS patient we could identify a similar pattern: perplexity about the unknown origin of the disease, rebellion caused by the absence of cure, fear of its progressive deterioration, and despair in the face of the inevitability of a premature death. It is patients' suffering in the emotional response to ALS that is the concern of this chapter. Psychological considerations in the care of the ALS patient will be presented from a developmental framework. Observations concerning emotional care based on the clinical experience of the author will be presented.

283

THE CONFLICT OF DEPENDENCE-INDEPENDENCE

The deepest needs of the human being make him dependent on others. Birtchnell describes dependency as "the extent to which an individual relies on another for his existence."[1] Through complex developmental processes the individual crosses from infantile dependency on the mother and the tender nurturing she offers, to the specialization of adult biological and psychological functioning.

The mother's nurturing allows the child to deal with anxiety, and to eventually achieve a loving and self-confident personality of his own.[2] Progressive maturation results in the evolution of a mature person who is a separate, autonomous, and independent individual, yet who is also able to establish intimate relationships. These relationships facilitate feelings of self-fulfillment without feelings of restriction or control by others. However, some interpersonal dependence is a lasting feature of human life. It is in the context of interpersonal relationships that we satisfy higher levels of human needs.

For healthy development, there is a dynamic and continual process of change in the individual's inner or internal self. Through this process there evolves the capacity to act autonomously, which enables an individual to adapt to or manage life crises.

The process of development, which Gesell referred to as one of "individuating maturation,"[3] results in a unique history for each human being.

THE DEVELOPMENTAL PERSPECTIVE OF RESPONSE

As health care workers, somehow we tend to focus on the unsuccessful resolutions of the process of human development. We are particularly eager to hear about the developmental history of those patients who present with a psychiatric problem or diagnostic label. Rarely do we attend to the developmental history in those patients presenting with physical illness. We seem to forget that our psychological *present* in part a historical summary that has all the resolved developmental contingencies *and* our unresolved conflicts and unfulfilled plans and aspirations. Misfortune, disease, and fear of dying open the door wide to the historical content of our minds, which is often saturated with infantile emotions and feelings.

Seldom do we include in our assessment observations of the patient's personality structure and functioning from a developmental perspective. We may even label patients in strict accordance with physical illness. It has been assumed that various diseases are associated with different types of personality. It is almost an "if A then B" type of spurious argument: here is the diagnosis, then you have already identified the psychological disturbance. However, research does not support this claim.[4] A psychological study of ALS patients by Houpt and co-workers in 1977 did not show any characteristics that distinguish them from any other organically sick patients.[5]

Neither the initial nor the ongoing emotional reaction of patients to ALS is merely a "here and now" response. It contains remnants of assimilation of experiences, intensification of personality traits, defensive postures to manage reality, and so on. Disease does not add anything new to the personality structure. For example, for many of our patients the maturation process has not been so well and satisfactorily accomplished. Developmental history may contain examples of traumatic events such as early abandonment, affective deprivation, denied tenderness, and other factors that prevent, in the words of Winnicott, "the self becoming complete."[6] The failure of completion in maturation paralyzes the individual in a dependent phase. Thus he may be unable to achieve full differentation of ego and object. The person then may have only a limited capacity to acquire an integrated self-concept, to achieve the ability to evaluate and accept himself, and to be able to give as well as receive affectively.

This impoverished emotional evolution tends to make such individuals continue through their life cycle overdepending on external objects and circumstances. In this mode there emerges a belief that respect comes from attaining a certain position, love of others derives from providing for them, acceptance comes only from "good behavior"—nothing, in other words, relates to one's self per se. What happens, then, if a disease such as ALS occurs? When the disease takes away aspects of social functioning, it takes away the external support for those persons. Then early and primitive questions related to self-worth and the meaning of one's existence, fear of isolation, and anguish that one does not belong take place and invade patients' inner reality.

This point is essential to consider when we provide emotional care. It is a questionable practice to label patients as "normally depressed." The full exploration of their developmental history is an irreplaceable component of emotional assessment. Identification of psychological strengths as well as weaknesses or disorders will enable us to determine the most effective therapeutic approach. That approach may be psychotherapy, psychopharmacology, or a combination of both treatment modalities.

As the disease process of ALS progresses, one may see a kind of vicious circle of psyche–soma interaction at work. Thus, as the patient preceives that his physical condition is deteriorating, the possible resultant emotional disturbance may intensify the pain and suffering. In turn, the heightened negative emotional response itself becomes psychologically painful.

Physical threat or life-threatening illness can be an eliciting factor in the occurrence of depression and/or anxiety. The manifestation of the depressed/anxious response has been recognized as highly influenced by previous life experience. This observation was recently corroborated by a study of depressed twins.[7] In light of the preceding discussion, it seems obligatory that the health care team caring for ALS patients include a person or persons with expertise in comprehensive clinical psychiatry care.

DENIAL AND ITS CONTRIBUTION TO COPING

In the reaction of the patient to his disease, we often perceive *denial*. Denial as a defensive mechanism essentially implies "rejecting and keeping something out of counsciousness."[8] The information is there, but because it is perceived as a threat to life or one's integrity, it is converted in a fashion. This conversion then substitutes the consequences of the "reality" and establishes a kind of intellectual acceptance of what has been repressed. Working with the patient's denial is an extremely delicate aspect of emotional care. We must consider that denial is part of a more complex intrapsychic process closely allied to resistance. Fairbain and Guntrip, among others, note the defensive aim of resistance. They describe resistance as serving to maintain the patient's internal world as a closed system, a static internal situation. These self-contained situations in inner reality may persist unchanged indefinitely so long as they remain self-contained.[9]

From the foregoing discussion, denial is seen not merely as a refusal of the patient to agree with the caregiver, to cooperate, collaborate, follow suggestions, or comply with a treatment plan. Neither is it some sort of "truth" that the patient avoids to tell us or will not accept from us. It appears that denial is a protective and primarily unconscious method of retaining psychological equilibrium. The disorganizing effects of overwhelming anxiety are thus averted. Denial is a closed system that protects the individual from the fears that arise out of having to "cope with life when one feels that one is just not a real person, that one's ego is basically weak, perhaps that one has hardly got an ego at all."[10]

The intervention at the level of denial must consider this assumed connection with resistance. If the health professional uses too much pressure, or the intervention is delivered with misunderstanding of the dynamics of denial and resistance, it may reinforce the patient's defense rather than help in its resolution.

Understanding and managing what we often refer to as denial or resistance is a significant example of the need for an open and comprehensive communication among members of the health care team. In the delicate equilibrium of life versus disease and its consequences, sometimes one professional can subtly and inadvertently undo what is being done by another member of the team. But most importantly, team communication can strengthen the understanding of the patient's global situation and his psychological processes.

PREPARATION FOR DYING

A pervasive component of the emotional response to ALS is fear of dying and preparation for dying. With the intensification of weakness and muscle atrophy, the patient is faced with increasing evidence of the ultimate outcome of his illness.

Each person experiences the inevitability of death in a unique, individual way. The possibility of understanding the patient's circumstances depends on what data are accessible to us from the person's history, how he experiences life, and the meaning he attributes to existence. Clinical observations of this author have pointed toward an existential component to the commonly noted fear of dying experienced by those with terminal illness. Thus, many patients exhibit a fear that their life has been worthless—that neither their life nor their death had meaning or would have meaning to anyone. The fear of dying alone and the loneliness of death increases, and if not dealt with may reach the point of an anguished obsession.

The development of inner resources to face death has been interfered within the socialization process of our society which exalts youth and seldom encourages understanding of death as belonging to the life cycle. It is then not surprising that a rather magic notion of what Yalom calls "one's own inviolability"[11] is found among us. This notion of inviolability may be a part of the mechanism operative when explanations and teaching about illness can not be processed.

EMOTIONAL CARE FOR THE DYING

The timing of teaching and listening to the ALS patient can not be "scheduled." Some patients, as Yalom notes "face death anxiety in a staccato fashion: a brief moment of awareness, brief terror, denial, internal processing and then preparedness for more information."[12] Other patients are more tentative in their approach to death anxiety. They may process information and observations much more slowly. Some of this information may have been present since the beginning of the diagnostic phase of illness, but was repressed because it has been assimilated through the underlying stratum of primitive emotions and experiences.

As previously discussed, denial serves as a resource to reduce anxiety. The information, nevertheless, is there. The core of emotional care is to assist in its reprocessing, moving the patient away from the anguish of isolation. It is intervention with the ingredients of compassion, caring, "extending one's self, touching the patient at a profound level."[13]

A vital need of the health worker caring for the ALS patient is understanding of the meaning of death to the patient. We must be cognizant of the meaning of death and the fears of death to individuals. We can not postpone this for "when things get worse." As with other physically ill patients, emotional care of ALS patients has as an aim helping them in whatever circumstances they are found, no matter what state of despair they are in. A prime goal is the promotion of self-care, helping the patient to discover his own strengths. For the patient in an advanced disease state, recapture of the positive experiences of the past (through recall or reminiscence) may help the patient assimilate those experiences constructively. This expression of his humanness may go far in banishing the patient's feelings of worthlessness as he reviews his life.

An overall aim of care for the ALS patient, from the very beginning of our contact with him, is to help the patient integrate the stage of death in his developmental continuum. In view of this consideration, beginning with these early contacts with the patient, discussion and listening to the patient about the limiting nature of the illness must begin. This, at the time, is one of the resources available to the health team to help the patient with the anguish of his condition and his coming to terms with it.

As the disease progresses, the patients can be helped to experience some continuity of their power, freedom, and autonomy. It is imperative to encourage them in the exploration of their wishes and choices and to help them make their decisions about death. The possibilities to do so are within the individual. As an example, the patient may decide that at some phase of his illness the prolongation of life through use of respirators would not be desired. The psychotherapeutic intervention is simply facilitating such consideration by the patient and his family, without imposition of one's own will. The health care worker seeks to support the patient and his family in discovering what they want, at a time in the course of illness when those decisions can most reasonably be made.[14] It is crucial to attend to this matter of choice before an emergency situation puts the burden of a final decision on a family member or a primary physician.

REALITY AND HOPEFULNESS

There is a sensitive balance between our ethical commitment to be realistic and the no less moral duty to nurture hopefulness in caring for ALS patients. Reality is perceived in a personal fashion. Patients with ALS, like other human beings, experience their human condition with the specific uniqueness of their being. In the name of loyalty to a reality that may not be congruent with the patient's reality, we may interfere with or destroy their hope. We can not forget that even though disease may have imprisoned the body, the patient's values, feelings, and will may be intact. Control and a sense of autonomy in dealing with one's own destiny is the essence of hope. It is a responsibility of the health care team to nurture that hope in the living and in the dying.

REFERENCES

1. Birtchnell J: Dependence and its relationship to depression. Br J Med Psychol 57:218, 1984.
2. Guntrip H: Personality Structure and Human Interaction. International Universities Press, New York, 1961, pp. 276–335.
3. Ames LB, Gillespie C, Haines J, Ilg FL: The Gesell Institute's Child from One to Six. Harper & Row, New York, 1979.
4. Cassileth BR, Lusk EJ, Strouse TB: Psychosocial status in chronic illness: A comparative analysis of six diagnostic groups. N Eng J Med 311:506–511, 1984.
5. Houpt JL, Gould BS, Norris FH: Psychological characteristics of patients with amyotrophic lateral sclerosis. Psychosom Med 39:299–303, 1977.
6. Winnicott DW: Collected Papers: Through Paediatrics to Psychoanalysis. Basic Books, New York; Tavistock, London, 1958, pp. 158–160.
7. Torgersen S: Developmental differentiation of anxiety and affective disorder. Acta Psychiatry Scand 71:304–310, 1985.
8. Freud S: General Psychological Theory (Papers on Metapsychology). Collier Books, New York, 1963, pp. 213–217.
9. Guntrip H: Personality Structure, p. 421.
10. Guntrip H: Personality Structure, p. 424.
11. Yalom ID: Existential Psychotherapy. Basic Books, New York, 1980, p. 118.
12. *Ibid.*
13. Yalom ID: Existential Psychotherapy, p. 12.
14. Maslow AH: The Farther Reaches of Human Nature. Viking Press, New York, 1971, p. 15.

CHAPTER TWENTY-ONE

ROLE OF THE VOLUNTARY HEALTH CARE AGENCY IN AMYOTROPHIC LATERAL SCLEROSIS

Rochelle L. Moss

Historically, people diagnosed as having amyotrophic lateral sclerosis (ALS) have been advised to go home and wait to die. In response to this attitude and based on our personal experience with ALS, The ALS Association was formed. The Association is the nonprofit voluntary health agency solely devoted to finding the cause and the cure of ALS. Our program includes funding research, patient services, public and professional education, chapter development, and the establishment of ALS clinics across the country. The ultimate goal of The ALS Association is to go out of business having solved ALS, which as one patient explains, is "like being given a ring-side seat to your own dissolution." The role of the voluntary health care agency is to see to it that ALS is properly addressed by scientists, rehabilitation specialists, and all those who are fortunate enough not to suffer the indignities of the disease.

RESEARCH

The ALS Association supports both biomedical research to determine the cause of ALS as well as clinical research to find a treatment. This support is provided through research grants and postdoctoral fellowships. Research grants are given to established investigators who are studying the etiology and treatment of ALS, and postdoctoral fellowships are given to young scientists entering the field of ALS research. Support is based on the recommendations of the Association's Scientific Review Committee. This Committee is comprised of neurologists with expertise in clinical neurology, immunology, chemistry, pharmacology, epidemiology, virology, and genetics. Understanding the familial form of ALS may

291

prove to be an important key to the sporadic form, as well. The ALS Association's greatest responsibility is to ensure that scientists who are studying the cause and the cure of ALS have the support necessary to pursue their investigations. To quote Dr. Murray Goldstein, Director of the National Institute of Neurological and Communicative Disorders and Stroke, a branch of the National Institutes of Health, the 1980s is "the decade of neurology." Based on tremendous progress being made in basic neuroscience as well as specific ALS research, we are now more certain than ever before that we can and will solve the problem. Research provides hope for ALS victims and their families, who unfortunately experience a tremendous sense of isolation when dealing with the disease.

PATIENT SERVICES

The Association acts as a clearinghouse for information on ALS and provides referrals and counseling to patients and families. This includes a national referral list of home health care agencies, a reference list of equipment for the handicapped, information on communication aids, and equipment for loan to ALS patients when available.

A pamphlet entitled *Home Care for the Patient with Amyotrophic Lateral Sclerosis* is available to patients and scientists free of charge. This handbook provides basic information about home care and is intended as a general guide. It should be used only in conjunction with professional medical care.

The ability to communicate, a common symptom of ALS, is often the most frustrating aspect of the disease. To address this problem, in addition to information on various communication devices, for example, computer systems, the Association distributes the ETRAN Communicator, an eye transfer communication system developed for those people whose voluntary muscle action, except for eye movement, no longer exists (Figs. 21–1 and 21–2). It was developed by an engineer who designed the Board after observing the terrible frustration of a friend who had reached the nonverbal state of ALS. The name ETRAN is used because these five letters are the most frequently used in the English language. The ETRAN Board can be obtained from The ALS Association for a nominal charge which covers the cost.

PUBLIC AND PROFESSIONAL EDUCATION

The ALS Association works toward creating an ALS identity in this country. Though the exact incidence of ALS is unknown, it is not rare

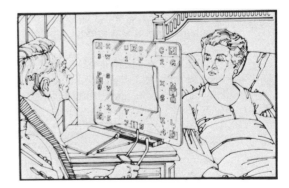

Figure 21-1. A bedridden ALS patient using the ETRAN Board.

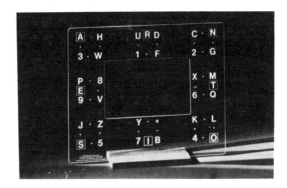

Figure 21-2. The ETRAN Board.

and indeed occurs throughout the world with no racial, ethnic, or socioeconomic boundaries.

The Association participates in the major scientific meetings held each year, that is, those of the American Academy of Neurology, the American Neurological Association, and the Society for Neuroscience. These meetings provide the scientific community with the opportunity to share their experience and research ideas with their peers, and provides The ALS Association with the opportunity to distribute material and request that patients be referred to our program for ongoing information and support. Reprints of professional articles are also distributed to the scientific community upon request. Support of professional seminars and workshops to encourage the exchange of information relative to the study of ALS is an important part of this program.

The Association publishes *The ALS Association Newsletter,* a quarterly publication which updates our constituency including patients, corporations, foundations, individual contributors, neurologists, and the media on progress being made. The newsletter includes reports on the current status of ALS research, human interest stories, reports from chapters, fundraising events, and a contribution envelope. The newsletter helps to encourage support and provides the encouragement that ALS patients and families must have.

Public education is accomplished through the distribution of television, radio, and print public service announcements which include visuals of former Senator Jacob Javits, an ALS patient, baseball stars Reggie Jackson and Kent Hrbek, and patients who are willing to participate.

The ALS Association is a member of the National Committee for Research in Neurological and Communicative Disorders (NCR) which is a coalition of voluntary and professional agencies working together to insure adequate federal funding for neurological research. Our role as a health care agency is not only to ensure funding through the private sector, but increased funding through the federal government for the National Institute of Neurological and Communicative Disorders and Stroke, one of the National Institutes of Health, as well.

CHAPTER DEVELOPMENT

The development of chapters across the United States is the key to a successful grassroots program. Chapters are extensions of the national office, responsible for fundraising, providing patient services, and creating an awareness of ALS in their individual areas. They are staffed by volunteers, many of whom have had a personal experience with ALS. Chapters solicit memberships, organize special events, hold support meetings for patients and families, publish chapter newsletters, and help to support the overall research and clinical services program of the Association. They provide the network necessary to develop an awareness of ALS. Patients who are dealing with ALS in areas where there are chapters are provided with the support and understanding that is necessary in coping with the disease.

In addition to chapters, individuals interested in working with The ALS Association can be designated as ALS representatives. These individuals solicit contributions, distribute information, and act as a liason between the national office and the local constituency.

AMYOTROPHIC LATERAL SCLEROSIS CLINICS

In 1978, The ALS Association provided a pilot grant to the Mount Sinai Medical Center in New York to develop a multidisciplinary team approach to the care of the ALS patient. Since then, additional clinics have been established at the University of Chicago Medical Center, the

University of Miami Medical Center in Florida, and Hahnemann University Hospital in Philadelphia. These programs offer a complete network system to insure that the quality of life and the integrity of the patient is maintained. These ALS clinics not only provide support and counseling for ALS patients; they also increase visibility for the disease which in turn encourages and stimulates scientific interest and generates clinical research to develop a treatment. Although the staffs may vary, they consist basically of clinical neurologists, social workers, occupational therapists, physical therapists, nurse specialists, speech pathologists, pulmonary and respiratory therapists, nutritionists, and psychologists.

To summarize, the role of the voluntary health care agency in ALS is to find the cause and the cure of amyotrophic lateral sclerosis and to provide the support systems and information essential to coping with the disease. Amyotrophic lateral sclerosis has been a closet disease for too long. The ALS Association is not only confronting the problem but working toward the solution while providing a climate of optimism and an expression of caring for those who are afflicted.

For additional information, please contact:

The ALS Association
185 Madison Avenue
New York, New York 10016
(212) 679-4016

The ALS Association
15300 Ventura Boulevard
Sherman Oaks, California 91403
(818) 990-2151

INDEX

Abiotrophy theory, 5
Acetylcholinesterase, 80
Acquired immune deficiency syndrome (AIDS), 35
Acute denervation, scores (scattergram), 28
Acute respiratory failure, 50–53
Adaptive aids. *See* Assistive devices
Adolescence, neurologic disorders in, 90
Age and aging, 5, 39, 46
Airway obstruction, masking from asthma, 70
Alpha motor neurons, 17
Alternative therapies, 110
Aluminum, toxicity, 94
Ambulation
  intervention, 231–234
  with limited endurance, 250
  problems during, 176
  requiring assistance, 251
Ambulatory aids, 14, 231–234
  recommendations, 250–251
Amitriptyline, 12, 270
Ammonia, in spinal cord, 89
Amyotrophic lateral sclerosis (ALS)
  age, 39–40
  assistive devices, 189–217
  biochemical factors, 89–91
  case studies, 182–184
  clinical features, 6–9
  communication problems, 257–265
  defined, 3–15
  diagnosis, 9–11, 33–43
  emotional response and patient care, 283–289
  ethical issues, 105–111
  etiology and research trends, 85–102

exercise in, 219–230
family interactions, 12, 39, 267–271
feeding difficulties, surgical management, 79–83
functional profiles, 173–187
home care, 247–255
incidence of, 6
life support decisions, 108–110
and neuromuscular disorders, 61–77
nursing care, 113–134
pathology, 3–5
patient assessment, 113–120
physical therapy, 219–244
progression, 39–40
psychosocial impact, 273–280
rehabilitation of patients, 163–171
respiratory failure in, 45–59
signs and symptoms, 6–9
staff reactions, 267–271
swallowing difficulties in, 155–161
survival analysis, 11
treatment, 11–14
trophic factors, 91–93
viral factors, 85–87
voluntary health care agency, role of, 291–295
ALS Association, 291–295
ALS Association Newsletter, 293
Anarthria, 262–263
Androgen receptors, damage or loss of, 5
Anhidrosis, sweat test for, 38
Animal models, research goals, 96
Ankle-foot orthosis, 166–231
Antibodies, to neural antigens, 87–88
Antidepressants, 130–270
Antispastic drugs, 130, 168
Antiviral agents, 95

Arm supports, 253
Arterial blood gases, 13, 71
Arthritis, 38
Articulation loss. *See* Anarthria
Aspiration pneumonia, 8
Assistive devices
  acceptance of, 195
  community resources, 214–215
  cost and availability, 214–215
  evaluation of, 190–195
  in functional enhancement, 176
  home care recommendations, 250–254
  patient and family involvement, 195–196
  safety factor, 193–194
  selection of, 189–217
  setting priorities, 192–195
  support services, 214–215
  weight factor, 197
Asthma, 70
Atelectasis, 47
Atropine, 12, 130
Autoimmune disorders, 88
Autopneumonectomy, 62
Azathiaprine, 89

Baclofen, 130
Balancing exercises, 225, 226
Barium swallowing, "modified," 157–158
Bathroom, assistive devices for, 200, 254
Beds, 254. *See also* Hospital beds
Behavior patterns, 268
Benzodiazepine, 92, 269
Betz cells, 3
Biochemical factors, 89–91
Blenderized foods, 158
Bowel dysfunction, 39
Brain stem, 23, 76
Breathing
  difficulty, treatment of, 13
  exercises, 235–241
  nursing care, 118, 121
  "paradoxical" pattern, 49
Bulbar disease, ventilatory failure in, 76
Bunina bodies, 3

Calcium
  abnormal, 41, 90, 94
  deficiency, 5
  in soil and water, 94
Cancer, 10
Carbohydrate, in dysphagia management, 147–148
Cerebrospinal fluid
  examination, 37
  toxicity, 95
Cervical arthritis, with severe spondylitis, 39
Cervical collars, 192–193
Chamorro Indians, 4, 94
Chest
  bellows disorders, 62–64
  x-rays, 13
Choline acetyltransferase, 92
Chronic respiratory failure, 54–58
Cinefluoroscopy, 157
Clavicle supports, 198
Clinics
  ALS—supported, 294–295
  lack of, 163
Cobalt, 95
Colace, 130
Communication
  aids, 194, 202, 208–214
  augmentative devices, 211–214
  defined, 257
  problems, 257–265
Compensatory mechanisms, in functional enhancement, 175–176
Computed tomography, 34
Conditioning exercises, 220–225
Congestive heart failure, pulmonary emboli and, 8
Connective tissue disease, 38
Constipation, 126, 151
Contracture prevention, 228
Copper, in spinal cord, 95
Corticospinal tracts, 23–24
Coughing, 238–239
Cranial nerves, involved in eating mechanics, 139
Creative phosphokinase (CPK), 10–11
Creutzfeld-Jakob disease, 85–86
Cricopharyngeal myotomy, 159
Crying, uncontrollable, 8
Cuirass ventilator, 51–52, 54

Cyanosis, 50
Cytoxan, 89

Daily living, determining activities of, 191–192
Death and dying, 287–288
Deconditioning, 225–227
Deformity, and level of functioning, 165–166
Deglutition, phases of, 137–139
Dehydration, 53
Dementia, Alzheimer-type, 9
Demyelination, and gliosis, 3
Denial
    and coping, 286–287
    patient use of, 274
Deoxyribonucleic acid (DNA)
    abnormal, in motor neurons, 5
    altered synthesis, 89–90
    repair enzymes, 90
Depage-Janeway gastrostomy, 80
Dependency, 274–276, 284
Depression, 274
Despair, patient reactions of, 276
Diabetes, 38
Diagnosis, 9–11
    differential, 33–43
    patient understanding of, 116–117
    referral practice, 106–107
    telling patients of, 105–107
Diet therapy, for dysphagia, 148–150
Disability, extent of, 165–166
Discharge planning, 133
Distal wasting, in motor neuropathy, 34
Disuse weakness, as exercise problem, 225–227
Dressing aids, 199, 205
Drop-arm commonde, 194
Ducolax, 130
Dysarthria, communication problems, 258–260
Dysphagia, 7–8, 155–161
    communication problems, 264
    evaluation of, 142–146, 156–158
    history and physical examination, 142–145
    nutritional management of, 137–153
    pathophysiology, 140–142
    radiologic studies, 145–146

surgical management of, 79
terminology, 159–160
treatment, 12, 158
Dyspnea, 8
    and neuromuscular disorders, 66
    treatment, 13

Eating
    equipment, 204
    mechanics of, 139
Elavil, 130
Electrolytes, 53
Electromyography, 10, 26, 33, 41
Electrophysiology, 25
Emotional response, and patient care, 283–289
Endocrine, abnormalities, 90
Endurance training, 220–221
Enzymes, 37, 91
Ethical issues, 105–111
Etiology, and research trends, 85–102
Exercise, 219–230
    metabolic studies, 230
    problems, 225–230
    program design, 220
    therapeutic, 174–175
    types of, 170, 220
Expiration, 238
    muscle conditioning exercises, 238–241
    pressure tests, 64–66
Explosive cough, 238

Familial spastic paraplegia, 37
Family
    assistive devices, involvement with, 195–196
    behavior patterns, 268–269
    feelings, legitimizing of, 276
    history, 39–40
    interviews, 248
    reactions, 267–271
Fasciculation, 29, 41
Fat, in dysphagia management, 147–148
Fatigue, 49, 54
    rehabilitation and, 169
Feeding
    aids, 199, 204
    alternative methods, 124

feeding (*continued*)
gastrostomy, 79–83
surgical management of, 79–83
Feelings, legitimizing of, 276
Fiberoptic bronchoscopy, 53
Flow rates, and pulmonary function, 70–71
Fluoroscopy, in swallowing difficulties, 157
Focal atrophies, 36
Follow-up evaluation, in nursing care, 132–133
Foods, soft or blenderized, 158–159
Footdrop, orthotics for, 231–232
Forearm crutches, 232–233
Formulas, and tube feedings, 151–152
Fractures, calcium related, 94
Fringe medicine, 110
Functional enhancement, 174–177
Functional profiles, 177–187
F-wave amplitude measurement, 26

Gag reflex, jaw jerk and, 8
Gait training, 14
Gastrointestinal, abnormalities, 90
Gastrostomy
feeding, 79–83
percutaneous endoscopic, 83
surgical technique, 79–81
Gliosis, demyelination and, 3
Global hypoventilation, 71
Glucose, abnormalities, 90
Glycine receptors, 92
Golgi tendon organs, 21
Grab bars, in bathroom, 194
Guam, 4–5
Guillain-Barre disease, immunologic factors, 87

Hahnemann University Hospital (Philadelphia), 295
Headaches, 50
Heavy metal intoxication, 35, 93
Hereditary motor neuropathy, family pedigree, 36
Hexosaminidase deficiency, 9, 89
History, and physical examination, 114–116
Home care, 247–255
assessment of, 248

assistive equipment recommendations, 250–254
follow-up visits, 249
patient history and, 247–248
vs. self-care, 247
"specialist effect," 249
therapist visits, 247–248
treatment methods, 249
Home Care for the Patient with Amyotrophic Lateral Sclerosis, 292
Homemaking, and meal preparation, 199
Hopefulness, reality and, 289
Horizontal-grip canes, 232
Hospital beds, 200
full electric, 251, 254
Human leukocyte antigen (HLA), 88
Hypercapnia, 50, 55
Hypernasality, 260–262
Hyperparathyroidism, 94
Hypophosphatemia, 53
Hypoxemia, 47

Imipramine, 12, 131
Immune mechanisms, therapeutic trials, 95
Immunoblot techniques, 87
Immunoglobulins, abnormalities in, 41
Immunologic factors, 87–89
genetically determined, 88
Immunosuppression, 95
Incontinence, 8
Inflammatory polyneuropathy, chronic relapsing, 36
Infrared switch, 213
Innervation, of swallowing mechanism, 138–139
Inspiration, 236
muscle conditioning exercises, 236–237
pressure tests, 64–66
spirometry and flow-volume curves, 66–68
Institutionalization, 279
Interferon, 95
Intermittent positive-pressure breathing (IPPB), 13
Intervention
ambulation, 231–234
in nursing care, 120–131
patient acceptance of, 121

Iron lung, 51
Isokinetic exercises, 222, 224
Isometric exercises, 221–224
Isotonic exercises, 222, 224

Japan, 5
Jaw jerk, and gag reflex, 8

Laughing, uncontrollable, 8
Laxatives, dosage instructions, 130
Lead, 5, 9
Life support decisions, 108–110
Linoleic acid, 148
Liquid diet, in feeding gastrostomy, 81–82
Living wills, 109
"Lou Gehrig's disease," 3
Lower motor neurons
  columnar cell diagram, 18
  cortical inputs, 24
  findings, 34–36
  localization of, 18
  monosynaptic excitatory connections, 20–21
  morphology of, 17
  peripheral inputs to, 20–21
  physiology of, 25
  signs, 33
  suprasegmental inputs to, 22–24
Lung, vital capacity of, 62, 63
Lymphocytic choriomeningitis, 86
Lymphoma, 35

Macroglobulinemia, 9
Magnesium, 5, 94
Magnetic resonance imaging (MRI), 34
Male, predisposition, 7
Malecot catheter, 80–81
Manganese, in spinal cord, 94
Mattresses, foam and water, 254
Maximal expiratory flow-volume (MEFV), 67–68
Maximum voluntary ventilation (MVV), 69
Mechanical ventilation
  in acute respiratory failure, 50–53
  control modes, 52
  family interaction, 55
  home programs, 56–57

intermittent use, 54–55
  negative-pressure devices, 51, 54
  patient selection, 56
  positive-pressure devices, 51, 54
Medical equipment, recommended, 200
Medications, frequently used, 130–131
Mentation, preservation of, 9
Mercury, in amyotrophic myelopathy, 93
Metabolic factors, 89
Misdiagnosis, 9, 10
Mobility aids, 200, 207
Monoclonal gammopathy, 89
Mononeuritis multiplex, 38
Motorized stair lift, 251
Motorized wheelchairs, 207–208, 250
Motor neuron disease (MND)
  functional profiles, 177–187
  lead toxicity and, 93
  normal properties and physiologic changes, 17–31
  type and incidence, 6–7
  see also Amyotrophic lateral sclerosis
Motor neuropathies, 34–36, 91
Motor scooters, safety considerations, 208
Motor units, 17–31
  evaluation in patient care, 27–29
  histochemistry, 19
  muscle fiber distribution, 19–20
  oxidative enzyme activity, 19
  size and function, 25
  types of, 19–20
Mt. Sinai Medical Center (New York), 294
Mucus, nutritional management, 151
Multiple sclerosis, 37
Multisystem atrophies, 37–38
Muscarinic receptors, 92
Muscle
  conditioning exercises, 221–225, 236–241
  cramps during rehabilitation, 169
  nerve fibers to, 20
  paralysis and hypoxia, 8
  protease activity, 90
Muscular Dystrophy Association, 164
Myelin antibodies, 41
Myelography, 34
Myelopathies, 9

Nasogastric tube, feedings, 53
Neck and shoulder weakness, assistive equipment recommendations, 252–253
Neck collars, 167, 198, 252
Neoplasia, 35
Nerve conduction studies, 25, 37
Nerve growth factor (NGF), 91
Neural antigens, antibodies to, 87–88
Neurological and Communicative Disorders, National Committee for Research in, 294
Neurologic disorders, 90
Neuromuscular disorders
    maximal static respiratory pressures, 64–66
    mechanical ventilation, 54
    pulmonary function in, 61–77
    respiratory failure in, 61–77
Neuronal attrition, and synaptic development, 91
Neuropeptides, in spinal cord, 92
Neurotransmitters, altered levels in blood, 90
Neurotrophic hormone, lack of, 5
No-touch telephones, 253
Nursing care, 113–134
    clinic admission chart, 114–115
    common diagnoses, 120
    follow-up evaluation, 132–133
    history and physical examination, 114–116
    intervention in, 120–131
    patient understanding of diagnosis, 116–117
Nutrition
    deficiencies, 53
    and dysphagia, 137–153
    nursing intervention, 119, 123–125
    teaching plan, 123–124

Obesity
    and chest bellows insufficiency, 62
    and rehabilitation, 170
Object manipulation, assistive devices, 205–206
Occupational therapy, 164–165
Oligoclonal binding, 37
Onufrowicz nucleus, 9
Oral hygiene, 159
    nursing intervention, 127–128

Ornithine, in spinal cord, 89
Orthotics, 166–168, 198–203
    ambulatory, 231–232
    commonly used, 198
    patient selection, 168
    see also Assistive devices
Over-the-door pulleys, 229
Overwork, as exercise problem, 228–230

Pain, nursing intervention, 129
Palatal lifts, 260–262
Pap smear, 119
Paraplegia, 64, 69
Paraproteinemias, 35
Parkinsonism, 37
Patients
    abandonment by physician, 107
    assessment of, 113–120
    assistive devices for, 189–217
    communication problems of, 257–265
    denial, use of, 274
    dependency, struggling with, 274–276
    discharge planning, 133
    elective or forced treatment, 107–108
    emotional response, impact on medical care, 283–289
    exercise for, 219–230
    feeding difficulties, surgical management of, 79–83
    feelings, legitimizing of, 276
    follow-up evaluation of, 132–133
    functional profiles, 173–187
    history and physical examination, 114–116
    home care, 247–255
    in hospitals, 106
    hydraulic lift, 254
    individual practice setting, 106
    interviewing, 248
    life support decisions, 108–110
    living alone, 196
    "normally depressed," 285
    nursing care, 113–134
    physical therapy for, 219–244
    reactions, 267–271
    rehabilitation of, 163–171
    services, ALS-supported, 292
    wheelchair or bedridden, 166
Peripheral neuropathy, 9

Personal computers, 212, 263, 292
Personal hygiene, assistive devices, 199, 205
Pharmacologic treatment, of respiratory failure, 53
Phonation aids, 264
Physical disability, 14
Physical examination, history and, 114–116
Physical therapy, 164, 219–244
  intervention, 14
  pulmonary, 235–242
Physicians
  diagnosis withheld by, 105
  interpersonal skills of, 106
  moral obligations of, 106
  negative emotional responses of, 107–108
  responsibility to patients, 108
Physiology
  in motor neuron diseases, 17–31
  in swallowing, 137–138
Plasmapheresis, 36, 95
Platform crutches, 232–233
Plexopathies, 38
Poliomyelitis, 42, 55
Polio virus, 86
Polyclonal gammopathy, 89
Portable intercoms, and buzzers, 210
Positioning, 191, 199
Postural drainage, 241–242
Postural exercises, 225, 226
Prednisone, 89
Primary lateral sclerosis (PLS), 6–7, 37
  case studies, 186
Pro-banthine, 131
Professional education, ALS-supported, 292–294
Progressive bulbar palsy (PBP), 6–7
  case studies, 185–186
  functional profiles, 181
Progressive muscular atrophy (PMA), 6–7
  case studies, 184–185
  functional profiles, 180
Pronunciation problems. *See* Dysarthria
Propantheline bromide, 12
Protein, in dysphagia management, 147–148
Psychiatric illness, 41
Psychoses, 270

Psychosexual behavior, 268
Psychosocial impact, 273–280
  patient assistance, 163
  of social workers, 277–279
  of support groups, 277
Psychotropic medications, use of, 269–270
Public education, ALS-supported, 292–294
Pulmonary function
  abnormal, prevalence of, 67
  clinical features, correlation of, 71–72
  findings, 66–71
  loss of, 75
  in neuromuscular disorders, 61–77
  prognosis and mortality, 73
  progression of changes, 72
  slope of decline and neuromuscular score, 73, 74
  tests, use of, 72–75

Quadriplegia, 64, 69
Quinine, dosage instructions, 131

Radiculopathy, 9
Radioautography, 92
Radiography, 34
Radioimmunoassay studies, 92
Raised toilet seat, 251
Range of motion exercises, 225, 228
Reading aids, 202, 209
Reality, and hopefulness, 289
Reclining wheelchair, 253
Regressive behavior, 267–268
Rehabilitation, 163–171
  attitudes toward, 170
  disability and level of functioning, 165–166
  facilities, 163–164
  and fatigue, 169
  home programs, 165
  main goals of, 164
  and muscle cramps, 169
  obesity and, 170
  orthotic prescription, 166–168
  spasticity and, 168–169
  treatment team, 164
  types of exercise, 170
Repetitive nerve stimulation, 26

Research trends
  etiology and, 85–102
  future goals, 96
  therapeutic trials, 95–96
Resistive exercises, 224–225
Respiration, 61
  muscles in, 45–47
  pressures by sex and age, 46
  therapy, 56
Respirators, 13
  ethical issues, 108
  for home care, 55–56
Respiratory failure, 45–59
  additional treatment, 53
  clinical recognition, 48–50
  mechanical ventilation in, 50–53
  mechanisms of, 48, 61
  in neuromuscular disorders, 61–77
  pharmacologic treatment, 53
  treatment of, 50–53
Restrictive ventilatory impairment, 62–64
Ribonucleic acid (RNA), 87, 90
Rolling walkers, 232–233

Safety, in home, 193–194
Saliva
  nutritional management, 150
  pooling and choking, 12
Sarcoidosis, 38
Scattergrams, in patient care, 27–29
Schizophrenia, 270
Selenium, 41, 93
Sensory disturbance, 37–39
  absence of, 9
  nerve action potentials, 33
  nursing assessment, 118
  "significant," 37
Serum
  protein electrophoresis, 35
  toxicity, 95
Sexual dysfunction, 9, 119
  nursing intervention, 129–131
Shoulder-elbow orthosis, 167
Signaling devices, 210
Single-fiber electromyography, 26
Sitting, problems during, 177
Skin care, 118
  nursing intervention, 128–129
Sleep problems, drugs for, 270
Snake venom, 110

Sneakers, and shoes, 231
Social workers, role of, 277–279
Spasticity
  and rehabilitation, 168–169
  treatment for, 13–14
Speech
  difficulty, 8, 14
  nursing assessment, 119, 125
  pathologist, 257–258
  problems, 257–258
  therapy, 164
  see also Communication
Sphincter control, 9, 119
  nursing intervention, 126–127
Spinal cord
  afferent fiber connections, 21, 22
  ammonia and ornithine in, 89
Spinal disorders, static respiratory pressures, 64
Spirometry, 13, 66–68
Sprouting factor, motor nerve, 92
Staff
  behavior patterns, 268–269
  reactions, 267–271
Stair lift, motorized, 251
Static lung volume, 69
Static respiratory pressures
  clinical limitations, 64
  in neuromuscular disorders, 64–66
  test apparatus, 64–66
Stationary cycling, 221–223
Steroids, 36
Subacute sclerosing panencephalitis, measles-related, 86
Suction machine, 12
Suicide, 276
Support cushions, 252
Support groups, 14
  function of, 277
Sural nerve, biopsy and medial necrosis, 39
Surgical management, of feeding difficulties, 79–83
Suspension slings, 200
Swallowing
  muscle weakness, patterns of, 155–156
  nursing assessment, 118
  physiology in, 137–138
  see also Dysphagia
Sweat test, 38
Swimming, patient response to, 221

Tay-Sachs disease, 90
Telephoning aids, 209–210
Teletypewriters, 210
Theophylline, in respiratory failure treatment, 53
Therapeutic trials, 95–96
Thiamine, in plasma and cerebrospinal fluid, 90
Thioridazine, use of, 270
Thyrotropin-releasing hormone (TRH), 5
immunocytochemistry, 92
therapeutic trials, 96
Tilorone, 95
Tissue culture, future goals, 96
Tofranil, 131
Total lung capacity, 63
Toxic factor, 93–95
Trace metals, 93–94
Tracheostomy, 13, 54
communication problems, 263–264
Transcutaneous electrical nerve stimulation (TENS), 169
Treatment, 11–14
of acute respiratory failure, 50–53
elective or forced, 107–108
Tricyclic drugs, 12
Trophic factors, 91–93
therapeutic trials, 96
Trunk and hip weakness, 176, 251
Tube feedings, formulas and, 151–152

University of Chicago Medical Center, 294
University of Miami Medical Center, 295

Upper extremity weakness, assistive equipment recommendations, 253
Upper motor neuron
findings, 37
signs, 33
Upper respiratory infection, 118

Velopharyngeal incompetence, 260–262
Ventilation. See Mechanical ventilation
Ventilatory failure, 75–76
Videofluoroscopy, 157, 158
Viral factors, 85–87
Viruses
mechanisms, 5
therapeutic trials, 95
types of, 86
Visiting nurse service, 122, 132
Vital capacity, of lung, 62, 63
Vocational rehabilitation, 164

Walking
difficulty, 14
or fast walking, 221
Water beds, 254
Weakness
muscles affected, 8
as principal symptom, 7
West New Guinea, 5
Wheelchairs
full-reclining, 201
selection of, 207
standard and motorized, 250
Wrist supports, 198, 253
Writing aids, 202, 209